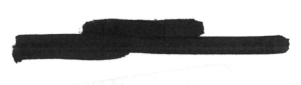

D0762353

Aging
and **male sexuality**

As the proportion of older people grows, and increased attention is paid to the quality of life in the aging population, there is greater awareness of the importance of sexuality and its disorders in this age group. Most reports on sexuality in older men adopt a disease model, focusing on functional deficits and impaired sexual performance. This book, by contrast, takes a broader view, including psychological and relationship issues in sexual satisfaction, based in part on the author's clinical experience and research at Mount Sinai Medical Center in New York.

It presents an up-to-date overview of the sexuality of aging men in health and illness, within a multidimensional conceptual framework, and takes account of physiological, psychological, interpersonal and social influences. Also discussed are the impact of medical illness, psychopathology and drugs, with a review of coping strategies in shaping individual sexual responses to aging and disease. Many case studies and vignettes are incorporated, and a chapter is devoted to the sexuality of older gay men. A balanced account of medical and psychosocial evaluation and treatment concludes the book, which will be of broad interest to clinicians and students interested in sexuality and aging.

Raul C. Schiavi is Emeritus Professor, Department of Psychiatry, Mount Sinai School of Medicine, New York. He is former President of both the Internationl Academy for Sex Research and the Society for Sex Therapy and Research, and a former member of the Board of Directors of the US Sex Information and Education Council.

Aging
and **male sexuality**

Raul C. Schiavi

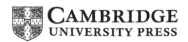

CAMBRIDGE
UNIVERSITY PRESS

PUBLISHED BY THE PRESS SYNDICATE OF THE UNIVERSITY OF CAMBRIDGE
The Pitt Building, Trumpington Street, Cambridge, United Kingdom

CAMBRIDGE UNIVERSITY PRESS
The Edinburgh Building, Cambridge CB2 2RU, UK   http://www.cup.cam.ac.uk
40 West 20th Street, New York, NY 10011–4211, USA   http://www.cup.org
10 Stamford Road, Oakleigh, Melbourne 3166, Australia

First published 1999

Printed in the United Kingdom at the University Press, Cambridge

Typeset in Adobe Minion 10.5/14 pt. in QuarkXPress® [SE]

A catalogue record for this book is available from the British Library

Library of Congress cataloguing in Publication data
Schiavi, Raul C.
     Aging and male sexuality / Raul C. Schiavi.
     p.   cm.
     Includes bibliographical references and index.
     ISBN 0 521 65391 6 (pbk.)
     1. Aged men – United States – Sexual behavior.   2. Aged men – United
States – Physiology.   3. Aged men – Health and hygiene – United States.
4. Sex (Psychology) – United States.   5. Sexual disorders – United
States.   I. Title.
     HQ1064.U5 S34 1999
     305.26–ddc21   98-44551 CIP

ISBN 0 521 65391 6 paperback

Every effort has been made in preparing this book to provide accurate and up-to-date information which is in accord with accepted standards and practice at the time of publication.
Nevertheless, the authors, editors and publisher can make no warranties that the information
contained herein is totally free from error, not least because clinical standards are constantly
changing through research and regulation. The authors, editors and publisher therefore disclaim
all liability for direct or consequential damages resulting from the use of material contained in
this book. Readers are strongly advised to pay careful attention to information provided by the
manufacturer of any drugs or equipment that they plan to use.

Contents

Preface

Sexual anatomy and function have become frequent subjects of discussion in the media following the recent approval and commercial availability of a new oral agent for the treatment of male erectile difficulties. Behind the decline of the taboo concerning sexual topics and humorous comments, there is the clinical reality that, increasingly, older men approach health-care professionals with the hope of enhancing their sexual function. Demographic and social changes as well as advances in sexual knowledge have led to a more open attitude by the aged about their sexual lives. The age structure of the Western World population, which is gradually evolving from a young to an aging society, has been accompanied by an evolution in the experience of adulthood and old age. The prolongation of life, improvements in health-care and a more proactive attitude concerning quality of life, reinforced by the American 'baby boom' generation now beginning to reach later adulthood, have all contributed to the increased importance of sexuality for contentment as age progresses. In parallel with these developments, considerable progress has been made, over the last twenty years, in our knowledge of sexual physiology and the deleterious effects of disease and drugs on male sexual function. Although this information has permitted valuable therapeutic interventions, it has also contributed to a distorted picture of aging and sexuality centred on medical illness and organic pathology. The original emphasis on the psychological determination of erectile difficulties has given ground to the current and equally undocumented view that most erectile disorders have an organic basis and to an evolving armamentarium of laboratory and biomedical approaches to diagnose and correct erectile failure. This 'medicalization' of sexual problems, fostered by significant technological advances, has led to the neglect of social, psychological, and relationship influences and their interaction with physical processes, a development that has consequences for our views about the sexuality of aging males.

Much of the medical literature is characterized by lack of clarity about the distinction between the natural, age-related changes in sexual function and sexual pathology and by simplistic, dichotomous notions about causation driven by the narrow focusing of the various disciplines that have addressed the sexual concerns of the aging male. There is a tendency to view the sexuality of older men through the lenses of youth, focusing on performance and erectile capacity, while overlooking psychological and interpersonal dimensions. Fortunately, a paradigm shift is beginning to take place with emphasis on the integration of physiological and psychosocial aspects of sexual function and dysfunction, and on multifactorial conceptual models that orient the interpretation of research and clinical findings.

This book is guided by a multidisciplinary perspective and is based on an up-to-date overview of empirical information and clinical experience. It will be of interest to psychiatrists, gerontologists, behavioral scientists, psychologists, sex researchers and, in general, to all professionals concerned with basic and clinical processes underlying sexuality and aging. Chapter 1 places the topic of aging sexuality within a broad conceptual framework, taking into consideration methodological issues on sex research and aging. Chapter 2 reviews data on the sexuality of older men with specific attention to health and illness. The following section, which includes chapters 3 to 7, focuses on nonpathological aging with emphasis on sexual variability. It provides a selective review of physiological, psychological, interpersonal, and social forces that mediate, influence or are associated with age-related changes in male sexuality. Chapters 8 to 12 present clinical evidence concerning the sexual disorders of older men. They consider the impact of medical illness, psychopathology, the effects of drugs and medication and the role of appraisal and coping in shaping individual responses to disease. Chapters 13 and 14 discuss the assessment, management and treatment of men with sexual problems, taking a balanced account of biomedical and psychosocial influences on the sexual satisfaction of older individuals. The concluding chapter reviews the most salient research and clinical findings that have helped to broaden our understanding of the sexuality of older men in health and illness. Most of the sections contain brief narrative individual sketches selected to illustrate the clinical relevance of the various topics discussed.

This book was stimulated by the results of research on the sexuality of the aging male conducted in our laboratories and by clinical experience in the Human Sexuality Program at Mount Sinai Medical Center over a period of close to twenty years. It reflects the valuable collaboration of our research team and the creative discussion of members of our faculty and trainees as we attempted to respond to the sexual problems of the many older patients who came to us for assistance. I would like to convey my appreciation to the Mount Sinai Medical Center that provided a clinical base for our work, to the National Institutes of Health that supported our research, and to the generative interactions with members of two organizations: the International Academy of Sex Research and the Society for Sex Therapy and Research (SSTAR). Above anything else my gratitude to Marvin Stein who inspired my initial fascination with research, and to my wife and daughters for all the pleasure and satisfaction they have brought to my life.

1   Aging and sexuality: concepts, issues, and research methods

Population dynamics and socioeconomic developments during the second half of this century have had a profound impact on the aged. The substantial increase in the rate of growth of elderly populations has been accompanied by an enhanced awareness of the aged as a distinct demographic group. The rapid change in social structures with emphasis on economic development and productivity has brought about a redefinition of how the aged are characterized. The view of old age as a repository of wisdom, tradition, and cultural memories has been replaced by a conceptualization of the aged as a problematic social group. The aged have been variously described as disengaged from the community, lacking in self-esteem, sexless and unattractive, burdened by physical and mental disorders, as well as dependent and passively expecting economic and social support (Brown, 1990a).

These stereotypical notions are being challenged by a wealth of information from social scientists, psychologists, biologists, and clinical investigators working in the field of gerontology, a relatively new discipline devoted to the study of aging processes. Models of aging characterized by physical and mental decline and emotional isolation are being replaced by models that incorporate concepts such as growth, competence, successful adaptation, and personal satisfaction. Increasing attention is given to factors that promote health, prevent disease and disability, and contribute to the self-esteem and quality of life of the aged.

It is in this context that changes in societal attitudes about sexuality need to be considered. The prevailing emphasis on sex, driven in part by our youth-oriented culture, has not been without consequences for the older population. The sexual concerns expressed by the growing number of older individuals seeking help from health-care professionals is indicative of evolving views and increasing expectations in this age group; it is shaped both by positive attitudes and by culturally ingrained misconceptions.

This section places the topic of sexuality within a broad conceptual framework. It provides a brief overview of gerontological information and methodological issues relevant to the understanding of clinical and research data on aging sexuality.

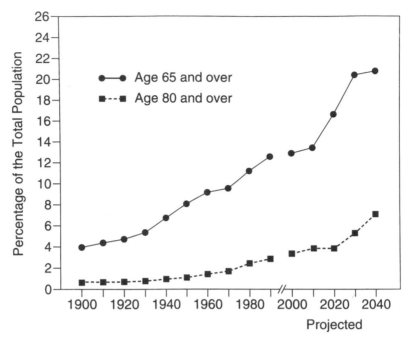

Figure 1.1   Demographic changes in the aging population in the USA, actual and projected 1900–2040. (Data from Schick and Schick, 1994.)

Demographic trends

Decreased fertility and declining death rates due to medical and public health advances in modern Western societies have resulted in marked changes in the age composition of the population. The proportion of the population in the USA aged 65 years or more, which was less than 5% at the beginning of the 1900s, had increased to 11. 3% in 1980 and is projected to raise above 16% by the year 2020 (Figure 1.1). The life expectancy at birth also increased markedly between 1900 and 1985 from 46 to 71 years for men and from 48 to 78 years for women (National Center for Health Statistics, 1986) (Table 1.1). Due to the higher mortality of males over the life span, older women markedly outnumber older men regardless of race and socioeconomic status. The number of males for every 100 females (sex ratio) was calculated in 1980 as 67.5% in the over-65 age group and 55.2% in the population over 75. These figures correspond to an excess of five million women at age 65; estimates for the year 2000 project an excess of 7.6 million women or about 20% of the total population 65 years and over (Siegel and Davidson, 1984).

The gender imbalance in the aged population and the fact that men tend to marry younger women results in marked differences in the patterns of the marital status of older men and women. In a recent population survey, 77% of older men

Table 1.1. Life expectancy at birth and at 65 years of age

Year	At birth		At 65 years	
	Men	Women	Men	Women
1900	46.3	48.3	11.5	12.2
1950	65.6	71.1	12.8	15.0
1970	67.1	74.8	13.1	17.0
1990	72.1	79.0	15.0	19.4
Projected				
2000	73.5	80.4	15.7	20.3
2020	74.9	81.8	16.6	21.4

Note:
Schick and Schick (1994).

and 40% of women were listed as married, in contrast to 14% of men and 51% of women who were widowed. Of the 70 000 persons aged 65 years or older who were married in the USA in 1984, 25 000 were women and 45 000 were men (Butler, Lewis and Sunderland, 1993). These demographic statistics of the number, proportion, and gender balance of the aged population have profound social and interpersonal consequences that are only beginning to be elucidated.

Who are the aged?

Old age is a relative concept that has evolved over time with the aging of the population; personal definitions of old age are also likely to change as we ourselves grow older. Characterization of the aged as a definable group was largely irrelevant during the late part of the eighteenth century when the average life expectancy was 35 years. This stands in contrast with the present time when more than 30 million people are over 65 in the USA, with the over-75 and over-85 age groups having become the fastest growing segments of the world population (Kart, Metress and Metress, 1992a).

Age 65 has been traditionally identified as the beginning of old age; this designation is arbitrary and based on socioeconomic events dating back to the nineteenth century. It has been accepted as a useful demarcation point by gerontologists, some of whom further distinguish between early old age, i.e., 65 to 74 years, and advanced old age, i.e., 75 years and above. Within the context of adult development and aging research, Siegler, Nowlin and Blumenthal (1980) have applied the working definition of middle age as being between 45 and 65 years old and of old age as being between 65 and 85 years. Other investigators (Neugarten, 1974) have employed the categorization of young-old (55–74 years of age), the elderly (75–84 years) and the very old (85 years and over). The age range of the populations as well as the categorization of age groups vary widely in human sexuality studies, limiting the generalizability of results.

General perspectives on aging

Aging is a central but seldom defined concept in gerontological research. It is employed as an independent variable to explain associated phenomena as well as a dependent variable that changes in response to other processes (Birren and Birren, 1990). Aging is usually conceptualized in the medical literature along strict biological lines. This is reflected in the definitions included in a standard medical dictionary:

(1) the process of growing old, especially failure of replacement of cells in sufficient number to maintain full functional capacity and (2) the gradual deterioration of a mature organism resulting from time-dependent, irreversible changes in structure that are intrinsic to the particular species, and which eventually lead to decreased ability to cope with the stresses of the environment, thereby increasing the probability of death (*Stedman's Medical Dictionary*, 25th edn)

Only recently has research oriented by developmental theory and psychological and social approaches converged with biomedical information in the study of the aging process. Increased awareness of the importance of psychosocial forces on the health, morbidity and quality of life of the aged has shaped the growth of gerontology as a multidisciplinary endeavor (Birren and Birren, 1990). A challenging issue in this field, relevant to the interpretation of age-related changes in sexual behavior, concerns the differentiation between normal and pathological aging. The aging of the population has been accompanied by a reduction in the incidence of infectious diseases and an increase in chronic conditions. The blurring of the distinction between the normal, age-related biological changes and the consequences of chronic disease and disability has fostered the view that aging is a medical issue (Estes and Binney, 1991). Several authors have emphasized the importance of differentiating the genetically programmed, universal and inevitable physiological processes intrinsic to aging (primary aging) from the results of life-style, environmental influences and disease (extrinsic or secondary aging); normal aging refers to changes that are progressive and irreversible and that can occur even under optimal circumstances (Kohn, 1978; Brown, 1990b). There are marked intrinsic differences, however, in the onset, rate, and severity of functional decline among individuals as well as among organ systems within the same individual. The distinction between changes inherent to the aging process and those secondary to pathology, although at times difficult to define, has considerable heuristic and clinical value in studies of aging sexuality (Esser and Abisch, 1986). It has stimulated research strategies aimed at minimizing the confounding of normal age-related changes and the consequences of disease.

Individual heterogeneity and aging

The investigation of subjects carefully selected to eliminate pathological conditions is a common approach to the study of normal aging. The results show significant effects of age on important clinical parameters such as renal function, glucose tolerance, cardiovascular physiology, bone density, and sympathetic nervous system activity. They also demonstrate that, regardless of the system evaluated, there is increasing variability in aging even when the effect of disease is excluded. Cross-sectional physiological research on presumably healthy individuals shows an average decline in function which is attributed to aging, but overlooks the heterogeneity that exists among subjects within age groups (Rowe and Kahn, 1987). Longitudinal studies also demonstrate that while some healthy individuals have functional declines in specific physiological parameters, others do not show evidence of change and still others may even demonstrate enhanced functional capacity with advancing age (Rodeheffer et al., 1984; Lindeman, Tobin and Shock, 1985). Considerable individual differences in psychological and behavioral processes in the healthy aged are also evident. Schaie (1990) has documented, for example, that although some cognitive tests show an average decline with age, 20–30% of subjects in their eighties perform as well young adults. As will become apparent in the chapters that follow, there is also considerable individual variability in the changes in sexual function and behavior that occur with aging and in the sexual consequences of chronic illness and disability. Research on the sexuality of aging has tended to report mean age-related trends, overlooking psychological and social factors that, interacting with the biological substrate, contribute to the wide range of sexual expression. Rowe and Kahn (1987), among others, have discussed the limitations inherent in dichotomizing research findings into age-determined and disease-induced processes, neglecting the physiological and cognitive heterogeneity of older individuals.

The concept of successful aging

What factors contribute to the individual variability of aging even after identifiable pathology is excluded? Social and psychological characteristics and life-style are important forces, in addition to genetic influences and possible effects of still unrecognized medical disorders, which shape individual responses to aging. Successful aging is a provocative and apparently contradictory concept that has stimulated considerable research on notions such as plasticity, reserve capacity, and positive adaptation (Butt and Beiser, 1987; Baltes and Baltes, 1990). Rowe and Kahn (1987) have applied the concept of successful aging to designated individuals who demonstrate minimal or no changes in a particular physiological function in contrast to subjects who show the usual, age-related, nonpathological declines within the heterogeneous category of a normal, nondiseased group. They draw attention to the importance of psychosocial characteristics and extrinsic factors such as diet, exercise and personal habits as contributors to the difference between successful and usual aging. The authors review empirical information on autonomy, personal control, and social support to exemplify the significantly positive as well as adverse effects that psychosocial factors may have on physiological indicators and subjective well-being. These data, as the authors indicate, challenge the tendency to consider age as a sufficient explanatory variable, and draw attention to interdisciplinary research on the determinants of functional transitions among successful, usual and pathological aging. This approach permeates the orientation of this book by focusing on a range of, still poorly understood, interacting influences that model individual sexual experiences and satisfaction as age progresses.

Baltes and Baltes (1990) state that the search for markers of successful aging should be based on multiple criteria that, given a cultural context, include both subjective and objective indicators. They state that, '. . . both the objective aspects of medical, psychological and social functioning and the subjective aspects of life quality and life meaning seem to form a Gordian knot that none is prepared to break at the present time'. Biological and mental health, cognitive efficacy, social competence, and satisfaction with life are mentioned among the multiple criteria of successful aging. These investigators have outlined a set of empirically derived propositions about the nature of aging that are relevant to clinical and research approaches to aging sexuality:

- There are major differences between normal, optimal and pathological behavior.
- There is much heterogeneity in aging.
- There is much latent reserve: behavioral and cognitive intervention studies have documented the existence of considerable individual plasticity and the capacity of older persons for new learning and corrective compensation. The concept of reserve capacity refers to the potential of older individuals to retain or to further develop, under favorable circumstances, clinically relevant functional abilities.
- Aging limits the magnitude and scope of reserve capacity: cognitive research shows that, as with physiological variables, there are age-related decreases in functional capacity in older individuals when tested at the limits of their optimal performance.
- Knowledge and technology can offset declines in reserve capacity. Pragmatic knowledge and the strategic development of skills and social support can exert an

important compensatory role in addressing the age-related loss of behavioral plasticity.

- The balance between gains and losses becomes less positive with aging: the age-related decrease in reserve capacity results in an increasingly less favorable balance in both objective behavioral assessment and subjective expectations. This results in life demands that increasingly exceed the limits of reserve capacity.
- The self remains resilient in old age: despite preconceived notions, older individuals, on average, do not differ from those in younger age-groups in terms of reports of satisfaction with life or measures of self-control or efficacy.

The concept of selective optimization with compensation was developed by Baltes and Baltes (1990), based on the above framework of propositions, as a strategic approach that has a bearing on the changes in sexual function that occur with aging. This notion refers to: (1) recognizing that the general reserve potential is reducing, and adapting by focusing on high-priority domains based on individual motivations, skills, and biological conditions; (2) maximizing the functional capacity in the areas selected; and (3) developing compensation strategies for when the demands exceed the adaptive limits of the individual. Other contributory factors are making realistic adjustments to individual expectations as age progresses and creatively adopting selective domains, to enhance personal satisfaction as well as the sense of mastery and control.

The concept of selective optimization and compensation for successful aging is applicable to the challenge of adapting to chronic illness (Curb et al., 1990). Most reports about the effect of chronic illness on sexuality follow a disease model with emphasis on functional deficits and loss. They tend to overlook the important role that psychological determinants play in shaping the nature and effectiveness of individual adaptive responses to medical illness and disability (Anderson and Wolf, 1986). The literature on coping provides a useful theoretical approach for the understanding of individual variations in adaptation to chronic disease. Several investigators have studied the effect of coping strategies on psychological adjustment in the medically ill (Moos, 1977), but little has been written relative to sexual function. This topic will be addressed further when discussing coping and adaptation in relation to aging sexuality and the management of sexual dysfunction.

Aging, health, and behavior

The narrow focus on aging and chronic illness needs to be broadened to consider sociocultural influences on health and behavior. The sociocultural environment can markedly alter the context of aging as well as affect the individual's health, the appraisal and coping with illness, and the interaction with health-care professionals. Aging is presently viewed not as a static concept, but as a dynamic process that is closely intertwined with social structure and social change (Hamburg, Elliot and Parron, 1982). Studies of aging, chronic illness, and sexual behavior, mostly bio-medically oriented, have neglected the importance of sociocultural factors. Behavioral research on sexual function is largely cross-sectional and, therefore, cannot distinguish changes intrinsic to aging from the effect of cohort differences in social background. The apparent decrease in sexual behavior in cross-sectional investigations of older-age cohorts, for example, may merely reflect the more restricted upbringing that prevailed in earlier eras rather than an age-related lowering in sexual expression.

Gerontologists study health-related behavior through the examination of health beliefs, perceived health status, psychosocial influences in the use of medical services, and compliance with medical advice. The interpretation given by older men and their sexual partners to age-related changes in sexual behavior, the nature of their interaction with health-care delivery systems and the role of health professionals in defining and addressing changes in sexual function have clinical and research consequences that are only beginning to be explored. Within the field of behavioral medicine, epidemiological studies have underscored the relationship between behavioral risk factors and disease. Life-style practices such as cigarette smoking, alcohol consumption, obesity and sleep patterns, for example, have significant long-term health, and possibly sexual, consequences extending well into the seventh decade of life (Ory, Abeles and Lipman, 1992). Behavioral risk analysis provides an important perspective on neglected life-style contributors to individual variability of age-related changes in sexual function.

The biomedicalization of aging

We know little about the determinants of the health-care-seeking behavior of older individuals relative to sexual function. The social construction of aging as a medical problem has fostered the attribution of sexual difficulties to biological causes, neglecting psychosocial contributors to sexual well-being and satisfaction. As the above review indicates, biological changes do not occur in isolation but take place in a social context that gives meaning and significance to aging. The unidimensional focus on biological processes, which characterizes much ongoing sexual research summarized in this book, carries the risk of distorting our perception of aging sexuality as being a medical problem (Kart, Metress and Metress, 1992b). The medical model orientation towards the assessment of signs and symptoms for diagnosis and treatment frequently overlooks the emotional aspects of health and well-being. Estes and Binney (1991) have written about the medicalization of aging and the social, professional and public policy consequences that stem from this view. Self-assessment and perceived control over health are as important predictors of general well-being and behavior in the aged as is medical status (Kart and Dunkle,

1989). In an epilogue to a book on aging and chronic disease, Kart, Metress and Metress (1992b) state that, 'professional care constitutes the minority of health provided to people to day regardless of age. . . Self evaluation of symptoms and self treatment are the basic and predominant forms of primary self care. They represent efforts on the part of people to retain and take control of health'. How the individual assesses health and interprets changes in body functioning determine, in large measure, the nature and the extent of the interaction with health providers. Older people are prone to attribute changes to internal physical processes rather than to external factors such as interpersonal problems or stressful events (Janis and Rodin, 1979). They may misattribute the natural effects of aging to pathology and seek medical solutions or, conversely, they may overlook disease or environmental factors and attribute all negative changes to the inevitability of growing old. Men, regardless of age and sexual function, are likely to welcome a prescription that would enhance sexual performance and improve quality of life. The development of oral drugs with erectogenic action addresses these expectations, reinforcing a medical view of male sexuality. The availability of oral drugs, if proven safe and effective, may represent a significant breakthrough in the treatment of sexual dysfunction. It shall be, nevertheless, important to maintain a broader perspective that does not neglect the relevance of psychological aspects for the sexual satisfaction of older individuals.

Methodological considerations on sexual research and aging

Several methodological problems, some stemming from the above conceptual discussion, need to be considered in the evaluation of studies of sexuality and aging. They include issues of sampling, research strategies and the scope of sexual measures and assessment procedures (Gurland and Gurland, 1980). A pervasive question is the contribution of disease to the sexual changes noted in studies of aging individuals. The relationship between aging and disease, and the extent to which they are considered as separable versus inseparable constructs have important implications for research strategy. The view that illness is an intrinsic component of aging leads to design studies where subjects are included without regard to health status or to the assessment of age-related changes on a healthy–unhealthy continuum. In contrast, the view that aging and disease are distinct constructs leads to studies where individuals are screened for all identifiable medical illness with the expectation that age-related differences or changes represent 'normal' or non-pathological aging. The study of such an elite group of older individuals provides valuable information but is not generally applicable to the population at large (Siegler and Costa, 1990). Most recent studies of aging and sexual behavior gather health status data but many fail to take full account of this information in the analysis and interpretation of results.

Studies of aging and sexual behavior are largely cross-sectional in design, sampling different age cohorts and interpreting changes as a longitudinal trend. This approach confounds the effects of the widely divergent cultural and developmental experiences of younger and older cohorts with the effects of aging. Similarly, individuals older than 65 are frequently considered as a single older cohort, ignoring the cultural heterogeneity within this group. Longitudinal studies, in which serial assessments are carried out on a given group of subjects at specified intervals, have their own limitations, however, since they confound the effect of aging and the temporal changes in societal attitudes concerning sexuality (Rowe, Wang and Elahi, 1990).

Two major problems in sexological research, including studies of aging, are the inadequate characterization of the populations investigated and the drawing of conclusions from small, nonrepresentative and nonrandom samples. There is controversy as to the magnitude and direction of participation bias in studies that explore sensitive issues such as sexual behavior. In general, people who volunteer for sexual studies have higher levels of education and less conservative sexual attitudes than nonvolunteers. The extent to which the results of studies of aging sexual behavior are influenced by a differential, age-dependent participation bias is not known.

Studies of the sexual behavior of aging men focus predominantly on coital activity and erectile capacity. They tend to be unidimensional and oriented towards sexual performance, neglecting the importance of motivational, cognitive, and affective factors. Phenomenologically, relevant aspects of the sexuality of older individuals such as sexual interest, sexual expectations and beliefs, satisfaction, and enjoyment are frequently ignored (Libman, 1989; Riportella-Muller, 1989). There is a need to operationally define and measure these constructs as they evolve and influence the sexual experiences of those who are growing old. Several sexual measures have been applied to the study of aging and sexuality, but the validity of some of these tests, developed in studies of younger subjects, needs to be reestablished in samples of older members of the population.

The chapters that follow will be guided by a multidimensional perspective of aging and sexuality. They are oriented by a biopsychosocial approach with emphasis on the biological and psychological interactions that shape individual sexual responses to advancing age during health and illness.

References

Anderson, B. J. and Wolf, F. M. (1986). Chronic physical illness and sexual behavior: psychological issues. *Journal of Consulting and Clinical Psychology* 54, 168–75.

Baltes, P. B. and Baltes, M. M. (1990). Psychosocial perspectives on successful aging: the model of selective optimization with compensation. In *Successful Aging. Perspectives for the Behavioral Sciences*, ed. P. B. Baltes and M. M. Baltes, pp. 1–34. New York: Cambridge University Press.

Birren, P. B. and Birren, B. A. (1990). The concepts, models and history of the psychology of aging. In *Handbook of the Psychology of Aging*, ed. J. E. Birren and K. W. Schaie, pp. 3–20, San Diego: Academic Press.

Brown, A. S. (1990a). The emergence of aging: an important area of study. In *The Social Processes of Aging and Old Age*, ed. A. S. Brown, pp. 1–11. Englewood, NJ: Prentice Hall.

Brown, A. S. (1990b). Physical and psychological aspects of aging. In *The Social Processes of Aging and Old Age*, ed. A. S. Brown, pp. 27–39. Englewood, NJ: Prentice Hall.

Butler, R. N., Lewis, M. and Sunderland, T. (1993). Who are the elderly? In *Aging and Mental Health. Positive Psychosocial and Biomedical Approaches*, 4th edn, pp. 3–28. New York: MacMillan.

Butt, D. S. and Beiser, M. (1987). Successful aging: a theme for international psychology. *Psychology and Aging* 2, 87–94.

Curb, J. D., Guralnik, J. M., LaCroix, A. Z., Korper, S. P., Deeg, D., Miles, T. and White, L. (1990). Effective aging meeting the challenge of growing older. *Journal of the American Geriatrics Society* 38, 827–8.

Esser, K. and Abisch, L. (1986). Is there a functional difference between normal and pathological aging? In *Dimensions in Aging, The 1986 Sandoz Lectures in Gerontology*, ed. M. Bergener, M. Ermini and H. B. Stahelin, pp. xvii–xx. San Diego: Academic Press

Estes, C. L. and Binney, A. A. (1991). The biomedicalization of aging: dangers and dilemmas. In *Critical Perspectives on Aging*, ed. M. Minkler and C. L. Estes. New York: Baywood Publishing.

Gurland, B. J. and Gurland, R. V. (1980). Methods of research into sex and aging. In *Methodology in Sex Research*, ed. R. Green and J. Wiener, pp. 67–92. Rockville, MA: National Institutes of Mental Health.

Hamburg, D. A., Elliot, G. R. and Parron, D. L. (1982). *Health and Behavior: Frontiers for Research in the Biomedical Sciences (Institute of Medicine Publication 82-010)*. Washington DC: National Academy Press.

Janis, I. and Rodin, J. (1979). Attribution, control and decision making: social psychology and health care. In *Health Psychology, a Handbook*, ed. C. G. Stone, F. Cohen and N. E. Adler. San Francisco: Jossey-Bass.

Kart, C. S. and Dunkle, R. E. (1989). Assessing capacity for self care among the aged. *Journal of Aging and Health* 1, 430–50.

Kart, C. S., Metress, E. K. and Metress, S. P. (1992a). Population aging and health status: the aged come of age. In *Human Aging and Chronic Disease*, ed. C. S. Kart, E. K. Metress and S. P. Metress, pp. 25–44. Boston, MA: Jones and Barlett.

Kart, C. S., Metress, E. K. and Metress, S. P. (1992b). The biologizing of aging: some precautionary notes. In *Human Aging and Chronic Disease*, ed. C. S. Kart, E. K. Metress and S. P. Metress, pp. 301–11. Boston, MA: Jones and Barlett.

Kohn, R. R. (1978). *Principles of Mammalian Aging*. Englewood Cliff, NJ: Prentice Hall.

Libman, E. (1989). Sociocultural and cognitive factors in aging and sexual expression: conceptual and research issues. *Canadian Psychology* 30, 560–7.

Lindeman, R. D., Tobin, J. and Shock, N. (1985). Longitudinal studies in rate of decline in renal function with age. *Journal of the American Geriatrics Society* 33, 278–85.

Moos, R. (1977). *Coping with Physical Illness*. New York: Plenum Press.

National Center for Health Statistics. (1986). *DHHS Publication No (PHS) 87–1232*. Washington, DC: Department of Health and Human Services.

Neugarten, B. (1974). Age groups in American society and the rise of the young-old. *Annals of the American Academy* 48, 187–98.

Ory, M. G., Abeles, R. P. and Lipman, P. D. (1992). Introduction: an overview of research on aging, health and behavior. In *Aging, Health and Behavior*, ed. M. G. Ory, R. P. Abeles and P. D. Lipman, pp. 1–23. Newbuty Park: Sage Publications.

Riportella-Muller, R. (1989). Sexuality in the elderly: a review. In *Human Sexuality The Societal and Interpersonal Context*, ed. K. McKinney and S. Sprecher, pp. 210–36. Norwood, NJ: Ablex Publishing Co.

Rodeheffer, R., Gerstenblith, G., Becker, L. C., Fleg, J. L., Weisfeldt, M. L. and Lakatta, E. G. (1984). Exercise cardiac output is maintained with advancing age in healthy human subjects: cardiac dilatation and increase stroke volume compensate for a diminished heart rate. *Circulation* 69, 203–13.

Rowe, J. W. and Kahn, R. (1987). Human aging: usual and successful. *Science* 237, 143–9.

Rowe, J. W., Wang, S. Y. and Elahi, D. (1990). Design, conduct and analysis of human aging research. In *Handbook of the Biology of Aging*, 3rd edn, ed. E. L. Schneider, G. F. Martin and E. J. Masoro, pp. 63–71. San Diego, CA: Academic Press.

Schaie, K. W. (1990). The optimization of cognitive function in old age: predictions based on cohorts-sequential and longitudinal data. In *Successful Aging. Perspectives for the Behavioral Sciences*, ed. P. B. Baltes and M. M. Baltes, pp. 94–117. New York: Cambridge University Press.

Schick, F. K. and Schick, R. (1994). *Statistical Handbook on Aging Americans*, Phoenix, AR: Oryx Press.

Siegel, J. S. and Davidson, M. (1984). Demographic and socioeconomic aspects of aging in the United States. *Current Population Reports. Special Study Series P-23, No. 138*. Washington DC: US Department of Commerce, Bureau of Census.

Siegler, I. C. and Costa, P. T. (1990). Health behavior relationships. In *Handbook of the Psychology of Aging*, ed. J. E. Birren and K. W. Schaie, pp. 144–66. San Diego, CA: Academic Press.

Siegler, I. C., Nowlin, J. B. and Blumenthal, J. A. (1980). Health and behavior: methodological considerations for adult development and aging. In *Aging in the 1980's. Selected Contemporary Issues*, ed. L. W. Poon, pp. 599–612, Washington, DC: American Psychological Association.

Stedman's Medical Dictionary, 25th edn. Baltimore, MD: Williams & Wilkins.

2   Sexuality in the aged male; research evidence

A point of departure from the exploration of the sexuality of aging males is an overview of the evidence of age-related changes in sexual behavior. This review incorporates a range of approaches: quantitative analysis of the frequency of sexual acts; phenomenological descriptions derived from nonrepresentative surveys based on nationally distributed questionnaires; systematic assessments of representative samples from the community at large; and objective measurement of sexual responses in the laboratory. The most relevant methodological aspects of these studies are summarized elsewhere (Schiavi and Rehman, 1995). This overview concludes with a brief discussion of the main findings on male aging and sexual behavior.

Aging and sexual behavior

Sexual activity in nonrandom subject samples

In the USA, the scientific approach to research into human sexual behavior started with Kinsey's pioneering studies in the 1940s. Kinsey, Pomeroy and Martin (1948) included over 14 000 men in their cross-sectional survey of male sexual behavior, but only 106 were over 60 years old. A progressive decline in sexual activity beginning at adolescence was noted, with nearly 30% of men completely inactive by the age of 70. The weekly frequency of total 'sexual outlets' (intercourse, masturbation, nocturnal emissions) in the active population decreased from a mean of 3 at ages 26–30 to 1 at ages 61–65, and to 0.3 in those aged 71–75 years. There was considerable variability in the frequency and range of sexual behaviors within every age group. Some of the men continued to report masturbation and nocturnal emissions well into the 76–80 age group. The percentage of erectile impotence remained less than 7% until the age of 60, when 18% of white males reported erectile failure. After that age the percentages markedly increased to 25%, 55%, and 75% at ages 70, 75, and 80 respectively. The authors acknowledged the lack of representation of older individuals in the total sample and speculated that biological, psychological, and social influences may all contribute to individual variability and to age-related changes in sexual behavior. Among the factors mentioned but not investigated were: general health, hormone levels, nutrition, lack of sexual variety, and work-related pressures.

Two major multidisciplinary, longitudinal studies conducted at Duke University on the biological, and psychosocial determinants of adaptation in late life confirmed and extended Kinsey's behavioral research findings. In the first study, initiated in 1954 (Pfeiffer, Verwoerdt and Wang 1968, 1969; Verwoerdt, Pfeiffer and Wang, 1969), 123 community male volunteers, aged 60–94 at the start, were evaluated on three occasions, each separated by an interval of three to four years. At the initiation of the survey, approximately two-thirds of the men in this sample were Caucasian and married. In the second study, which began in 1969 (Pfeiffer, Verwoerdt and Davis, 1972), 261 white, married men, aged 45–69, were assessed every two years during a ten-year period. The subjects, chosen randomly from an insurance membership list, were representative of the community's upper-middle socioeconomic strata. The data, which were analyzed cross-sectionally in both studies, provided mostly consistent and complementary findings:

- There was a gradual age-related decline in the frequency of sexual intercourse.
- The intensity of sexual interest also decreased with age, although to a lesser degree than sexual activity.
- At all ages men reported higher levels of sexual interest and activity than women.
- The proportion of individuals who were sexually active declined with advancing age: 40–65% of men between the ages of 60 and 71 years had intercourse in contrast to 10–20% of subjects over 78 years.

The questions about sex included in both Duke studies were few and limited to sexual interest and intercourse; masturbation and other sexual activities were not explored and there was no explicit inquiry about sexual dysfunction. The medical evaluations and laboratory tests were extensive, but provided limited information about the specific effect of illness on age-group differences, as well as on individual variations in sexual activity. The fact that in the 1954 study 41% of the initial sample had died by 1967 indicates that health issues need to be taken into account in the behavioral changes previously mentioned. Pfeiffer and Davis (1972) evaluated, by multiple regression analysis, the determinants of individual differences and found that subjective and objective health ratings contributed significantly and independently to the total variance in sexual behavior, after age and previous sexual experience were taken into account.

The Baltimore Longitudinal Study of Aging is another large, multidisciplinary project; it began in 1967 and explored some of the determinants of sexual function in aging males (Martin, 1975). There were 628 subjects, typically white, married, upper-middle-class, well-educated urban residents, aged 20–95 years and in good health at the beginning of the study. Participants in the program underwent a battery of physiological and psychological testing at the Gerontology Research Center at 12- to 24-month intervals. In one of the visits to the center the subjects were interviewed about marriage and sexual activity. Cross-sectional analysis of the data revealed that coital and total sexual activity decreased with age, as shown by Kinsey's data. As in the Duke studies, considerable individual variability within the age groups was noted. Recalled frequency of sexual behavior in earlier years emerged as a significant predictor of current sexual frequency, in keeping with the notion that, through their lives, men maintain a relatively stable level of sexual activity in relation to other men. The percentage of men who reported adequate erectile function or only incidental erectile failures decreased from 93% in the 20–39 age group to 43% at ages 70–79 (Martin, 1975). Martin concluded, based on the observation that several physiological measures were significantly associated with sexual behavior frequency, that physical well-being contributes importantly to maintaining sexual activity into old age (Martin, 1977). However, the specific effects of medical illness on sexual differences between and within age groups were not reported.

Analysis of the data from the 60- to 79-year-old men in the Baltimore study showed that frequency of sexual activity was independent of demographic features, marital adjustment, perceived sexual attractiveness, and sexual attitudes (Martin, 1981). Lack of sexual motivation was viewed as an explanatory factor in older men who, despite significant erectile difficulties, did not feel sexually deprived or deficient in self-esteem, described their marriages as highly successful and did not perceive the need for help to enhance their 'sexual vigor'. Martin stated that, 'the vast majority of subjects were apparently functioning at a level commensurate with their feelings of desire and, because few were lacking in other resources for maintaining self esteem, what losses did occur did not produce the emotional trauma that is often encountered in clinical practice'.

Several additional studies of nonrandom samples of convenience have been carried out in recent years. Weizman and Hart (1987) commented on the possible confounding effects of chronic illness and medication on the sexual function of the aged. They evaluated, using a self-report scale, the sexual behavior of 81 married volunteers from two community health clinics in Israel. The subjects, aged 60–71 years, were physically healthy and had been screened to rule out the effects of drug, psychopathology, and marital problems. A total lack of sexual desire was reported by only 14% of the men; 64% continued to engage in intercourse and about one-half of the total group acknowledged regular masturbatory activity. Sexual expression appeared to change with age, as shown by the lower frequency of intercourse and the higher rate of masturbation in those aged between 66 and 71 years compared to the subjects aged 60–65. Over one-third of the total sample experienced erectile dysfunction with no difference between the two age subgroups. Mulligan and Moss (1991) also explored the effect of aging on sexual behavior in a much larger subject sample and within a wider age range. They surveyed by mail 1249 randomly selected male veterans, registered at a medical center, stratified by age between the ages of 30 and 99. The authors found that sexual interest decreased significantly with age, but less than the frequency of intercourse. No-one reported a complete lack of sexual activity. The frequency of sexual intercourse for men with partners decreased from a mean of once-a-week for 30–39 year olds to once per year for men aged 90–99 years. Erectile capacity decreased markedly and significantly with age, with few subjects in the oldest age groups reporting regular intercourse. Alternative forms of sexual expression (caressing, oral sex, and masturbation) declined with age, in a similar fashion to intercourse.

The lack of a compensatory increase in noncoital sexual experiences, despite continued sexual interest and diminished coital capacity, contrasts with the results of a study of healthy, upper-middle-class volunteers living in residential facilities in Northern California, USA (Bretschneider and McCoy, 1988). Their sample included 100 men aged 80–102 years, 53 of whom had regular partners. Touching and caressing were reported by 82% of men to be the most common sexual experiences, followed by masturbation and intercourse which were reported by 72% and 63% of the subjects respectively. In keeping with Martin (1975), retrospective estimation of the value of sex in earlier years was significantly correlated with the frequency and enjoyment of intercourse and noncoital sexual experiences at the time of the evaluation.

Cross-sectional investigations are limited by the confounding of the effects of aging with those attributable to the social and cultural characteristics of the groups or cohorts included in the study. Pfeiffer, Verwoerdt and Wang (1969) reported a longitudinal assessment of 20 men drawn from the first Duke study who were evaluated four times over a ten-year period beginning at the mean age of 68. While the proportion of men with continuing sexual interest was relatively stable, remaining at 75% over the course of the investigation, the percentage of subjects still reporting sexual activity (intercourse) fell from 70% at the start of the study to 25% ten years later. The analysis of these data, which was based on aggregate values, does not allow individual behavioral changes over time to be identified. George and Weiler (1981) reanalyzed the results of the 1969 study of 278 persons (170 men) with a statistical approach that permitted assessment of aggregate *and* intraindividual patterns of sexual activity. The majority of men had stable levels of intercourse over a six-year period; approximately 20% indicated a decrease or cessation of sexual activity and about 5% reported actual increases in sexual behavior. The investigators emphasized the importance of not extrapolating from group or average statistics to estimate individual patterns of sexual activity.

Nonrepresentative sexual surveys based on nationally distributed questionnaires

In the winter of 1978 *Consumers Report*, a monthly magazine published in the USA, announced a study of family and social relationships and human sexuality for people aged 50 years and older (Brecher, 1984). Out of the 9800 questionnaires sent, there were 4246 replies from 2402 men and 1844 women; 79% of the men were married and 25% were 70 years of age and older. This self-selected sample was characterized by a better than average income, education, and general health. Responses to the questionnaire, which consisted of multiple-choice and open-ended queries, indicated a broad spectrum of beliefs and practices. There was a strong association, for both men and women, between the quality of marital relationships and sexual enjoyment. Analyses of age-related sexual trends for both genders showed that sexual desire, ease of sexual arousal, frequency of masturbation, as well as sex and orgasm with their partner all decreased with age. Generally, impaired health and specific medical conditions, such as reported heart attacks, antihypertensive medication, diabetes mellitus, and prostate surgery, had a measurable adverse impact on sexual function, but to a lesser degree than the effect of age per se on sexuality. Brecher comments that sexual pleasure can, and sometimes does, increase with age, even though the mean frequency of various sexual activities declines. Among the compensatory strategies used to maintain and occasionally enhance sexual enjoyment, reported in descriptive detail by some of the respondents, were the use of sexual fantasy, erotic materials, nudity, fondling and cuddling, oral, genital or anal stimulation, adjustment of coital positions, and manually assisted penetration of the nonerect penis.

Following the popular success of the Hite Report on female sexuality, Hite conducted a similar survey of males (1978). This report is based on responses to a broad questionnaire distributed to various population groups selected to approximate census statistics in the USA. The overall response rate was 6% and among the 7239 completed questionnaires, 6% of the men were 65 years of age or over. The author's impressionistic conclusions, illustrated by the florid, descriptive statements of older respondents, challenge the stereotypical notions of aging and sexuality. For most respondents, sexuality continued into their seventies and eighties, but its physical expression was varied and intimately linked to the emotional attraction and feelings for their partners.

Starr and Weiner (1981) challenged the narrow focus on quantitating performance and emphasized the value of a phenomenological approach that would explore the meaning and significance of sexuality in aging individuals. They conducted a study in several centers for senior citizens selected to encompass a wide demographic range in four regions of the USA and, therefore, to minimize the high degree of selection bias inherent in magazine surveys. Following a discussion of the problems of aging, Starr and Weiner (1981) distributed a 50-item open-ended questionnaire to be returned anonymously in a self-addressed envelope. The investigators received 800 complete replies representing a 14% response rate: 35% of the respondents were men aged 60–91 years and 64% of them were married. They were mostly retired, in good health and of above average socioeducational status. Sexuality was a valued aspect of the lives, attitudes, and experiences of this group. Ninety per cent of the men stated that they liked sex or that they would prefer to have it if it were available; 84% considered touching and cuddling important, 75% reported sexual arousal when looking at erotic books and movies, and 50% indicated a desire for greater sexual freedom, and more variety of sexual experience and partners. The average frequency of intercourse in the male sample was 1.44 times per week; 44% masturbated and 73% reported that having orgasms was an important aspect of their sexuality. Despite a progressive decrease in coital frequency and an increase in erectile problems with aging, 64% indicated that sexual satisfaction was the same or better compared with when they were younger. A cross-sectional national survey in the USA was recently conducted by Janus and Janus (1993), who also attempted to include a sample that would conform with the demographic characteristics of the US population. From the 4550 questionnaires distributed, the authors obtained 2765 satisfactory responses. Sixteen per cent of the 1347 male replies were from men 65 years of age or older; they were mostly married (57%), and with a high-school or college education. In keeping with Starr and Weiner's (1981) observations, the older subjects in the sample reported a remarkably broad range of sexual activities and a small decline in sexual satisfaction when compared with younger men.

Probability sampling studies from the community

The self-selected nature of the participants and wide differences in sample characteristics limit the generalizations that may be drawn from the studies just described. There are several surveys of representative samples of the population at large. Regrettably, a comprehensive sexual survey recently published by Laumann et al. (1994) did not include subjects older than 59 years. Persson (1980) investigated a representative, systematic sample of 70-year-old individuals born in 1901–1902 in Gothenburg, Sweden. Eighty-five per cent of the subjects agreed to participate in the study, which included a physical examination, a psychological evaluation, and an interview with questions on sexual development and sexual activity. Of 128 married men, 52% reported that they continued to have intercourse; among the variables that emerged as significantly associated with sexual activity were better global ratings of mental health, positive attitudes towards sexual activity, and the reported strength of sexual drive in younger years. Ratings of physical health were not associated with the frequency of intercourse in this investigation. No information about masturbation or other noncoital sexual behaviors was obtained.

Marsiglio and Donnelly (1991) assessed the frequency of sexual behavior among married persons selected from a US national probability sample of over 13000 adults carried out in 1987–1988. Sixty-six per cent of the 807 respondents who were

60 years old or more at the time of the survey provided adequate information. Among the respondents who reported having had sex at least once during the preceding month, 65% were aged 60–65, 45% were aged 71–75 and 24% were 76 years and older. Regression analysis demonstrated that the monthly incidence and overall frequency of sex were negatively related to age but that they were not associated with gender, race or, surprisingly, to self-reports of health status. Frequency of sex was significantly and positively linked, however, to the individual's sense of self-worth and competence and the partner's own health status. Although this study was restricted to only one question about the frequency of sexual activity and did not verify health status, it is one of the first representative surveys of a national sample of married persons older than 60. Diokno, Brown and Herzog (1990) conducted an epidemiological and clinical survey of individuals aged 60 years and older identified by a probability sampling of over 13000 households in Michigan. Trained evaluators interviewed 65% of the subjects from the initial 2993 eligible persons. Gender and marital conditions were significantly related to sexual activity: 73% of married men and 55.8% of married women were estimated to be sexually active; the respective percentages of unmarried men and women were 31.1% and 5.3% respectively. There was a highly significant decline in the sexual activity of both genders with increasing age, as well as an age-related increase in sexual difficulties frequently associated with medical disorders. Helgason et al. (1996) surveyed the sexual activity of 435 randomly selected Stockholm male residents, aged 50–80 years, with a response rate of 73%. Eighty-eight per cent reported sexual desire and 68% indicated that they were able to achieve erectile stiffness, 'usually sufficient for intercourse'. Although there was an overall age-related decrease in erectile function, 51% of the 70- to 80-year-old men continued to have adequate morning or spontaneous erections and 46% reported orgasms at least once per month. In those men who had unimpaired sexual desire and orgastic pleasure, most were distressed by a decrease in their erectile function. Erectile capacity appeared to be influenced by health status and medication, but physiological and psychological factors were not assessed in this study.

The Massachusetts Male Aging Study, a landmark multidisciplinary investigation conducted in the late 1980s, expanded the range of inquiry to sexual preferences, attitudes, and satisfaction, to add to the psychosocial and biological data. One aim of this epidemiological investigation was to obtain information about the factors associated with cross-sectional variations in sexual activity in men aged 40–70 living in the community (Gray, Jackson and McKinlay, 1991; Feldman et al., 1994; McKinlay and Feldman, 1994). Introductory letters were sent to over 5000 men chosen at random from randomly selected communities in the Boston area and, among the successful contacts, 1709 subjects agreed to participate, giving a response rate of 53%. Of the 1709 subjects, 1290 (75.5%) completed all the questions about sexual function. Comparisons between the volunteers and the

Erectile Function

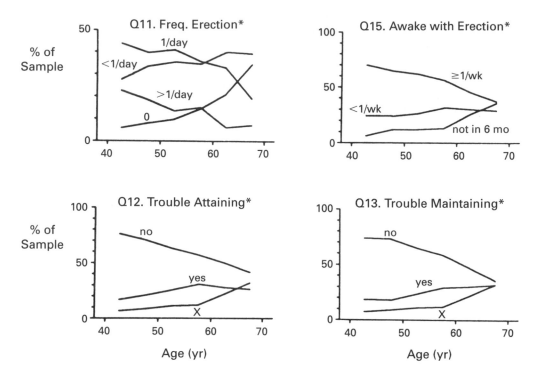

Figure 2.1   Erectile function assessed by self-report in the Massachusetts Male Aging Study.
*Statistically significant cross-sectional age trend, $p<0.0025$. X indicates no intercourse in the last six months. (Reproduced with permission from McKinlay and Feldman, 1994. *Sexuality Across the Life Course*, ed. A. S. Rossi, pp. 261–85. Chicago, IL: The University of Chicago Press.)

men who declined to participate did not provide evidence of response bias. Trained field technicians interviewed each subject in his home, administered psychological tests, including measures of dominance, anger and depression, and obtained two blood samples, drawn 30 minutes apart, to determine hormone levels. Health status was assessed by asking the participants to indicate from a list those diseases that they did *not* suffer from, as well as those that were and were not treated. The interviewer listed the medications taken. The participants then completed the sex questionnaire in private.

The results, reported by McKinlay and Feldman (1994), reveal that there is a consistent and statistically significant decline in erectile function with age (Figure 2.1), a similar decrease in the frequency of intercourse and ejaculation as well as an increase in ejaculatory difficulties with age (Figure 2.2). Sexual desire and fre-

Intercourse and Ejaculatory Function

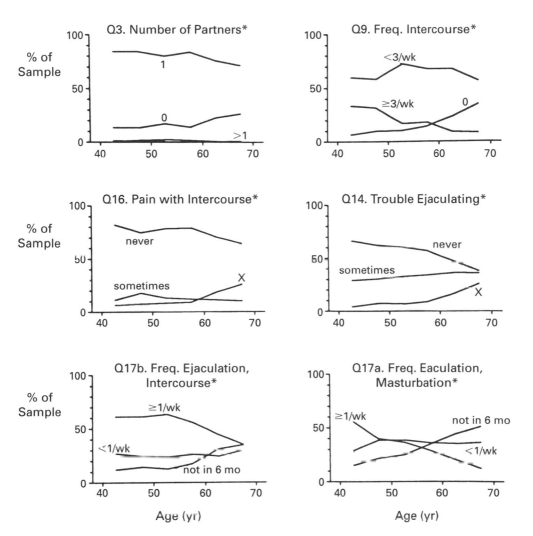

Figure 2.2   Intercourse and ejaculatory function by self-report in the Massachusetts Male Aging Study. *Statistically significant cross-sectional age trend, $p < 0.0025$. X indicates no intercourse in the last six months. (Reproduced with permission from McKinlay and Feldman, 1994. *Sexuality Across the Life Course*, ed. A. S. Rossi, pp. 261–85. Chicago, IL: The University of Chicago Press.)

Subjective Aspects of Sexuality

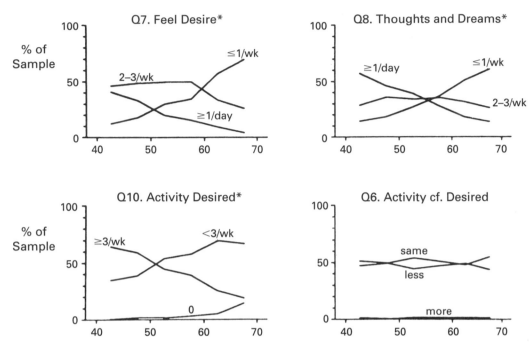

Figure 2.3   Subjective aspects of sexuality in the Massachusetts Male Aging Study. *Statistically significant cross-sectional age trend, $p < 0.0025$. (Reproduced with permission from McKinlay and Feldman, 1994. *Sexuality Across the Life Course*, ed. A. S. Rossi, pp. 261–85. Chicago, IL: The University of Chicago Press.)

quency of sexual thoughts and dreams also decreased with age, a change that closely paralleled the decrease in sexual activity (Figure 2.3). In contrast with the decrease in sexual desire and activity, sexual satisfaction did not change with age (Figure 2.4).The authors speculated that the age-related decrease in expectations about sexual activity, reflected in the subjects' response to one of the questionnaire items (Figure 2.4, question 21), may explain the continued level of sexual satisfaction despite diminished sexual function.

Multivariate statistics were used to reduce the large set of sociodemographic, psychological, and biomedical variables that might influence male sexuality. Regression analysis demonstrated that aging was strongly and negatively associated with 'sexual involvement' (a measure of sexual desire and activity); health status was positively related with sexual involvement and satisfaction, while emotional depression was associated with increased sexual difficulties and less sexual satisfaction. The investigators emphasized the importance of obtaining normative data

Satisfaction and Expectation

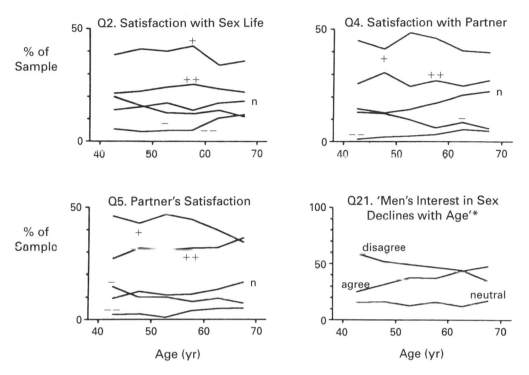

Figure 2.4   Sexual satisfaction assessed by self-report in the Massachusetts Male Aging Study. ++Extremely satisfied; +somewhat satisfied; nneither satisfied nor dissatisfied; ¯somewhat dissatisfied; ¯¯extremely dissatisfied. *Statistically significant cross-sectional age trend, $p < 0.0025$. (Reproduced with permission from McKinlay and Feldman, 1994. *Sexuality Across the Life Course*, ed. A. S. Rossi, pp. 261–85. Chicago, IL: The University of Chicago Press.)

about the usual and *nonmodifiable* changes in sexual interest and activity attributable to aging in order to provide a baseline for evaluating the *modifiable* social, psychological and life-style effects on sexual function.

Age and sexual responsiveness

An organizing principle orienting research on sexual responsiveness is that a predictable, cyclical sequence of physiological events can be identified during sexual arousal. Masters and Johnson (1966) divided this sequence into four, by now well known, phases: excitement, plateau, orgasm, and resolution characterized by genital and extragenital changes. Their physiological studies were limited to 39 men, only 20 over 60 years of age. They reported that older men, during the excitement and plateau phases, had slowly developing and less rigid erections, reduced scrotal sac and testicular vasocongestion, minimal preejaculatory fluid and an increased need for direct genital stimulation. The intensity of the orgastic release and ejaculatory volume was decreased, ejaculatory control was increased, detumescence during the ejaculatory phase occurred at a faster rate and the refractory period following ejaculation was prolonged in comparison to younger men. Extragenital responses such as hypotonia, nipple erections and sex flush were similarly reduced in intensity with age. The age-related losses of sexual responsiveness were attributed to physical and mental disorders, and to psychological factors such as boredom, career preoccupation, fatigue or fear of poor sexual performance. Masters and Johnson (1966) described modal changes; they gave no quantitative information about individual arousal patterns, and neither did they pay any attention to the psychological correlates of the sexual experience. This lack of information about individual variability contrasts with the previously reviewed information on the wide range of behavioral responses within age groups.

Increasingly, published research details objective evidence of individual patterns of sexual arousal, measured using psychophysiological methods under controlled laboratory conditions (Rosen and Beck, 1988). This research has been stimulated in part by the need to develop diagnostic tests that assess decrements in erectile capacity. Two approaches have frequently been used to evaluate sexual arousal in men: measuring waking erectile responses to erotic stimulation and the recording of nocturnal penile tumescence (NPT) during sleep. Remarkably few psychophysiological studies have obtained quantitative information that complements the behavioral reports of the sexuality of aging men.

Arousal responses during wakefulness

Solnick and Birren (1977) compared the rate of penile circumference increase over time between two physically healthy groups of men, 19–30 and 48–65 years of age, when exposed to the same erotic movie. The erectile response of the younger group was almost six times faster than that of the older group under controlled experimental conditions. Rowland et al. (1993) broadened the scope of this research to include several self-reported and laboratory-measured physiological responses during the sexual arousal of a group of healthy, sexually functional men aged between 21 and 82 years. Erectile function was measured by penile circumference changes during erotic films and self-induced fantasy. Although sexual interest among older men remained high, and there were no differences in self-reported erectile function with age, there were age-related decreases in erectile capacity and increases in latency to erection. Penile vibrotactile and electrical sensitivity and local autonomic function, measured by penile responses to ischemia, also decreased with aging. It is noteworthy that age-related changes in physiological function were not limited to the genitals. Older men had less sensitive fingers, decreased vascular reactivity to ischemia of the finger, and diminished tibial-evoked responses, suggesting that the decrements in sexual function are part of the generalized aging process. The significance of these findings will be elaborated in the next chapter.

Nocturnal penile tumescence during sleep

Research conducted in the 1960s (Oswald, 1962; Fisher, Gross and Zuch, 1965; Karacan et al., 1966) identified that regularly occurring episodes of penile tumescence accompany the cyclical presence of what is presently known as rapid eye movement (REM) sleep, a physiologically distinct and universally present sleep pattern characterized by bursts of bilateral, synchronous, rapid eye movement. NPT monitoring has frequently been used when diagnosing erectile disorders in older men (see Chapter 13), but still little is known about age-related variability in NPT in healthy individuals. Karacan et al. (1975), in an ontogenetic study, recorded penile tumescence changes during sleep in healthy men and found that the frequency and duration of tumescence episodes reach their maximum at puberty and then gradually decline. Older men, compared to younger adults, had shorter periods of tumescence during REM sleep, had less frequent and shorter periods of maximum tumescence, as well as more frequent erections during nonREM sleep. Schiavi and Schreiner-Engel (1988) verified the degree of erections by direct observation, in addition to recording the penile circumference of healthy, sexually nondysfunctional men aged 23–73 when asleep. Total sleep time and the ratio of total sleep time to time in bed (sleep efficiency) decreased significantly with age. The frequency and duration of NPT decreased progressively with age, independent of variations in sleep. In contrast to men in the younger age groups, most men older than 60 did not have full sleep erections even though they and their partners reported regular intercourse. We speculate that decrements in NPT reflect age-dependent changes in central neurophysiological mechanisms that mediate sexual arousal. In older individuals spontaneous sleep-generated tumescence may not be associated with adequate rigidity, and erections sufficient for intercourse are only achieved when the penis is stimulated directly. This may explain the apparent discrepancy between inadequate nocturnal erections and adequate sexual function during wakefulness in the older group of men. The need to gather systematic information from healthy aging men on the relationships between sexual behavior, sexual function and psychobiological measures led to a study conducted in our laboratories which is described in Chapter 4.

Conclusions

It is difficult to draw secure overall conclusions from the many studies of aging and its effects on male sexuality, because of the considerable diversity in their aims, the populations sampled and the methods used. A review of the literature does suggest that with aging there is a decrease in the frequency of sexual behavior, a lesser diminution in sexual desire and an increased prevalence of sexual dysfunction. Marked variability in sexual behavior is consistent within age groups, and there is some evidence, albeit retrospective, that individual differences may partly reflect characteristics that remain relatively stable as the men age. Medical illness, psychopathology, and drugs, although not systematically evaluated, are undoubtedly important determinants of these age-related changes *and* the individual variability in male sexual activity. Most studies have not included the sexual partner when assessing the effects of age on male sexuality. Partner availability, the nature and quality of the relationship over time and the partner's own health status probably, although this is largely unexplored, contribute to the range of sexual experiences of aging men. Studies of the effects of aging mainly involve white, middle-class, well-educated populations and there is minimal information about the role that race, education and socioeconomic conditions play in determining sexuality. The paucity of prospective studies means that it is difficult to draw definite conclusions. As most of the studies summarized in this chapter have a cross-sectional design, it is not possible to rule out cohort effects and to confidently assume that the age-related changes reflect a longitudinal trend.

It is important to note that statistical analysis of behavioral frequencies does not necessarily capture the changes in sexual meaning and expression as men age. Several studies, including the Massachusetts Representative Aging Survey, have shown that, while coital frequency and erectile capacity decrease with age, sexual satisfaction may not. Although the nonrepresentative surveys are methodologically flawed, they do provide potentially valuable qualitative information that needs to be considered when interpreting the results.

The contribution made by psychophysiological methods that provide objective evidence, under controlled conditions, of the effects of aging on male sexual function has yet to be fully explored. There are measurable age-related decreases in erectile capacity during wakefulness in response to erotic stimuli, and during REM sleep. A proportion of aged, healthy, volunteers and their partners report continuing sexual activity and regular intercourse despite marked decrements in erectile function as measured by NPT (Schiavi et al., 1990). It would appear that, for these individuals, the value placed on sexuality during their life, the frequency and range of their past sexual behaviors, their motivation and ability to develop compensatory sexual strategies and the supportive attitude of their partners are instrumental to their continuing sexual activity and sexual satisfaction and to the perception of not being sexually dysfunctional. Psychological and interpersonal characteristics in conjunction with biological factors, to be explored in the following chapters, all determine whether men age in a 'usual' or 'successful' way.

References

Brecher, E. (1984). *Love, Sex and Aging: A Consumer's Union Report.* Boston, MA: Little, Brown.

Bretschneider, J. G. and McCoy, N. L. (1988). Sexual interest and behavior in healthy 80- to 102-year olds. *Archives of Sexual Behavior* 17, 109–29.

Diokno, A. C., Brown, M. B. and Herzog, A. R. (1990). Sexual function in the elderly. *Archives of Internal Medicine* 150, 197–200.

Feldman, H. A., Goldstein, I., Hatzichristou, D. G., Krane, R. J. and McKinlay, J. B. (1994). Impotence and its medical and psychosocial correlates. Results of the Massachusetts male aging study. *Journal of Urology* 151, 54–61.

Fisher, C., Gross, J. and Zuch, T. (1965). Cycle of penile erection synchronous with dreaming (REM) sleep. *Archives of General Psychiatry* 12, 29–45.

George, L. K. and Weiler, S. J. (1981). Sexuality in middle and late life; the effects of age, cohort and gender. *Archives of General Psychiatry* 38, 919–23.

Gray, A., Jackson, D. N. and McKinlay, J. B. (1991). The relation between dominance, anger and hormones in normally aging men: results from the Massachusetts Male Aging Study. *Psychosomatic Medicine* 53, 375–85.

Helgason, R., Adolfsson, J., Dickman, P., Arver, S., Fredikson, M., Gothberg, M. and Steineck, V. (1996). Sexual desire, erection, orgasm and ejaculatory functions and their importance in elderly Swedish men: a population-based study. *Age and Ageing* 25, 285–91.

Hite, S. (1978). *The Hite Report on Male Sexuality.* New York: Alfred A. Knopf.

Janus, S. S. and Janus, C. L. (1993). *The Janus Report on Sexual Behavior.* New York: McGraw Hill.

Karacan, I., Goodenough, D. R., Shapiro, A. and Starker, S. (1966). Erection cycle during sleep in relation to dream anxiety. *Archives of General Psychiatry* 15, 183–9.

Karacan, I., Williams, R. L., Thornby, J. I. and Salis, P. J. (1975). Sleep-related penile tumescence as a function of age. *American Journal of Psychiatry* 132, 932–7.

Kinsey, A. C., Pomeroy, W. B. and Martin, C. R. (1948). *Sexual Behavior in the Human Male.* Philadelphia: WB Saunders.

Laumann, E. O., Gagnon, J. H., Michael, R. T. and Michaels, S. (1994). *The Social Organization of Sexuality.* Chicago, IL: University of Chicago Press.

Marsiglio, W. and Donnelly, D. (1991). Sexual relations in later life: a national study of married persons. *Journal of Gerontology* 46, S338–S344.

Martin, C. E. (1975). Marital and sexual factors in relation to age, disease and longevity. In *Life History Research in Psychopathology*, vol. 4, ed. R. D. Wirdt, G. Winokur and M. Roff, pp. 326–47. Minneapolis: University of Minnesota Press.

Martin, C. E. (1977). Sexual activity in the aging male. In *Handbook of Sexology*, ed. J. Money and H. Muraph, pp. 815–24. New York: Excerpta Medica.

Martin, C. E. (1981). Factors affecting sexual functioning in 60–79 year old married males. *Archives of Sexual Behavior* 10, 399–420.

Masters, W. H. and Johnson, V. E. (1966). *Human Sexual Response*. Boston, MA: Little, Brown.

McKinlay, J. B. and Feldman, H. A. (1994). Age-related variation in sexual activity and interest in normal men: results from the Massachusetts Male Aging Study. In *Sexuality Across the Life Course*, ed. A. S. Rossi, pp. 261–85. Chicago, IL: The University of Chicago Press.

Mulligan, T. and Moss, C. R. (1991). Sexuality and aging in male veterans: a cross-sectional study of interest, ability and activity. *Archives of Sexual Behavior* 20, 17–25.

Oswald, I. (1962). *Sleeping and Waking, Physiology and Psychology*. Amsterdam, Elsevier.

Persson, G. (1980). Sexuality in a 70-year old urban population. *Journal of Psychosomatic Research* 24, 335–42.

Pfeiffer, E. and Davis, G. C. (1972). Determinants of sexual behavior in middle and old age. *Journal of the American Geriatrics Society* 20, 151–8.

Pfeiffer, E., Verwoerdt, A. and Wang, H. S. (1968). Sexual behavior in aged men and women. *Archives of General Psychiatry* 19, 753–8.

Pfeiffer, E., Verwoerdt, A. and Wang, H. S. (1969). The natural history of sexual behavior in a biologically advantaged group of aged individuals. *Journal of Gerontology* 24, 193–8.

Pfeiffer, E., Verwoerdt, A. and Davis, G. C. (1972). Sexual behavior in middle life. *American Journal of Psychiatry* 128, 1262–7.

Rosen, R. and Beck, J. G. (1988). *Patterns of Sexual Arousal. Psychophysiological Processes and Clinical Applications*. New York: The Guilford Press.

Rowland, D. L., Greenleaf, W. J., Dorfman, L. J. and Davidson, J. M. (1993). Aging and sexual function in men. *Archives of Sexual Behavior* 22, 545–57.

Schiavi, R. C. and Rehman, J. (1995). Sexuality and aging. *Urological Clincs of North America* 22, 711–26.

Schiavi, R. C. and Schreiner-Engel, P. (1988). Nocturnal penile tumescence in healthy aging men. *Journal of Gerontology* 43, M146–150.

Schiavi, R. C., Schreiner-Engel, P., Mandeli, J., Schanzer, H. and Cohen, E. (1990). Healthy aging and male sexual function. *American Journal of Psychiatry* 147, 766–71.

Solnick, R. and Birren, J. E. (1977). Age and male erectile responsiveness. *Archives of Sexual Behavior* 6, 1–9.

Starr, B. D. and Weiner, M. B. (1981). *The Starr–Weiner Report on Sex and Sexuality in the Mature Years*. New York: McGraw Hill.

Verwoerdt, A., Pfeiffer, E. and Wang, H. S. (1969). Sexual behavior in senescence. II. Patterns of sexual activity and interest. *Geriatrics* 24, 137–54.

Weizman, R. and Hart, J. (1987). Sexual behavior in healthy married elderly men. *Archives of Sexual Behavior* 16, 39–44.

3   The neurobiology of aging males' sexuality

Age-related physiological changes contribute to the variability of the sexual function and behavior of older individuals, even when the confounding effects of medical illness and drugs are considered. There is little information on the mechanisms that mediate age-dependent differences in the sexual function of healthy individuals. This chapter provides a brief update on the neurobiology of male sexual function, and discusses the role of neurological, hormonal, and vascular processes possibly involved in sexual changes during nonpathological aging. It also summarizes the results of a multidisciplinary study of healthy aging men conducted in our laboratories.

The biology of sexual function

Sexological research has been oriented by conceptual models that help organize information about processes and mechanisms that underlie behavior. Sexual arousal is an encompassing concept implicit in Kinsey's research (Kinsey, Pomeroy and Martin, 1948) that unifies all physiological phenomena, central as well as peripheral. Masters and Johnson (1966) elaborated this notion further by structuring their observations along a progressive sequence of phases: excitement – plateau – orgasm – resolution, which they labeled the sexual response cycle. Kaplan (1979), based primarily on clinical evidence, incorporated a cognitive/motivational component in what she called the 'triphasic' model of sexual desire, arousal and orgasm, postulating that each of these phases is subserved by separate but interrelated physiological systems. Everitt and Bancroft (1991) criticized the validity of this model because of a lack of scientific evidence and the difficulty of operationally distinguishing between sexual desire and arousal. Despite these limitations, Kaplan's model has had important heuristic consequences, helping to organize research along clinically relevant dimensions which have been incorporated in a broadly used nosological system of sexual disorders (American Psychiatric Association, *Diagnostic and Statistical Manual of Sexual Disorders*, 1994).

Sexual desire

Sexual desire is a subjective state characterized by cognitive and affective components. It is usually considered within a motivational model which, like hunger and other appetitive functions, has a biological substrate that drives the organism towards behavioral expression. Sexual desire and sexual arousal are closely related and the distinction between both raises considerable conceptual and methodological problems. Measuring sexual desire requires both objective as well as subjective information. Individuals may engage in sexual behavior for reasons that are other than sexual, i.e., a wish to please the partner or fear of rejection, or, conversely, they may not behaviorally express their desire because of restraining psychosocial causes. In some investigations sexual desire has been measured based on reported frequencies of all sexual activity, the subjective desire to engage in any sexual behavior and the spontaneous occurrence of sexual thoughts and fantasies (Schreiner-Engel and Schiavi, 1986).

Androgens, mainly testosterone, play a necessary role in sustaining sexual desire. Men with abnormally low testosterone levels because of hypogonadism or following castration show a lack of sexual interest and associated sexual activity, whereas androgen replacement therapy markedly increases sexual thoughts and re-establishes sexual desire within a few weeks (Skakkebaek et al., 1981; Davidson, Kwan and Greenleaf, 1982; Kwan et al., 1983). The important effects of endogenous testosterone on sexual behavior was also recently demonstrated in a study of normal men (Bagatell et al., 1994). Inducing an androgen-deficient state, with a gonadotrophic-releasing hormone (GRH) antagonist that suppresses testosterone production, resulted in marked decreases in sexual desire, sexual fantasies and intercourse after four weeks of treatment; normal sexual function was restored in parallel with testosterone levels at the end of pharmacological intervention.

There are broad differences in the circulating levels of testosterone in normal adult men, but there is no solid evidence that testosterone levels account for individual variations in sexual drive and behavior. Administration of testosterone to eugonadal individuals has no marked behavioral effects. It has been postulated (Bancroft, 1989) that the circulating testosterone level necessary for behavioral activation is below the normal adult range. This may explain why, above this threshold level, normal individual hormonal differences do not measurably affect behavior. The possibility that androgen variability in eugonadal men may be associated with more subtle cognitive or affective characteristics requires further study. Presently there is little information on the minimal testosterone concentration necessary for adequate sexual function. Studies of hypogonadal men have shown that the threshold testosterone concentrations required to maintain normal sexual desire and arousal range between 144 and 346 ng/dl (Salmimies et al., 1987; Gooren, 1987). Most of the testosterone circulates tightly linked with a sex-hormone-binding globulin (SHGB) and is without physiological effect; approximately 4% is free and 40% is loosely bound to plasma albumin and both fractions are available for brain uptake.

Evidence, primarily from animal research, suggests that testosterone needs to be converted to dihydrotestosterone, by the enzyme 5α-reductase, or aromatized to estrogen, by the enzyme aromatase, to exert its biological and behavioral actions (Swerdloff et al., 1992). These effects take place following coupling at receptor sites located in central and peripheral tissues. A major advance in androgen physiology has been the cloning of the genes for the androgen receptor, the α-reductase enzyme and the aromatase enzyme. Despite this progress we remain largely ignorant of the neurophysiological and molecular events that mediate the effects of androgens on sexual drive and behavior. Sex steroid receptors have been located primarily in the preoptic and anterior hypothalamic regions, amygdala and hippocampus, areas within the hypothalamic–limbic system that participate in the regulation of motivated behaviors and the integration of endocrine and visceral functions (Kupfermann, 1991). Animal research discussed by Everitt and Bancroft (1991) is beginning to elucidate the hypothalamic–limbic structures that mediate the appetitive components of sexual behavior. Although the specific neurochemical processes that mediate testosterone's action on sexual function have yet to be identified, neurotransmitters, such as dopamine and serotonin, and neuropeptides are probably involved in these effects. Due to the difficulty in differentiating the neurochemical substrates of sexual drive from sexual arousal they will be discussed jointly in the next section.

Uncontrolled clinical information suggests that other steroids such as estrogen and nonsteroidal hormones such as prolactin may be implicated in the modulation of sexual desire and arousal in men (Segraves, 1988). Elevated prolactin levels, for example, can be associated with low sexual interest independently from decreases in circulating androgens; this may be a direct effect of prolactin or it may reflect reduced dopaminergic activity.

Sexual arousal

Sexual arousal is characterized by a cognitive–affective state associated with sexual excitement, genital responses, peripheral psychophysiological changes and mediating cerebral and spinal neurophysiological processes (Rosen and Beck, 1988a). Each one of these components and their interactions needs to be taken into account in the assessment of sexual arousal. Penile erections may occur without the subjective experience of sexual excitement, as during rapid eye movement (REM) sleep, and cardiovascular and respiratory systems may be activated by other emotional states such as anxiety or anger. Since no predictable pattern of peripheral nongenital changes has been identified as characteristic of sexual arousal, most psychophysiological research has focused on the recording of erectile responses. Work in this area has been stimulated further by the current interest in the medical treatment of erectile disorders.

The physiology of erectile function

Penile erection is under the control of two synergistic neurophysiological pathways: a sacral, mainly parasympathetic component that mediates reflexogenic erections; and a thoracolumbar, mainly sympathetic pathway that mediates psychologically induced sexual stimulation. Somatic innervation, by the pudendal nerve, provides input from sensory receptors in the penis and efferent fibers to the striated perineal muscles (De Groat and Booth, 1980; Murphy, 1993a). The autonomic nervous system regulates the hemodynamic events responsible for erection and detumescence. Penile tumescence is the result of the relaxation of the smooth muscle within the corpora cavernosa of the penis and the dilation of the cavernosal and helicine arteries that supply the blood to the lacunar spaces within the sponge-like cavernosal tissue. Expansion of the trabecular walls against the nondistensible tunica albuginea that surrounds the corpora cavernosa compresses the venous drainage and leads to increase corporeal pressure and penile rigidity. The endothelial cells that line the trabeculae of the corpus cavernosum play an important role in the physiology of erection. The relaxation of the cavernosal smooth muscles is thought to be influenced by cholinergic and nonadrenergic, noncholinergic nerves which control the release of endothelium-derived mediators, primarily nitric oxide and possibly vasoactive intestinal polipeptide (VIP) (Rajfer et al., 1992; Lerner, Melman and Christ, 1993). At the cellular level, activation of adenylate cyclase/adenosine 5'-cyclic monophosphate (cAMP) and guanylate cyclase/guanosine 5'-cyclic monophosphate (cGMP) pathways by nitric oxide elevates intracellular second messenger concentrations and causes an efflux of intracellular calcium leading to smooth muscle relaxation.

Detumescence occurs as the result of the sympathetically induced contraction of the helicine arteries and the corporeal smooth muscles resulting in diminished arterial inflow, decompression of the subtunical venules and increased venous outflow from the cavernosal spaces (Krane, Goldstein and de Tejada, 1989). Contraction of the trabecular smooth muscle, leading to detumescence and maintenance of the flaccid state, is mediated by α_1-adrenergic receptor stimulation. There is new evidence that oxygen tension regulates the nitric oxide pathway. A lowering of oxygen tension in the corpora by decreased arterial inflow may contribute to detumescence by inhibiting nitric oxide and increasing the synthesis of endothelin-1, which is a potent vasoconstrictor (de Tejada, 1995). The reverse process may, in turn, contribute to the development of tumescence.

Our knowledge of central mechanisms is restricted mainly to animal research

(Everitt and Bancroft, 1991). There is evidence that the brain has both excitatory and inhibitory actions on the spinal mechanisms that control erections. The brain regions primarily implicated in sexual arousal include the limbic–hypothalamic structures, the medial preoptic–anterior hypothalamic area and descending pathways in the medial forebrain bundle and the ventral tegmentum of the midbrain (Murphy, 1993b; Giuliano et al., 1995).

Neuroendocrine aspects

Recent studies have attempted to clarify the degree to which testosterone may influence erectile function independently from a primary effect on sexual drive. Androgen's mechanism of action has been explored by recording sleep-related erections and by measuring erectile responses to controlled presentation of erotic stimuli and to sexual fantasy. Sleep-related erections, which are usually impaired in hypogonadal men, are restored by exogenous testosterone (Kwan et al., 1983; O'Carroll, Shapiro and Bancroft, 1985; Carani et al., 1992). Conversely, administration of medroxy progesterone acetate (MPA), an antiandrogen that reduces total testosterone levels, significantly decreases the amplitude of the nocturnal penile tumescence (NPT) response. Erections in response to visual erotic stimuli in untreated hypogonadal men are no different from those of normal subjects and are not affected by androgen replacement. In contrast, fantasy-induced erections appear to depend on androgen (Bancroft and Wu, 1983; Kwan et al., 1983; O'Carroll, Shapiro and Bancroft, 1985). Bancroft (1989) has proposed that androgens, in addition to sustaining sexual desire and spontaneous erections during sleep, are involved in brain systems that mediate cognitive processing of sexual information (Bancroft, 1989). An alternative explanation is that the primary effect of androgens is peripheral, acting through the enhanced perception of pleasure from peripheral sexual responses (Davidson, Kwan and Greenleaf, 1982). Limited data are available on the effect of castration on erectile function in older men. Greenstein, Plymate and Katz (1995) assessed the relationship between testosterone and erectile responses to erotic visual stimulation in castrated older men with metastatic prostatic cancer. There was a marked decrease in sexual desire, no reported spontaneous erections and a total lack of sexual activity in all patients after castration. However, 4 out of 16 men (25%) had functional erections after visual erotic stimulation. The mean circulating free testosterone levels in these men were significantly greater, albeit within the range typical of castrated men, than those of the subjects who did not achieve an erection.

Central neurotransmitter mechanisms

Animal research has shown that several central monoamines, primarily dopamine, serotonin and noradrenaline, and neuropeptides such as endogenous opioids participate in the regulation of sexual behavior (Everitt and Bancroft, 1991). The relevance of these studies is underscored by the significant effects that centrally active monoaminergic drugs have on human sexual function. Although the clinical literature on this topic is extensive (see Chapter 10) we remain largely ignorant of the specific neurochemical systems involved in the mediation of human sexual responses. Recent reviews have discussed central neurotransmitter mechanisms in considerable detail (Murphy, 1993b; Giuliano et al., 1995), and this topic will only be briefly mentioned here. In general, dopaminergic activation enhances, and decreased dopaminergic transmission depresses, sexual behavior in rodents. Activation of different brain sites has differential behavioral effects, however. Pharmacological activation of the dorsal striatum and the medial preoptic/anterior hypothalamic regions modifies primarily copulatory responses, whereas drugs that act on ventral striatal dopamine receptors influence predominantly the appetitive aspects of male sexual behavior. The modulating role of dopaminergic transmission on motivated behavior also involves related limbic structures such as the amygdala and the hippocampus.

Drugs that increase central serotonergic transmission depress sexual activity whereas inhibition of serotonergic synthesis enhances sexual behavior. The central site of action and specificity of these effects remain unclear. Central serotonergic transmission influences not only sexual behavior but also feeding, sleep and mood states. Several families of serotonin receptors that participate in the mediation of physiological effects have been identified: $5HT_{1a}$, $5HT_{1b}$, $5HT_{1c}$, and $5HT_2$. Some receptors subtypes such as $5HT_{1c}$ mediate erectogenic effects and there is evidence that serotonergic agents have differential actions on sexual appetite and arousal depending on the different receptors involved (Murphy, 1993b).

Although central noradrenergic mechanisms have been the focus of less attention, recent information points to their important role in sexual drive and erectile capacity. α_2-Adrenoceptor agonists and antagonists have marked effects on several sexual behavior components in animals and possibly men. Finally, endogenous opioid peptides such as β-endorphin and enkephalin appear not only to affect sexual drive but also to disrupt genital reflexes. The combination of naloxone, an opioid antagonist, and yohimbine, an α-adrenergic blocking agent, was reported to induce full and sustained erections in normal volunteers (Charney and Heninger, 1986). This synergistic effect points to the largely unexplored interactions among brain neurochemical systems that control sexual behavior, and suggest, specifically, that central opioid and noradrenergic systems are functionally related in the mediation of penile erection.

Orgasm

Orgasm is characterized by an acme of sexual pleasure variously associated with rhythmic contractions of perineal and reproductive organ structures, autonomically mediated cardiovascular and respiratory changes and a release of sexual tension. The physiological changes in reproductive structures during orgasm in men may be divided into two phases: during the emission phase the smooth muscles of the vas deferens, prostate and seminal vesicles contract, propelling the seminal fluid into the bulbar urethra. Closure of the internal sphincter prevents the backflow of semen into the bladder. During the ejaculatory phase, the external bladder sphincter relaxes and the striated bulbocavernosus and ischiocavernosus muscles that surround the bulbar urethra contract rhythmically, projecting the semen out of the urethra. The emission phase is thought to be under thoraco-lumbar sympathetic control and mediated by noradrenaline release interacting with α-adrenergic receptors. The ejaculatory phase is controlled by a sacral–spinal reflex with afferents and somatic efferents traveling along the pudendal nerve (Lipshultz, McConnell and Benson, 1981; Newman, Reiss and Northup, 1982).

The participation of supraspinal processes in the orgasmic responses has been the focus of limited experimental research. Limbic structures involved in penile erection and ejaculation have been identified in primates with deeply implanted electrodes but, for obvious reasons, this approach has not been applied to healthy humans. Electroencephalography (EEG) studies with scalp electrodes during arousal and orgasm have provided conflicting findings. Cohen, Rosen and Goldstein (1976) reported a left-to-right shift in hemispheric dominance during self-induced orgasm in both sexes but Graber et al. (1985) failed to replicate this finding.

Considerable controversy surrounds the question of what constitutes the physiological underpinnings of the orgastic experience in men. The emission phase may be interfered with by surgery, medical pathology or α-adrenergic blocking drugs without eliminating the sensation of orgasm (Rosen and Beck, 1988b). Subjectively, deficient accumulation of seminal fluid in the bulbar urethra caused by abnormalities in the emission phase may result in the lack of sensation of 'ejaculatory inevitability' that usually precedes by seconds the ejaculation proper. The rhythmic contraction of striated pelvic muscles during the expulsive phase contributes to pleasurable orgastic sensations. Total interruption of the ascending fibers that carry sensory input from sexual structures to the brain eliminates the capacity for orgasm. Some paraplegic men with complete spinal cord injury do report experiencing orgasm during sleep; they have been labeled 'phantom orgasms' for they are thought to occur as a mental representation in the context of dreaming (Money, 1960). The extent to which central neurophysiological events are related to the nature and intensity of orgastic experiences and to male–female differences in the refractory period is not known.

During arousal culminating in orgasm peripheral changes in cardiovascular and respiratory function are frequently noted. Heart rate, systolic and diastolic blood pressure and respiration rate may markedly increase followed by rapid deceleration after the sexual climax (Rosen and Beck, 1988b). These changes are not solely due to physical exertion during sexual activity. Analysis of the relationship between subjective orgastic duration, intensity or satisfaction and peripheral psychophysiological measures have provided inconsistent results. The clinical significance of these autonomic changes during high arousal and orgasm in men with cardiovascular pathology will be discussed in Chapter 9.

Neuroendocrine studies have shown that secretion of oxytocin, a neuropeptide hormone, is linked to the orgasm but its functional role in men remains uncertain. Carmichael et al. (1987) found a significant positive relationship between perineal contractions, systolic blood pressure elevations and increases in plasma oxytocin levels during orgasm in both men and women. Murphy et al. (1987) also observed a specific link between oxytocin and orgasm as well as an increase in vasopressin secretion during arousal but not during orgasm. Some investigators have reported increases in testosterone, luteinizing hormone (LH) and prolactin secretion during sexual arousal and orgasm but these findings are not consistent and it is likely that they have limited physiological significance to humans (Stearns, Winter and Faiman, 1973; Lee, Jaffe and Midgley, 1974; Hellhammer, Hubert and Schurmeyer, 1985). Androgen secretion, by its action on the secretory activity of the prostate and seminal vesicles, is necessary for ejaculation but it is not clear whether the amount of ejaculatory fluid is linked to the quality of the orgasmic experience.

Physiological aspects of nonpathological aging

Aging and reproductive hormones

There is considerable evidence that aging is associated with decreased free and biologically active, circulating testosterone levels (Vermeulen, 1991). Hormonal assessments in the Massachusetts Aging Study described in the preceding chapter demonstrate that there is a decline in free and albumin-bound testosterone of approximately 1% per year for a total decrease of about 30% in a healthy subsample of men 40–70 years of age (Gray et al., 1991b). Total plasma testosterone diminished less because of the significant age-dependent increase in SHBG, the main protein carrier of androgens in plasma. In addition, several studies have shown that the normal circadian variation of the circulating testosterone level is attenuated or diminished with aging (Marrama et al., 1982; Bremner, Vitiello and Prinz, 1983). The concentration of adrenal androgens also decreases, but that of serum 5-dihydrotestosterone changes little, whereas levels of estradiol either increase or do not change in older individuals (Gray et al., 1991b; Vermeulen, 1996). The inconsistencies noted in earlier studies of the relationship between age and testosterone levels are probably due to methodological problems such as the confounding effects of medical illness or drugs, inadequate numbers of study subjects or blood samples, and a lack of consideration of diurnal hormonal changes (Gray et al., 1991a). The identification of age-dependent testosterone variations has been also obscured by the existence of high interindividual hormonal differences in healthy subjects. Some investigators have attributed circulating testosterone variations to still poorly studied environmental, behavioral, or socioeconomic conditions. Physical and emotional stress, dietary factors and obesity, for example, have been associated with decreases in plasma testosterone levels, whereas tobacco smoking has been reported to induce a rise in total and free testosterone levels (Vermeulen, 1993).

The primary cause of the age-dependent decrease in testosterone concentration is the gradual decline in testicular function as evidenced by a diminished Leydig cell mass, impaired testicular perfusion, reduced testosterone secretion in response to stimulation by human chorionic gonadotrophin (hCG) and a compensatory increase in circulating LH in older men (Nankin et al., 1981; Winters and Troen, 1982; Neaves et al., 1984). The LH increase is not, however, commensurate with the decline in circulating androgens suggesting that, in addition to testicular insufficiency, the hypothalamic–testicular axis is also compromised. The following indicate the existence of age-related alterations in central nervous system (CNS) pituitary mechanisms controlling gonadal function. Firstly, an increased sensitivity to sex steroid negative feedback, secondly the observation that naltrexone, an opioid antagonist, increases LH pulses in the young but has no effect in older men and thirdly the blunted CNS-controlled circadian rhythmicity of testosterone previously mentioned (Vermeulen and Kaufman, 1992; Mulligan et al., 1995). The effect of aging on prolactin secretion remains unclear. Serum values and circadian rhythmic variations of this hormone have been described as significantly increased, decreased or no different compared with those of younger individuals (Vekemans and Robyn, 1975; Rolandi et al., 1982). As with testosterone, differences in the timing and frequency of blood sampling and the confounding effects of illness and medication probably contribute to the discrepant findings.

The observation that aging is associated with a decline in gonadal function as well as decreased sexual behavior led to the notion that androgen deficiency contributes to the observed changes in the behavior of older men. This hypothesis rests on previously reviewed evidence, primarily derived from studies of hypogonadal patients, that testosterone is necessary to sustain sexual drive (Schiavi, 1996). However, remarkably few studies have evaluated the role of hormones on the sexuality of healthy older men. Tsitouras, Martin and Harman (1982), in the Baltimore longitudinal study of aging, observed a modest association between circulating testosterone levels and sexual behavior frequency. Weizman et al. (1983) noted a correlation between mild hyperprolactinemia and decrease sexual desire and activity in healthy men aged 60–70 years. Davidson et al. (1983) reported that there were low but significant correlations between the circulating free testosterone and LH levels and frequency of sexual thoughts, sexual activity and morning erections in older men aged 41–93 years recruited at a medical outpatient clinic. The hormonal evaluations were based on single samples and the behavioral assessment relied on retrospective information from a limited range of questions without partner validation. Sadowsky et al. (1993), in a cross-sectional study of 60 men aged 60–80 years, found an inverse association between age and sexual activity but no relationship between testosterone and prolactin concentrations and sexual activity. No attempt was made to screen-out patients with chronic medical conditions, and neither free nor bioavailable testosterone was measured.

It has been hypothesized that the threshold required for the behavioral action of testosterone may increase with age, resulting in a relative hormonal insufficiency for sustaining adequate sexual function (Bancroft, 1994). Indirect supportive evidence is provided by the observation that sleep erections are androgen sensitive and that they are impaired in healthy older men (Cunningham et al., 1990; Schiavi et al., 1990). A more direct approach to this question would be provided by investigating androgen-supplementation effects on the sexual function of aging individuals (see Chapter 14 on hormonal treatment). In younger, eugonadal, sexually nondysfunctional subjects, controlled androgen administration has variously resulted in increased sexual awareness and arousability but no changes in sexual behavior and mood (Anderson, Bancroft and Wu, 1992), in a modest increase in sexual drive in patients with low sexual desire (O'Carroll and Bancroft, 1984), or in enhanced sexual function only in impotent men with borderline levels of free testosterone (Carani et al., 1990). We recently conducted a double-blind, placebo-controlled study to assess the effect of biweekly injections of testosterone over a six-week period on sexual behavior and mood in a small group of healthy eugonadal men aged 46–67 years with erectile dysfunction (Schiavi et al., 1996). Testosterone administration resulted in significant increases in the frequency of masturbation, sexual activity with partner and early morning erections but had no effects on reported erectile rigidity. To the extent that the increase in sexual activity reflects sexual interest, these findings are consistent with prior studies suggesting that the primary effect of testosterone is on sexual desire rather than erectile function. There was no evidence that exogenous testosterone significantly affects the subjects' affective state or mood. There is a need for longer-term, controlled multidisciplinary research to address the effects of androgen supplementation on the sexuality and mood of aging men.

Aging and the nervous system

There is little evidence of neurological involvement in the mediation of the effects of aging on male sexuality, and that available is mostly indirect. There is ample documentation of anatomical, biochemical, and functional CNS changes during nonpathological aging. Structurally, cerebral neuronal loss occurs, the number of glial cells increases, and the number of dendrites and dendritic spines and synaptic alterations falls. The age-related neuronal loss does not occur uniformly throughout the brain but is selectively evident in specific regions such as the frontal cortex, hippocampus, amygdala, thalamus, locus ceruleus and substantia nigra (Creasey and Rapoport, 1985; Goldman, Calingasan and Gibson, 1994). Biochemically, these anatomical changes during normal aging are accompanied by significant modifications in the concentration and metabolism of brain neurotransmitters (Palmer and De Kosky, 1993). Of particular interest are age-related dopaminergic, serotonergic, and noradrenergic alterations because of their involvement in the processes that modulate sexual drive and arousal. Among the likely functional consequences of age-related changes in central monoaminergic activity are alterations of circadian endocrine secretion (McGinty, Stern and Akshohoff, 1988), sleep architecture and nocturnal penile tumescence (NPT). Emphasis on NPT for the diagnosis of organic impotence has detracted from considering sleep erections as a 'window' of brain neurophysiology. NPT decrements in older individuals may reflect, at least in part, changes in the central neurobiological processes that mediate the effects of age on sexual functioning (Schiavi and Schreiner-Engel, 1988).

Normal aging may also influence sexual function by its general effects on sensory, particularly somatosensory, systems. Most studies have documented a decrease in tactile sensitivity measured by an increased threshold to touch stimuli and a decline in sensitivity to vibrotactile stimulation at the glans penis (Zhong Cheng Xin et al., 1996). Somatosensory-evoked potential recordings also show an age-related diminution in amplitude and increase in latency which may reflect fiber loss, reduced myelinization and synaptic changes in peripheral and central sensory pathways (Allison et al., 1984). Few studies have explored the relevance of age-related changes in somatic sensory systems to sexual function. Edwards and Husted (1976) found an age-related decrease in penile vibrotactile sensitivity which correlated significantly with the frequency of sexual activity during the study period. Rowland et al. (1989) assessed genital sensitivity by vibrotactile and electrical stimulation at the finger tips and ventral surface of the penis and found markedly higher penile thresholds for both sensory modalities in men aged 56–75 years than in younger men. Differences in penile sensitivity accounted for a substantial portion of the variability in sexual activity and performance, suggesting that sensory mechanisms contribute to the effects of age on sexual functioning. A study involving somatosensory-evoked potential and sacral reflex latency measurements in men with no clinical evidence of neurological disease demonstrated that there is a relationship between subclinical, age-related, penile sensory deficits and erectile dysfunction (Benelmans et al., 1991). Penile sensory deficits may influence sexual function and behavior by interfering with reflex mechanisms that mediate erections as well as by modifying the pleasurable quality of the sexual experience. Further research is required to elucidate the significance of penile sensory receptivity in age-related changes in sexual activity.

Aging and the vascular system

Two lines of inquiry converge on the vascular mediation of age-induced changes in sexual function: the hemodynamic physiology of erection previously discussed and information on the vascular pathology associated with aging. The distinction between healthy and pathological aging is perhaps nowhere more difficult to determine than when assessing cardiovascular activity. Although the close interactions among age, life-style, and disease complicate the identification of the vascular effects of aging it is important to differentiate the natural arterial changes that occur as age progresses from those due to hypertension and abnormal blood lipid levels (Lakatta, 1993). At the vascular level, aging is associated with decreased inflow of blood into the cavernous tissue and a prolonged arterial response time following pharmacologically induced erections in physically normal men (Chung, Park and Kwon, 1997). At the cavernous smooth muscle level, aging is associated with a reduced response to nitric oxide and other endothelium-derived relaxing factors and with an enhanced effect of endothelin-1, a potent endothelium-generated vasoconstrictor. The level of prostacyclin, an agent secreted from endothelial tissues that mediates relaxation of vascular smooth muscle and inhibits thrombosis formation, decreases with age and may also contribute to the increase in vascular tone observed in older men. Structurally, endothelial dysfunction appears to promote an age-related subintimal accumulation of collagen, monocytes and smooth muscle cells and a decrease of elastin in the vascular walls. Changes in the extracellular matrix of the fibromuscular frame of the corpora involving collagen and glycation end-products may contribute to deficient penile rigidity in older men (Lerner, Melman and Christ, 1993). It has been suggested that age-related decreases in NPT may lead to corporal hypoxia and to increased release of growth factors and cytokines favoring corporal fibrosis (Broderick, 1996). Also affected by age is the capacity of the vascular smooth muscle to respond to endothelial bioactive agents as well as to cholinergic and adrenergic influences acting independently from endothelial function (Cooper, Cooke and Dzau, 1994). The age-dependent increased sensitivity of vascular smooth muscle from the corpus cavernosum of impotent men to α-adrenergic agents suggests, in addition, that elevated erectile smooth muscle tone in aging individuals may render the corpora less sensitive to endogenous vasorelaxation (Christ, Stone and Melman, 1991). It should be noted, however, that despite the growth of information on vascular physiology, our present knowledge of the effects of aging on erectile hemodynamics remains largely speculative.

In conclusion, accumulating data strongly suggest that neurobiological processes, as well as endocrine and vascular mechanisms all contribute to the effects of aging. This information is of considerable value when addressing the deleterious consequences of medical illness and medications for sexuality. In the context of

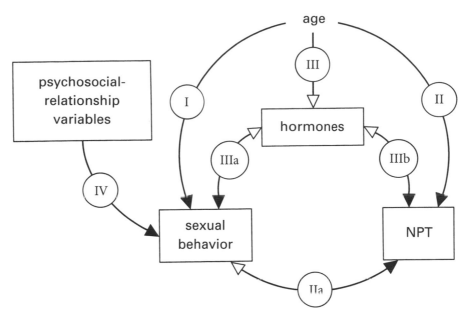

Figure 3.1   Diagram representing the conceptual framework of the cross-sectional, multidisciplinary study, on sexual function and behavior of healthy men aged 45–74 years. NPT, nocturnal penile tumescence.

nonpathological aging, the evidence tends to be atheoretical, unidimensional and does not integrate behavioral and psychological data. It does offer, however, an essential 'building block' for understanding the effects of aging on the sexuality of men.

A psychobiological study of the sexuality of aging males

Information on the sexual behavior of aging men and the physiological processes that mediate the effects of aging is frequently limited by the varied health status of the subjects, the narrow range of sexual questions without validation by the sexual partner, and the lack of a multidisciplinary approach that incorporates objective measures of erectile capacity, psychological, and marital dimensions. The objective of the following cross-sectional study was to gather behavioral, psychophysiological, hormonal, and psychosocial data on healthy men aged 45–74 years, living in stable sexual relationships. The methodological framework considered sexual behavior and associated psychological and marital measures in relation to age-related neurobiological changes reflected in sleep patterns, NPT, and pituitary–gonadal activity.

The major aims of the investigation, as indicated in Figure 3.1, were: (1) to assess age-related variations in sexual desire, behavior and satisfaction, and to identify the presence of sexual dysfunction (designated as I in the figure); (2) to assess age-related changes in NPT and to investigate the relationship of NPT to sexual functioning (II and IIa); (3) to assess age-related changes in circulating pituitary and gonadal hormones (III) and to evaluate the relationship between these endocrine variables and sexual behavior (IIIa) and NPT (IIIb); and (4) to explore the interaction of psychological and interpersonal measures along with behavioral changes in the sexual and marital satisfaction of aging men (IV). Methods and procedures, behavioral, sleep, psychophysiological, and hormonal findings will be summarized and briefly discussed below. The following two chapters will elaborate on the psychological and marital data. The reader is referred to published articles for a detailed discussion of the investigation (Schiavi, 1990; Schiavi, White and Mandeli, 1992; Schiavi et al., 1990, 1991, 1993).

Subject selection

The couples were selected from a pool of volunteers living in the New York city area who responded to announcements for a study on factors contributing to health, well-being and marital satisfaction in older men. Two hundred and five couples were screened by phone and considered ineligible because of illness, medication intake, lack of motivation or unwillingness of the partner to participate in the study. Seventy-seven couples completed the investigation, who had been married for a mean of 28.7 (range 2–50) years. Most of the men were predominantly white (94.8%), well educated, engaged in professional occupations (50.6 %) or retired (31.2%). Among those retired, 75% had retired from professional and 25% from clerical jobs. Male subjects met the following inclusion criteria: (1) they were aged between 45 and 75 years; (2) they were married or living in a stable relation with a sexual partner for at least one year; (3) they had obtained a high school diploma; and (4) English was their primary language. Exclusion criteria were: (1) evidence of medical disorders or surgical procedures that could compromise sexual function, drug intake, or substance abuse; (2) the presence of a major psychopathology; and (3) obesity (>20 % above ideal body weight).

Methods and procedure

Each subject and his sexual partner underwent, together and separately, a two-hour-long semi-structured interview, to gather psychosexual, medical, and psychiatric information. The male volunteers completed the Brief Michigan Alcoholism Screening Test (Selzer, 1971) for alcohol abuse, the MiniMental State Examination (Folstein, Folstein and McHugh, 1975) to rule out organic mental disorders and a sleep questionnaire to obtain clinical information about sleep patterns and problems. In following sessions they were given a comprehensive medical evaluation, a urological examination, the Schedule for Affective Disorders and Schizophrenia (Endicott and Spitzer, 1978) was applied to identify current psychopatholgy, and a battery of psychological tests was completed. In addition, penile vascular assessments were carried out by ultrasonic Doppler and mercury strain gauge plethysmography to identify vascular problems that may have contributed to erectile difficulties.

The male subjects were then studied in the sleep laboratory for four nights under similar conditions according to a protocol previously described (Fisher et al., 1979). EEG, eye movements, muscle tone, and penile tumescence were monitored throughout all the nights. In addition, during the first night's sleep, thermistors measured combined oro-nasal air flow, and bilateral anterior tibialis muscle activity was recorded electromyographically to identify occult sleep disorders. The effect of sleep disorders on the sexuality of aging males will be discussed in Chapter 9. Sleep was not disturbed during the first two recording sessions; during the third night, visual checks and photographic records were obtained during tumescence episodes to document the degree of erection in relation to the recorded increase in penile tumescence. Blood samples were collected from outside the subject's room at 20-min intervals during the fourth night for measuring hormone levels. All records were scored for sleep and sleep stages in 30-s epochs according to standardized criteria (Rechteschaffen and Kales, 1968). Analysis of the degree, frequency, and duration of penile tumescent episodes are described in detail elsewhere (Schiavi, 1988). Plasma testosterone, LH, and prolactin were measured in duplicate from each 20-min sample by established radioimmunoassay procedures. Bioavailable testosterone (bT) and estradiol in plasma pools formed from equal aliquots of each of the night's samples were measured in duplicate. Each subject was asked to keep a daily record of mood states, sexual activity, and sexual thoughts for the duration of the study period or at least 30 days. Questions were asked about the initiation and occurrence of sexual activity, the presence of erectile problems and sexual satisfaction.

Results

Relationship between age and behavioral variables

There was a consistent decrease with age of sexual desire, sexual arousal, and sexual activity. In keeping with previous reports, sexual interest, responsiveness, and activity were noted even among the oldest subjects in the study. Increasing age was positively correlated with the prevalence of erectile dysfunction but was not associated with hypoactive sexual desire or premature ejaculation. A nonparametric analysis compared the prevalence of sexual behavior among the 45–54, 55–64 and 65–74 age groups. As illustrated in Figures 3.2–3.4, several measures of sexual

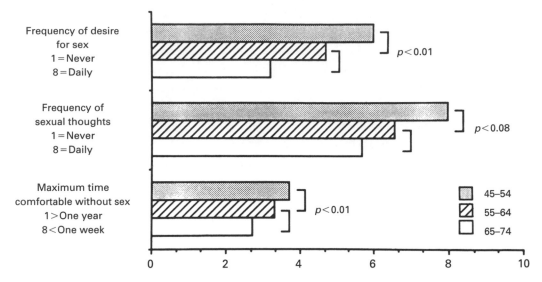

Figure 3.2   Relation between age and sexual desire variables in healthy men aged 45–74 years. Brackets indicate nonsignificance between groups according to multiple comparisons.

desire, sexual arousal, sexual activity and the total number of orgasms per month decreased with age, with differences observed mainly between the 45–54 and 65–74 age groups. In contrast, the degree of satisfaction with the men's own sexual functioning or enjoyment of marital sexuality did not change with age. Prospective data from daily records obtained for at least one month validated retrospective information from the psychosexual interview.

Relationship between age, sleep and NPT measures

The assessment of sleep erections provided an objective indicator of age-related changes in sexual function in men. There were significant decreases in total sleep time and sleep efficiency with aging but no differences in REM sleep (Figure 3.5). The frequency, duration, and degree of nocturnal erectile episodes markedly declined with age (Figure 3.6). The decrease in duration of tumescence remained significant after adjustment for the decrease in total sleep time associated with aging. As Figure 3.6 shows, multiple comparisons tests revealed that the oldest group had significantly lower mean tumescence values than the two other groups, which did not differ statistically from each other. Of the subjects younger than 65 years, 90% had at least one episode of maximum tumescence during the four study nights. In contrast, in only 19% of the subjects who were 65 or older was there clear evidence of penile rigidity during sleep.

The results only partially support the notion that NPT may reflect central neurobiological processes that are expressed subjectively by, for example, sexual desire, pleasure, or satisfaction (Figure 3.1, IIa). With the exception of sexual desire,

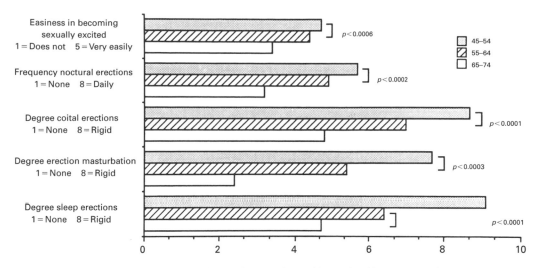

Figure 3.3   Relation between age and sexual arousal variables in healthy men aged 45–74 years. Brackets indicate nonsignificance between groups according to multiple comparisons.

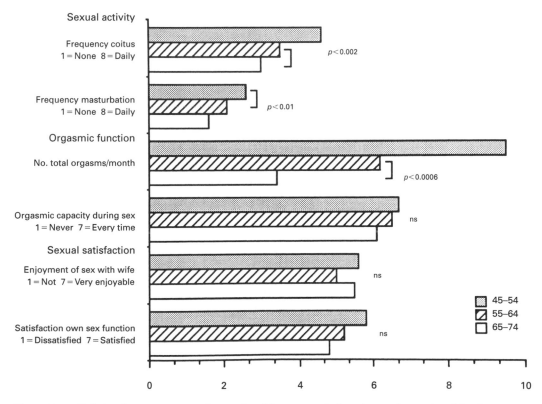

Figure 3.4   Relation between age and sexual activity, orgasmic function and sexual satisfaction variables in healthy men aged 45–74 years. Brackets indicate nonsignificance between groups according to multiple comparisons.

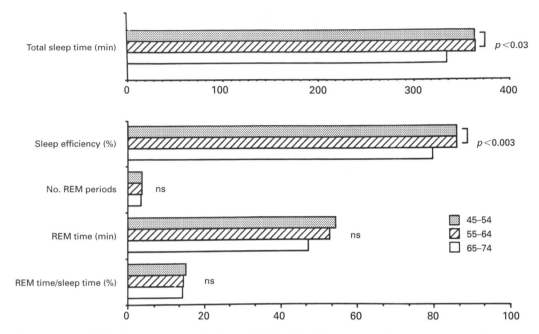

Figure 3.5   Relation between age and sleep variables in healthy men aged 45–74 years. Brackets indicate nonsignificance between groups according to multiple comparisons.

defined as the maximum time subjects said they were comfortable without sex, correlations between behavior and NPT lost their significance after age was controlled for.

Relationship between age, hormonal measures, and sexual behavior

The bT concentration decreased significantly with age, and the level of LH increased in compensation, consistent with the notion that aging is associated with a reduction in gonadal activity. A scatter plot illustrating the negative relationship between age and bT is shown in Figure 3.7. This age-related decline cannot be explained by the effects of medical illness or drug intake because of the rigorous inclusion/exclusion criteria and the extensive screening procedures. It should be noted that wide individual differences in hormonal and behavioral measures were observed within as well as across age groups. In contrast to bT, total testosterone, estradiol and prolactin levels did not vary with age, a finding noted by some but not all investigators.

Blood sampling every 20 min during the night permitted the characterization of patterns of hormone release during sleep. Abrupt testosterone, LH and prolactin peak fluctuations occurred irregularly with few age-related differences in the

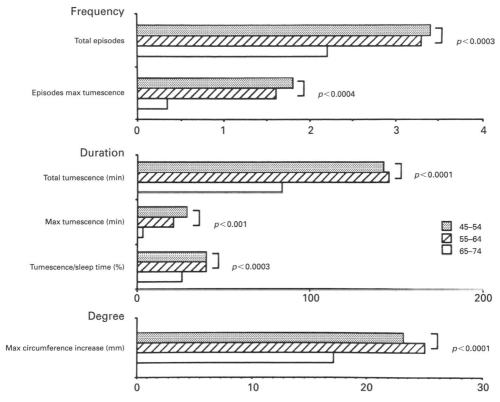

Figure 3.6   Relation between age and nocturnal penile tumescence variables in healthy men aged 45–74 years. Brackets indicate nonsignificance between groups according to multiple comparisons.

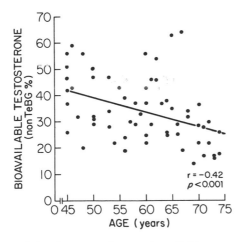

Figure 3.7   Relation between plasma bioavailable testosterone and age. (Reprinted from Schiavi et al., *Psychoneuroendocrinology* **17**, 599–609, 1992, with kind permission from Elsevier Science Ltd., The Boulevard, Langford Lane, Kidlington OX5 1GB, UK.)

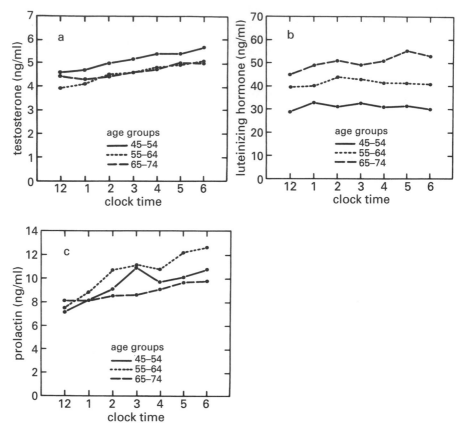

Figure 3.8   Time-related changes in plasma testosterone, luteinizing hormone and prolactin. Shown are means of all determinations made within each hour period. (Reprinted from Schiavi et al., *Psychoneuroendocrinology* **17**, 599–606, 1992, with kind permission from Elsevier Science Ltd., The Boulevard, Langford Lane, Kidlington OX5 1GB, UK.)

number and degree of hormonal peaks during the night. In order to compare slow endocrine variations during sleep, hormonal values were averaged hourly throughout the night between 2300 hours and 0600 hours. Figure 3.8 illustrates the time-related testosterone, LH and prolactin changes in the three age groups. Testosterone and prolactin concentrations increased significantly as the night progressed with no differences between the age groups. In contrast, the LH concentration increased significantly with age, but was not affected by the clock time.

The results of correlation analysis between pituitary and gonadal hormones, age and behavioral variables are presented in Table 3.1. bT levels, and the bT /LH ratio were significantly and positively associated with desire and arousal (but not sexual activity according to the psychosexual interview), and with the frequency of sleep erections reported prospectively during the course of the study. Total testosterone

Table 3.1. Correlations between plasma hormones, age, and sexual behavior

Psychosexual variable	Total testosterone	Estradiol	Bioavailable testosterone	LH	Bioavailable testosterone/ LH	Prolactin	Age
Retrospective assessment							
Desire							
Frequency of sexual thoughts	–	–	0.48 (0.008)	–	0.36 (0.03)	–	-0.50 (0.001)
Frequency of desire for sex	–	–	0.52 (0.001)	–	0.45 (0.006)	–	-0.52 (0.001)
Arousal							
Easiness in becoming aroused	–	–	0.26 (0.04)	–	0.24 (0.05)	–	-0.45 (0.0001)
Degree of masturbation erections	–	–	–	–	0.33 (0.03)	–	-0.38 (0.01)
Degree of coital erections	–	–	0.34 (0.01)	-0.33 (0.01)	0.35 (0.01)	–	-0.59 (0.0001)
Frequency of sleep erections	–	–	0.30 (0.01)	-0.24 (0.05)	0.33 (0.006)	–	-0.36 (0.002)
Activity							
Frequency of coitus	–	–	–	–	–	–	-0.40 (0.0004)
Frequency of masturbation	-0.34 (0.0005)	–	–	–	–	–	-0.34 (0.002)
No. of orgasms per month	–	–	–	–	–	–	-0.51 (0.0001)
Prospective assessment							
Frequency of sexual thoughts	0.31 (0.02)	–	–	–	–	–	-0.41 (0.28)
Frequency of sleep erections	–	–	0.28 (0.04)	-0.33 (0.01)	0.35 (0.01)	–	-0.44 (0.0004)
Frequency of coitus	–	–	–	–	–	–	-0.42 (0.001)
Frequency of masturbation	–	–	–	–	–	–	-0.22 (0.09)
Age	-0.09 (0.45)	-0.20 (0.10)	-0.60 (0.0001)	0.32 (0.008)	-0.51 (0.0001)	0.04 (0.76)	

Note:

Behavioral–hormonal correlations indicated only when significant. Reproduced in modified form from Schiavi et al. (1991). *Psychosomatic Medicine* **53**, 363–74.

and LH were not linked consistently with measures of sexual arousal and activity, while estradiol and prolactin were not associated with any measure of sexual behavior. Most associations between hormone levels and behavior lost their significance following statistical adjustment for the effect of age both on endocrine and activity measures.

Relationship between plasma hormones, age, and NPT

bT correlated significantly with NPT measures, while total testosterone, estradiol, LH, and prolactin were mostly unrelated to NPT (Table 3.2). bT and NPT no longer correlated significantly after adjustment for the effect of age on both correlates in the total subject sample. Analysis of the relationship between bT and the duration of NPT by age group revealed, however, a significant association between the two variables for men aged 55–64 years old, but not for the younger and older age groups.

Comparison of aging subjects with and without sexual dysfunction

Erectile dysfunction (ED) was operationally defined as an inability to achieve and maintain vaginal penetration until orgasm on at least 50% of the attempts during the preceding six months. The operational definition of hypoactive sexual desire disorder (HSDD) was based on the subjective desire and frequency of all sexual activities of less than twice per month for at least the previous six months. There were 17 men who met criteria for ED and 5 who met criteria for HSDD. This represents 22% and 6.5% respectively of the total group (n=77). The mean age of men with ED compared with the subjects who did not met criteria for ED was 64.5 versus 57.8 years, a statistically significant difference. There was also a significant difference in the mean age of men who did and did not have HSDD (70.8 versus 58.6 years, respectively). Comparison of the groups of men with and without ED, matched for age, was not significant for sleep, NPT, hormonal, and psychological measures. The small number of men with HSDD did not permit statistical comparison with nonHSDD volunteers.

Conclusions

A central aim of this investigation was to study the effect of aging on men carefully screened to minimize the possible effects of illness and medication on sexuality. The following conclusions may be drawn:

1. Sexual desire, sexual arousal, and sexual activity decreased significantly with aging. Although erectile difficulties were frequently reported by couples in the oldest age group, enjoyment of marital sex and men's satisfaction with their own sexuality did not change with age. This may reflect the particular characteristics of this sample of men in stable and committed relations who were, as a group, more

Table 3.2. Correlations between plasma hormones, age and nocturnal penile tumescence

NPT parameters	Total testosterone	Estradiol	Bioavailable testosterone	LH	Prolactin	Age
Frequency						
Total episodes	–	–	0.31 (0.01)	–	–	–0.35 (0.002)
Episodes during REM	–	–	0.34 (0.005)	–	–	–0.38 (0.0008)
Episodes with maximum tumescence	–	–	0.30 (0.02)	–	–	–0.45 (0.0001)
Duration						
Total tumescence	–	–	0.37 (0.002)	–	–	–0.40 (0.0003)
Simultaneous REM and tumescence						
Maximum tumescence	–	–	0.31 (0.01)	–	–	–0.43 (0.0002)
Tumescence/sleep time (%)	–	–	0.32 (0.008)	–	–	–0.35 (0.001)
Degree						
Mean increase in circumference	–	–	0.24 (0.055)	–0.33 (0.006)	–	–0.36 (0.001)
Maximum increase in circumference	–	–	–	–0.34 (0.006)	–	–0.36 (0.001)
Age	–0.09 ns	–0.20 ns	0.60 (0.0001)	0.32 (0.008)	0.04 ns	–

Notes:

Behavioral–hormonal correlations indicated only when significant. ns=p>0.05. Reproduced in modified form from Schiavi et al. (1991). *Psychosomatic Medicine* 53 363–74.

attracted to the study by the wish to learn about factors that contribute to health and well-being than by marital and sexual concerns.

2. The frequency, duration, and degree of NPT decreased significantly with age. The significance of the age-related decrements in tumescence after adjustment for sleep time support the existence of distinct ontogenetic changes in NPT independent of sleep architecture. The notion that NPT may reflect central neurobiological processes that are expressed in variations of sexual desire or behavior was only partially supported by the results; most associations between behavior and NPT lost their significance after controlling for age. The lack of evidence of full sleep erections in the majority of men older than 65 may be explained by the inhibitory effects of anxiety or embarrassment induced by the recording situation. An alternative explanation is that NPT decrements reflect age-related changes in central neurobiological processes that mediate endogenous sexual arousal. This may lead to an increasing dependence on the added synergistic effect of direct penile stimulation for the development of reflexogenic erections in aging men.

3. There was a highly significant decrease in bT and a compensatory increase in LH consistent with research previously reviewed, showing that aging is associated with decreased gonadal activity. The greater decrease in plasma concentrations of bT than total testosterone is probably caused by the age-related increase in SHBG concentration as documented in several laboratories. Sexual desire and reported sleep erections were the behavioral domains most closely related to the bT concentration. In contrast, the frequency of coitus, which is presumably influenced by each partner's own receptivity, was not significantly associated with hormone levels. These results are in keeping with evidence, primarily derived from hormonal replacement studies of hypogonadal patients (Davidson, Camargo and Smith, 1979; Kwan et al., 1983; O'Carroll, Shapiro and Bancroft, 1985), that androgens are more important for sustaining sexual desire and sleep-related erections than they are for maintaining erectile responses to external stimuli. The age-related effect of bT was, however, a more important determinant of reported variations in sexual behavior and sleep erections than were the effects of bT independent of age. When the hormonal concentrations were adjusted for the effect of age, the subjects with greater behavioral and sleep erection ratings continued to have higher bT levels than the less active group, but the differences were no longer statistically significant. These results support previous reports (Tsitouras, Martin and Harman, 1982; Davidson et al., 1983) that circulating androgens play a relatively small, independent role in age-related declines in sexual behavior in eugonadal men. There was no evidence that hormonal factors contribute to erectile dysfunction in aging subjects.

4. Aging may be associated with an increase in the threshold of activation of central receptor sites that mediate the behavioral effects of circulating androgens. Although older men may have plasma concentrations within the 'normal' range,

these levels may no longer be sufficient to sustain adequate sexual function. The finding that a significant association between bT and NPT, following age adjustment, was only observed in the middle age group is consistent with this hypothesis. Circulating androgens may be well above the threshold of activation of NPT responses in younger men, fall within the elevated threshold range of middle-aged individuals, and become no longer sufficient to sustain adequate NPT function in older men. Changes in receptor site sensitivity with aging may be reflected, therefore, in the observed age-dependent effect of bT and in the significant relationship between bT and NPT noted in the middle-aged but not in the two extreme groups.

5. The lack of statistical differences in physiological variables between two age-matched groups of men with and without ED may be due to a lack of power because of the relatively small number of dysfunctional subjects. The results raise, nevertheless, a note of caution against reaching premature conclusions about the pathogenic significance of atypical findings when age is not taken into account in the interpretation of results. A lack of evidence of low circulating testosterone levels, total and bioavailable, in the ED group is consistent with previously reviewed information that androgens are not directly involved in potency disorders in eugonadal individuals with adequate sexual desire.

6. Emphasis on sexual performance has been accompanied by neglecting sexual satisfaction in studies of aging sexuality. The results of this investigation suggest that clinical evaluation and therapeutic interventions should also consider psychological factors, as well as the quality of marital relationships. These important aspects will be elaborated in the two chapters that follow.

References

Allison, T., Hue, A. L., Wood, C. and Goof, W. R. (1984). Developmental and aging changes in somatosensory, auditory and visual evoked potentials. *Electroencephalography and Clinical Neurophysiology* 58, 14–24.

American Psychiatric Association. (1994). *Diagnostic and Statistical Manual of Mental Disorders*, 4th edn. Washington, DC: American Psychiatric Association.

Anderson, R.A., Bancroft, J. and Wu, F.C.W. (1992). The effects of exogenous testosterone on sexuality and mood in normal men. *Journal of Clinical Endocrinology and Metabolism* 75, 1503–7.

Bagatell, C. J., Heiman, J. R., Rivier, J. E. and Bremner, W. J. (1994). Effects of endogenous testosterone and estradiol on sexual behavior in normal adult men. *Journal of Clinical Endocrinology and Metabolism* 78, 711–16.

Bancroft, J. (1994). Androgens, sexuality and the ageing male. In *Endocrinology*, ed. F. Labrie and L. Proulx, pp. 913–16. Amsterdam: Elsevier.

Bancroft, J. (1989). *Human Sexuality and its Problems*, p. 95. New York: Churchill Livingstone.

Bancroft, J. and Wu, F. C. W. (1983). Changes in erectile responsiveness during androgen therapy. *Archives of Sexual Behavior* 12, 59–66.

Benelmans, B. L. H., Meuleman, E. J. H., Anten, B. W. M., Doesburg, W. H., Kerrebroeck, P. E. V. and Debruyne, F. M. J. (1991). Penile sensory disorders in erectile dysfunction: results of a comprehensive neuro-urophysiological diagnostic evaluation in 123 patients. *Journal of Urology* 146, 777–82.

Bremner, W. J., Vitiello, M. V. and Prinz, P. M. (1983). Loss of circadian rhythmicity in blood testosterone levels with aging in normal men. *Journal of Clinical Endocrinology and Metabolism* 56, 1278–81.

Broderick, G. A. (1996). Intracavernous pharmacotherapy. *Urology* 23, 111–25.

Carani, C., Zini, D., Baldini, A., Della Casa, L., Ghizzani, A. and Marrama, P. (1990). Effects of androgen treatment in impotent men with normal and low levels of free testosterone. *Archives of Sexual Behavior* 19, 223–34.

Carani, C., Bancroft, J., Granata, A., Del Rio, G. and Marrama, P. (1992). Testosterone and erectile function, nocturnal penile tumescence and rigidity, and erectile response to visual erotic stimuli in hypogonadal and eugonadal men. *Psychoneuroendocrinology* 17, 647–54.

Carmichael, M. S., Humbert, R., Dixen, J., Palmisano, G., Greenleaf, W. and Davidson, J. (1987). Plasma oxytocin increases in the human sexual response. *Journal of Clinical Endocrinology and Metabolism* 64, 27–31.

Charney, G. J. and Heninger, G. R. (1986). Alpha 2-adrenergic and opiate receptor blockade; synergistic effects on anxiety in healthy subjects. *Archives of General Psychiatry* 43, 1037–41.

Christ, G. J., Stone, B. and Melman, A. (1991). Age-dependent alterations in the efficacy of phenylephrine-induced contractions in vascular smooth muscle isolated from the corpus cavernosum of impotent men. *Canadian Journal of Physiology and Pharmacology* 69, 909–13.

Chung, W.K., Park, Y.Y. and Kwon, S.W. (1997). The impact of aging on penile hemodynamics in normal responders to pharmacological erections: a Doppler sonographic study. *Journal of Urology* 157, 2129–31.

Cohen, H. D., Rosen, R. C. and Goldstein, L. (1976). Electroencephalographic laterality changes during the human sexual orgasm. *Archives of Sexual Behavior* 5, 189–99.

Cooper, L. T., Cooke, J. P. and Dzau, V. J. (1994). The vasculopathy of aging. *Journal of Gerontology* 49, B191–6.

Creasey, H. and Rapoport, S. I. (1985). The aging human brain. *Annals of Neurology* 17, 2–10.

Cunningham, G. R., Hirshkowitz, M., Korenman, S. G. and Karacan, I. (1990). Testosterone replacement therapy and sleep related erections in hypogonadal men. *Journal of Clinical Endocrinology and Metabolism* 70, 792–7.

Davidson, J. M., Camargo, C. A. and Smith, E. R. (1979). Effect of androgen in sexual behavior in hypogonadal men. *Journal of Clinical Endocrinology and Metabolism* 48, 955–8.

Davidson, J. M., Kwan, M. and Greenleaf, W. J. (1982). Hormonal replacement and sexuality. *Clinical Endocrinology and Metabolism*, 11, 599–623.

Davidson, J. M., Chen, J. J., Crapo, L., Gray, G. D., Greenleaf, W. J. and Catania, J. A. (1983). Hormonal changes and sexual function in aging men. *Journal of Clinical Endocrinology and Metabolism* 57, 71–7.

De Groat, W. C. and Booth, A. M. (1980). Physiology of male sexual function. *Annals of Internal Medicine* 92 (Part 2), 329–31.

de Tejada, I. S. (1995). Commentary on mechanisms for the regulation of penile smooth muscle contractility *Journal of Urology* **153**, 1762.

Edwards, A. E. and Husted, J. R. (1976). Penile sensitivity, age and sexual behavior. *Journal of Clinical Psychology* **32**, 697–700.

Endicott, J. and Spitzer, R. L. (1978). A diagnostic interview: the schedule for affective disorders and schizophrenia. *Archives of General Psychiatry* **35**, 837–44.

Everitt, B. S. and Bancroft, S. (1991). Of rats and men: the comparative approach to male sexuality. *Annual Review of Sex Research* **2**, 77–117.

Fisher, C., Schiavi, R. C., Edwards, A., Davis, D., Reitman, M. and Fine, J. (1979). Evaluation of nocturnal penile tumescence in the differential diagnosis of sexual impotence. *Archives of General Psychiatry* **36**, 431–7.

Folstein, M. F., Folstein, S. E. and McHugh, P. R. (1975). 'Mini-Mental State'. A practical method for grading the cognitive state of patients for the clinician. *Journal of Psychiatric Research* **12**, 189–98.

Giuliano, F. A., Rampin, O., Benoit, G. and Jardin, A. (1995). Neural control of penile erection. *Urological Clinics of North America* **22**, 747–66.

Goldman, J. E., Calingasan, N. Y. and Gibson, G. E. (1994). Aging and the brain. *Current Opinion in Neurology* **7**, 287–93.

Gooren, L. J. G. (1987). Androgen levels and sex functions in testosterone-treated hypogonadal men. *Archives of Sexual Behavior* **16**, 463–73.

Graber, B., Rohbaygh, J. W., Newlin, D. B., Varner, J. L. and Ellingson, R. J. (1985). EEG during masturbation and ejaculation. *Archives of Sexual Behavior* **14**, 491–503.

Gray, A., Berlin, J. A., McKinlay, J. B. and Longcope, C. (1991a). An examination of research design effects on the association of testosterone and male aging: results of a meta-analysis. *Journal of Clinical Epidemiology* **44**, 671–84.

Gray, A., Feldman, H. A., McKinlay, J. B. and Longcope, C. (1991b). Age, disease, and changing sex hormone levels in middle-aged men: results of the Massachusetts male aging study. *Journal of Clinical Endocrinology and Metabolism* **73**, 1016–25.

Greenstein, A., Plymate, S. R. and Katz, P. G. (1995). Visually stimulated erection in castrated men. *Journal of Urology* **153**, 650–2.

Hellhammer, D. H., Hubert, W. and Schurmeyer, J. S. (1985). Changes in saliva testosterone after psychological stimulation in men. *Psychoneuroendocrinology* **10**, 77–87.

Kaplan, H. S. (1979). *Disorders of Sexual Desire*, New York: Brunner/Mazel.

Kinsey, A. C., Pomeroy, W. B. and Martin, C. R. (1948). *Sexual Behavior in the Human Male*. Philadelphia: WB Saunders.

Krane, R. J., Goldstein, I. and de Tejada, I. S. (1989). Impotence. *New England Journal of Medicine* **321**, 1648–59.

Kupfermann, I. (1991). Hypothalamus and limbic system: motivation. In *Principles of Neural Science*, 3rd edn, ed. E. R. Kandel, J. H. Schwartz and T. M. Jessel, pp. 750–60. New York: Elsevier Science.

Kwan, M., Greenleaf, W. J., Mann, J., Crapo, L. and Davidson, J. M. (1983). The nature of androgen action on male sexuality: a combined laboratory/self-report study on hypogonadal men. *Journal of Clinical Endocrinology and Metabolism* **57**, 557–62.

Lakatta, E. G. (1993). Cardiovascular regulatory mechanisms in advanced age. *Physiological*

Reviews 73, 413–67.

Lee, P. A., Jaffe, R. B. and Midgley, A. R. (1974). Lack of alteration of serum gonadotropins in men and women following intercourse. *American Journal of Obstetrics and Gynecology* 120, 985–7.

Lerner, S. H., Melman, A. and Christ, G. J. (1993). A review of erectile dysfunction: new insights and more questions. *Journal of Urology* 149, 1246–55.

Lipshultz, L., McConnell, J. and Benson, G. S. (1981). Current concepts of the mechanisms of ejaculation. *Journal of Reproductive Medicine* 26, 499–507.

Marrama, P., Carani, C., Baraghini, G. F., Volpe, A., Zini, D., Celani, M. F. and Montanini, V. (1982). Circadian rhythm of testosterone and prolactin in ageing. *Maturitas* 4,131–8.

Masters, W. H. and Johnson, V. (1966). *Human Sexual Response.* Boston, MA: Little, Brown and Co.

McGinty, D., Stern, N. and Akshohoff, N. (1988). Circadian and sleep-related modulation of hormone levels: changes with aging. In *The Endocrinology of Aging*, ed. J. R. Sowers and J. V. Felicetta. New York: Raven Press.

Money, J. (1960). Phantom orgasm in the dreams of paraplegic men and women. *Archives of General Psychiatry* 3, 373–82.

Mosko, S. S., Dickel, M. J., Paul, T., Latour, T., Dhillon, S., Ghahim, A. and Sassin, J. F. (1988). Sleep apnea and sleep-related periodic leg movements of community resident seniors. *Journal of the American Geriatrics Society* 36, 502–8.

Mulligan, T., Iranmanesh, A., Gheorghiu, S., Godschalk, M. and Veldhuis, J. D. (1995). Amplified nocturnal LH secretory burst frequency with selective attenuation of pulsatile (but not basal) testosterone secretion in healthy aging men. *Journal of Clinical Endocrinology and Metabolism* 80, 3025–31.

Murphy, M. (1993a).The neuroanatomy and neurophysiology of erection. In *Impotence: An Integrated Approach to Clinical Practice*, ed. A. Gregoire and J. P. Pryor, pp. 29–55. Edinburgh: Churchill Livingstone.

Murphy, M. (1993b). The pharmacology of erection and erectile dysfunction. In *Impotence: An Integrated Approach to Clinical Practice*, ed. A. Gregoire and J. P. Pryor, pp. 55–77. Edinburgh: Churchill Livingstone.

Murphy, M. R., Seckl, J. R., Burton, S., Checkley, S. A. and Lightman, S. L. (1987). Changes in oxytocin and vasopressin secretion during sexual activity in men. *Journal of Clinical Endocrinology and Metabolism* 65, 738–41.

Nankin, H. R., Linn, T., Murono, E. P. and Osterman, J. (1981). The aging Leydig cell. III. Gonadotropic stimulation in men. *Journal of Andrology* 2, 181–5.

Neaves, W. B., Johnson, L., Porter, J. C., Parker, C. R. and Petty, C. S. (1984). Leydig cell numbers, daily sperm production and serum gonadotropin levels in aging men. *Journal of Clinical Endocrinology and Metabolism* 59, 756–63.

Newman, H. F., Reiss, H. and Northup, J. D. (1982). Physical basis of emission, ejaculation, and orgasm in the male. *Urology* 19, 341–50.

O'Carroll, R. and Bancroft, J. (1984). Testosterone therapy for low sexual interest and erectile dysfunction in men: a controlled study. *British Journal of Psychiatry* 145, 146–57.

O'Carroll, R., Shapiro, C. and Bancroft, J. (1985). Androgens, behavior and nocturnal erections in hypogonadal men: the effects of varying the replacement dose. *Clinical Endocrinology* 23,

527–38.

Palmer, A. M. and De Kosky, S. T. (1993). Monoamine neurons in aging and Alzheimer's disease. *Journal of Neural Transmission (General Section)* **91**, 135–59.

Rajfer, J., Aronson, W. J., Bush, P. A., Dorey, F. J. and Ignarro, L. J. (1992). Nitric oxide as a mediator of relaxation in the corpus cavernosum in response to nonadrenergic, noncholinergic neurotransmission. *New England Journal of Medicine* **326**, 90–4.

Rechteschaffen, A. and Kales, A. (1968). *A Manual of Standardized Terminology, Techniques and Scoring System for Sleep Stages.* Washington, DC: U.S. Government Printing Office.

Rolandi, E., Magnani, G., Sannia, A. and Barreca, T. (1982). Evaluation of Prl secretion in elderly subjects. *Acta Endocrinologica* **100**, 351–7.

Rosen, R. C. and Beck, J. G. (1988a). Patterns of sexual arousal. In *Patterns of Sexual Arousal. Psychophysiological Processes and Clinical Applications*, pp. 23–52. New York: The Guilford Press.

Rosen, R. C. and Beck, J. G. (1988b). The psychophysiology of orgasm. In *Patterns of Sexual Arousal. Psychophysiological Processes and Clinical Applications*, pp. 134–57. New York: The Guilford Press.

Rowland, D. L., Greenleaf, W., Mas, M., Myers, L., Davidson, J. (1989). Penile and finger sensory thresholds in young, aging and diabetic males. *Archives of Sexual Behavior* **18**, 1–12.

Sadowsky, M., Autonovsky, H., Sobel, R. and Maoz, B. (1993). Sexual activity and sexual hormone levels in aging men. *International Psychogeriatrics* **5**, 181–6.

Salmimies, P., Kockott, G., Pirke, K. M., Vogt, H. J. and Schill, W. B. (1987). Effects of testosterone replacement on sexual behavior in hypogonadal men. *Archives of Sexual Behavior* **11**, 345–53.

Schiavi, R. C. (1988). Nocturnal penile tumescence in the evaluation of erectile disorders: a critical review. *Journal of Sex and Marital Therapy* **14**, 83–96.

Schiavi, R. C. (1990). Sexuality and aging in men. *Annual Review of Sex Research* **1**, 227–50.

Schiavi, R. C. (1996). Androgens and sexual behavior in men. In *Androgens and the Aging Male*, ed. B. O. Oddens and A. Vermeulen, pp. 111–25. New York: Parthenon Publishing Group.

Schiavi, R. C. and Schreiner-Engel, P. (1988). Nocturnal penile tumescence in healthy aging men. *Journal of Gerontology* **43**, M146–50.

Schiavi, R. C., Schreiner-Engel, P., Mandeli, J., Schanzer, H. and Cohen, E. (1990). Healthy aging and male sexual function. *American Journal of Psychiatry* **147**, 766–71.

Schiavi, R. C., Schreiner-Engel, P., White, D. and Mandeli, J. (1991). The relationship between pituitary-gonadal function and sexual behavior in healthy men. *Psychosomatic Medicine* **53**, 363–74.

Schiavi, R. C., White, D. and Mandeli, J. (1992). Pituitary-gonadal function during sleep in healthy aging men. *Psychoneuroendocrinology* **17**, 599–609.

Schiavi, R. C., White, D., Mandeli, J. and Schreiner-Engel, P. (1993). Hormones and nocturnal penile tumescence in healthy aging men. *Archives of Sexual Behavior* **22**, 207–15.

Schiavi, R. C., White, D., Mandeli, J. and Levine, A. (1996). Effect of testosterone administration on sexual behavior and mood in men with erectile dysfunction. *Archives of Sexual Behavior* **26**, 231–41.

Schreiner-Engel, P. and Schiavi, R. C. (1986). Lifetime psychopathology in individuals with low sexual desire. *Journal of Nervous and Mental Disease* 174, 646–51.

Segraves, R. T. (1988). Hormones and libido. In *Sexual Desire Disorders*, ed. S. Leiblum and R. C. Rosen, pp. 271–312. New York: The Guilford Press.

Selzer, M. L. (1971). The Michigan alcoholism screening test: the quest for a new diagnostic instrument. *American Journal of Psychiatry* 127, 1653–8.

Skakkebaek, N. E., Bancroft, J., Davidson, D. W., and Warner, P. (1981). Androgen replacement with oral testosterone undecanoate in hypogonadal men: a double blind control study. *Clinical Endocrinology*, 14, 49–67.

Stearns, E. L., Winter, J. S. D. and Faiman, C. (1973). Effects of coitus on gonadotropin, prolactin and sex steroid levels in man. *Journal of Clinical Endocrinology Metabolism* 37, 687–91.

Swerdloff, R. S., Wang, C., Hines, M. and Gorski, R. (1992). Effect of androgens on the brain and other organs during development and aging. *Psychoneuroendocrinology* 17, 375–83.

Tsitouras, P. D., Martin, C. E. and Harman, S. M. (1982). Relationship of serum testosterone to sexual activity in healthy elderly men. *Journal of Gerontology* 37, 288–93.

Vekemans, M. and Robyn, C. (1975). Influence of age on prolactin secretion in women and men. *British Medical Journal* 2, 738–9.

Vermeulen, A. (1991). Clinical review 24. Androgens in the aging male. *Journal of Clinical Endocrinology and Metabolism* 73, 221–4.

Vermeulen, A. (1993). Environment, human reproduction, menopause, and andropause. *Environmental Health Perspectives Supplements* 101 [Suppl. 2], 91–100.

Vermeulen, A. (1996). Declining androgens with age: an overview. In *Androgens and the Aging Male*, ed. B. J. Oddens and A. Vermeulen, pp. 3–12. New York: The Parthenon Publishing Group.

Vermeulen, A. and Kaufman, J. M. (1992). Editorial: role of the hypothalamo–pituitary function in the hypoandrogenism of healthy aging. *Journal of Clinical Endocrinology and Metabolism* 74, 1226A–C.

Weizman, A., Weizman, R., Hart, J., Maoz, B., Wusenbeek, H. and David, M. B. (1983). The correlation of increased serum prolactin levels with decreased sexual desire and activity in elderly men. *Journal of the American Geriatrics Society* 31, 485–8.

Winters, S. J. and Troen, P. (1982). Episodic LH secretion and the response of LH and FSH to LH-releasing hormone in aged men. Evidence for co-existing primary testicular insufficiency and an impairment in gonadotropic secretion. *Journal of Clinical Endocrinology and Metabolism* 55, 560–5.

Zhong Cheng Xin, Woo, S. C., Young, D. C., Do, H. S., Y, J. C. and Hyung, K. C. (1996). Penile sensitivity in patients with primary premature ejaculation. *Journal of Urology* 156, 979–81.

4 Psychological aspects of aging males' sexuality

The viewing of aging and sexuality through the prism of behavioral frequencies and erectile function inherent in much current research has led to the neglect of potentially important psychosexual determinants and correlates. Clinical and phenomenological reports emphasize the importance of studying the meaning and significance of sexuality for aging individuals, but there is little systematic research into the relevant motivational, cognitive, and affective influences on this population. While this chapter focuses on the psychology of aging and sexuality, we should remain aware of the pitfalls of viewing the psychological aspects separately from the biological, interpersonal, and sociocultural contexts that shape the individual experience.

Sexual interest and motivation

The terms sexual interest, desire, motivation, and drive are frequently mentioned without addressing their underlying conceptual underpinnings. Some investigators assume that an innate drive exists, mediated by neuroendocrine mechanisms that motivate sexual behavior, while others emphasize psychosocial factors to the exclusion of biological ones. Some retrospective investigations note that men, as they age, retain characteristic levels of sexual interest and activity compared with other men. While men's interest in sex declines overall with age, variation between individuals persists through life and thus accounts for a significant proportion of the variation of sexual functioning in the elderly (Pfeiffer and Davis, 1972; White, 1982; Botwinick, 1984a).

Assuming that prospective studies will validate these observations, why is it that the patterns of sexual activity remain consistent over time? We have already discussed the significance of androgens and their effects on sex drive and it is conceivable, although by no means proven, that their central action contributes to the observed variation in libido within the population. Martin (1981) reevaluated data obtained from interviews with 60- to 79-year-old married subjects from the Baltimore Longitudinal Study of Aging. He concluded that differences in motivation best explain the consistency in sexual function from middle to old age. While acknowledging that biology and personality influence sexual motivation, Martin emphasizes how continued exposure to erotic cues and erotic reactions to sexual stimuli both sustain men's sexual desire and motivation over time. The observation that some men, in our study of healthy couples, showed marked global decreases in sexual interest when their sexual partners were either not available or without sexual desire around the menopausal period, would be difficult to explain on the basis of biological determinants alone. It is not clear, however, why the sex drive of some men decreases as they get older or are exposed to fewer erotic stimuli, whereas other men become increasingly frustrated and dissatisfied. Perhaps a model that integrates the biology *and* psychology of aging and sexuality will be best able to explain the evidence obtained to date.

Sexual attitudes and knowledge

Sexual attitudes and knowledge are closely interwoven with sexual interest. There is little doubt that sociocultural influences, to be discussed in Chapter 7, conspire to minimize or deny the existence or value of sexuality for the aged. In an early study Cameron (1970) gave a questionnaire to groups of young (aged 18–25), middle-aged (40–55 years) and older (65–79 years) adults to assess their beliefs about sexuality. The old evaluated themselves, and were judged by the two other groups, as being the less knowledgeable about sex, less desirous and less capable. The extent to which the attitudes of the aged towards their own sexuality reflect cultural stereotypes may be related to the increased conservatism frequently noted in older individuals (Glamser, 1974). Differences in sexual permissiveness, however, are not only influenced by age but also by gender, socioeconomic level, and marital status. Snyder and Spreitzer (1976), for example, compared sexual attitudes towards the nontraditional sexual behavior of two age groups over and under the age of 65 from a US national probability sample. While the older respondents had more conservative attitudes to sex, background variables such as gender, educational level, marital status, and religiosity were significant predictors of sexual attitudes in both age groups even after controlling for age. These findings, although limited by a lack of data about generation effects, challenge the assumption that older men are a homogeneous group. Using validated psychometric methods, White (1982) assessed the sexual attitudes and knowledge of a sample of institutionalized aged people. Prior sexual history, retrospectively obtained, emerged as a strong predictor of current sexual activity, as it is for those who are not institutionalized. Sexual attitudes and knowledge are both significantly related to the frequency of sexual behavior but, unexpectedly, they were not statistically related to each other. At the turn of the twentieth century, when this group was growing up, there were few opportunities to learn about sexuality because of the attitudes that prevailed at that time. White (1982) speculates that this group has remained ill-informed regardless of any subsequent sexual permissiveness.

Inadequate knowledge of sex and sexuality has been repeatedly emphasized by clinicians as an important contributor to sexual problems (Kaplan, 1974). Aging men, ignorant of normal age-related changes in sexual function, may be particularly vulnerable to faulty expectations and concerns about performance. It is remarkable that there has been so little systematic research on how sexual knowledge influences the sexual experiences of aging individuals (Steinke, 1994). Despite the limited data, sex education has been included in therapeutic programs for the aged, resulting in their having more permissive sexual attitudes, increased sexual activity, and enhanced sexual satisfaction (White and Catania, 1982). Psychoeducational approaches to aging and sexuality will be discussed in Chapter 14.

Affective responses and self-esteem

The impact of age-related changes on sexual function should be considered in the context of underlying fears of growing old and apprehension about anticipated declines in intellectual and physical abilities. Those who are wrongly informed about the consequences of aging or who have inaccurate expectations of sex are at risk of reacting to decreases in erectile capacity with anxiety, fear of failure, and excessive concerns about performance. These emotional reactions, frequently linked with fears of rejection and obsessive self-monitoring of sexual responses, escalate what may be a limited sexual change into total sexual disability.

Much has been written by sex therapists about the central role that anxiety about sex plays in the development and maintenance of sexual dysfunction (Kaplan, 1990). Empirical evidence provided by Barlow and coworkers (Barlow, 1986) shows that demands for sexual performance have different effects on physically healthy sexually functional and dysfunctional men. Cranston-Cuebas and Barlow (1990) devised a working model based on this research. This model predicts that there is a positive feedback loop, in which demands for sexual performance generate positive affect and expectations which result in increasingly efficient attention being focused on erotic cues during enhanced autonomic arousal. In contrast, in sexually dysfunctional men, performance demands lead to negative affect and expectations and to attention being focused on nonerotic cues – a maladaptive process that is reinforced by increased autonomic activation. This pioneering research studied mostly college-aged males, and there is evidence that older men may have different sexual responses to the experimental manipulation of anxiety and performance demands (Beck and Barlow, 1986). It would be of considerable interest to apply this experimental model to the study of cognitive and affective processes in aging individuals.

Why do some men adjust to natural decreases in sexual function without apparent emotional distress while others respond with anxiety, embarrassment or shame? Personality characteristics, as well as what sexuality means to the individual are both likely to influence men's appraisal of sexual change and the nature of their reaction to it. Byrne and Schulte (1990) developed a heuristic framework for personality research aimed at integrating a set of psychological variables that influence how external stimuli affect behavior. The measures of disposition include: affect (emotion), evaluation (attitudes), cognition, expectations, imagination (fantasy), and physiological arousal. The authors reviewed evidence on the ability of these variables to predict several aspects of sexual function. They introduced the construct erotophobia–erotophilia, which is defined as, 'the disposition to respond to sexual clues along a negative–positive dimension of affect and evaluation'. Erotophobes report having negative emotional reactions to sexuality (including guilt and anxiety), respond negatively to or avoid sexual cues and have few sexual fantasies. Erotophiles, in comparison to erotophobes, report more sexual interest, more frequent and varied past sexual experiences and greater sexual satisfaction. This construct is associated with dimensions such as sexual permissiveness and conservatism, and may help to explain differences in sexual response within and across the age groups.

The meaning and significance of sexuality to the individual is an important determinant of the nature of their reaction to sexual changes. Perception and psychomotor skills decline as age progresses but they do not elicit the same degree of self-doubt as does diminution of erectile capacity. The culturally reinforced link between sexual ability and feelings of self-worth render older men vulnerable to a loss of self-esteem when faced with physiological decreases in sexual function. These changes have particular consequences because they challenge denial of aging and the retention of a more youthful self-image (see Case study 4.1 for illustration). A body of research shows that older persons look to the 'middle-aged' or even to the 'young' as a reference group rather than to their peers. Bultena and Powers (1978), in a study of persons 70 years and older, found that a substantial number of individuals continued to consider themselves as middle-aged. Those who thought that their health, physical independence, and need for help compared favorably to those of older persons most often thought of themselves as being middle-aged. The persistence of inappropriate standards or reference models may contribute to sexual dissatisfaction, to self-doubts and a lowering of self-esteem as the aged experience natural declines in sexual capacity. The significance of sexuality for men's self-esteem varies with age. Stimson, Wase and Stimson (1981) noted, for example, that for younger men it is the amount of sexual activity that is associated with sexual confidence and self-esteem, while for older men it is the perceived quality of sexual performance that is central to their feelings of self-worth. Similarly, in a study of married couples aged 50–77 years, it was the men's confidence about their capacity to perform adequately that emerged, together with their degree of sexual motivation, as the most significant predictor of the perceived quality of sexual experiences for both partners (Creti and Libman, 1989).

Coping and adaptation

A decline in the capacity to perform sexually is a pervasive source of concern for aging men. The reaction to this change is compounded by prevailing situations, such as retirement and decreased social participation, that challenge the sense of personal adequacy and self-worth. For some, as previously mentioned, it is associated with considerable anxiety and emotional distress. Cognitive appraisal and coping, considered at some length in Chapter 12, provide a useful conceptual framework for understanding individual responses to changes in sexual functioning. Cognitive appraisal means the individual's evaluation of an event and its impact on the person's well-being (Lazarus and DeLongis, 1983). How a man appraises a change in sexual function, whether it is perceived as a benign, threatening or challenging event, will determine the nature of his response as well as his emotional, physiological, and behavioral reactions. Coping has been defined, 'as the process of managing demands that are appraised as taxing or exceeding the resources of a person' (Cohen and Lazarus, 1983). Coping theory offers a framework for understanding the range of individual responses to age-related changes in sexual function, as well as to the impact of medical illness on sexual behavior. The appraisal of a decrease in erectile capacity as either a natural or a threatening event, and how men subsequently cope and adapt are all influenced by the following: how they have valued sexual expression over their lifetime, their personality characteristics, their personal beliefs and expectations and their belief in whether they can modify or improve their sexual situation. As Lazarus and DeLongis (1983) stated, '... *throughout life people struggle to make sense out of what happens to them and to provide themselves with a sense of order and continuity. This struggle is centered in divergent personal beliefs and commitments, shapes cognitive appraisals of stressful transactions and coping, and therefore has profound consequences for morale, social and work functioning, and somatic health. It is thus not age alone, but the significance of stressful events viewed within the continuity of a person's life that must be taken into account.*' The significance of coping and sexual expression in the face of obvious physiological limitations is illustrated in Case study 4.2.

Well-being and sexual satisfaction

The concentrated attention on behavioral changes in the aged has been accompanied by a neglect of assessing sexual satisfaction. Sexual satisfaction may best be considered within the broader context of well-being in late life. Aging is associated with a variety of personal, interpersonal, and social changes that challenge the adaptive capacity of the individual. Self-reported health is the variable that is most consistently related to well-being in stress and coping research (Larson, 1978); however, within the vast number of publications about life satisfaction few studies consider sexuality. Several studies have shown that life satisfaction does not appear to change with age (Kausler, 1982); however, Botwinick (1984b) points out that life satisfaction and well-being are not unitary concepts and that the sources of satisfaction change with age. In an analysis of twelve different areas that influence satisfaction with life, Cutler (1979) found that home, wealth, and area of residency were significant for persons aged 35–44 and that contentment with marriage and family were most important for the 65 to 74 year olds. Palmore and Kivett (1977), in one of the few longitudinal investigations of life satisfaction among the middle-aged and the 'young-old', studied 378 community residents, 46–70 years old, over a four-year period. Mean satisfaction with life for the total group did not change over the time of the study, and men and women were not significantly different. Significant predictors of life satisfaction were, mainly, self-rated health and to a lesser extent sexual enjoyment and the number of hours spent in social activity.

Recent literature reveals that sexual satisfaction does not necessarily decline with age despite decreases in sexual function and behavior. Martin (1981), in the previously cited report from the Baltimore Study on Aging, found that a large proportion of volunteers were sexually satisfied, did not experience sexual anxiety or feelings of deprivation and were not interested in seeking treatment despite significant sexual difficulties. He speculated that the persistence of sexual satisfaction despite a decline in sexual frequency and functional capacity was due to a corresponding decline in sexual motivation. He concluded that, '. . . *the vast majority of subjects were apparently functioning at a level commensurate with their feelings of desire, and, because few were lacking in other sources for maintaining self-esteem, what losses did occur did not produce the emotional trauma that is encountered in clinical practice.*' Although Martin's interpretation of results could be questioned because of the study's cross-sectional design and the retrospective nature of the analysis, it focuses the importance of including sexual satisfaction as a parameter of theoretical and clinical significance. McKinlay and Feldman (1994), in the Massachusetts Male Aging Epidemiological Study, provided additional information on aging and sexual satisfaction. They found no age-related changes in satisfaction with the men's own sexuality, their sexual relations with partners and their perception of the partner's own satisfaction, despite a significant decline in sexual activity and erectile function. There was, as summarized in the previous chapter, a strong relationship between the reported age-related decrease in sexual activity and diminution of sexual desire. While acknowledging the possibility of a cohort effect, the authors speculate that the stable levels of sexual satisfaction reflect a concordance between sexual interest and activity, as well as a decrease in sexual expectations as men age. Principal component analysis identified sexual satisfaction as one of four independent factors significantly related to sexual activity. Good health was strongly associated with sexual satisfaction while a scaled measure of depression was negatively related to it and strongly predicted sexual difficulties.

Research on the determinants of sexual enjoyment and satisfaction has been devoted primarily to female sexuality. There are virtually no systematic studies of factors that contribute to the sexual satisfaction of healthy older men. As described in the previous chapter, we found, consistent with the two studies already described, a significantly negative relationship between age and sexual desire, sexual arousal and activity, but no effect of age on sexual enjoyment and satisfaction. Case study 4.3 describes a couple who took part in our study, and remain sexually satisfied without having sexual intercourse. We evaluated (Schiavi, Mandeli and Schreiner-Engel, 1994), in a follow-up investigation of the same group of aging volunteers, changes in psychological and marital influences that are likely to be associated with the quality of sexual experiences. We also explored the predictive significance of psychosexual, marital, and behavioral variables and their effect on sexual satisfaction. Three dimensions of sexual satisfaction, rated by the subjects, were considered: *general sexual satisfaction, satisfaction with the individual's own sexual function*, and *enjoyment of marital sexuality*. It was hypothesized that individual psychosexual characteristics, the quality of the couple's relationship, and changes in sexual functioning would interact to determine men's sexual satisfaction as they aged.

The following independent variables were assessed:

Psychosexual measures. They are components of the Derogatis Sexual Function Inventory (DSFI), a self-report inventory that gathers information on several primary areas of sexuality. It includes subtests of sexual information, experience, drive, attitudes, psychological symptoms, affect, gender role definition, fantasy, and body image. The measure is adequately reliable, internally consistent and valid (Derogatis and Melisaratos, 1979).

Marital measures. They were obtained from two validated tests of marital adjustment and satisfaction: the Locke–Wallace Marital Adjustment Test (L–W) (Kimmel and Van der Veen,1974), and the Dyadic Adjustment Scale (DAS) (Spanier, 1976). Both measures were used to assess subjects and their partners independently.

Behavioral measures. They were selected, a priori, from a wide range of items included in the structured interview which was used to assess the subjects and their partners jointly and separately. The variables were: subjective arousal, degree of coital erections, coital frequency, number of orgasms per month, and problems with erections. Each of these behavioral measures significantly decreased with age.

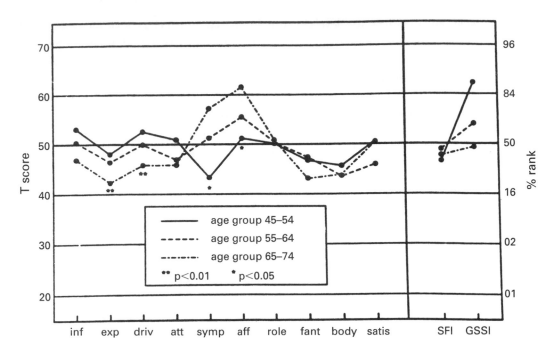

Figure 4.1   Derogatis Sexual Function Inventory (DSFI) score profiles of the three age groups of healthy men. inf, information; exp, experience; driv, drive; att, attitude; symp, symptoms; aff, affect; role, gender role; fant, fantasy; body, body image; satis, satisfaction; SFI and GSSI, global indices of sexual function. (Reprinted from Schiavi et al. 1994. Sexual satisfaction in healthy aging men. *Journal of Sex and Marital Therapy* **20**, 3–13, with permission from Brunner/Mazel, Inc., New York.)

Figure 4.1 is a graphic profile of the psychosexual measures included in the DSFI compared with the norms. Although the DSFI norms were derived from a younger population, the three age groups all had subtest scores within the normative mean, except for affect of those aged 65–74. A comparison of median *T*-scores among the three age groups revealed that the oldest age group had significantly lower scores in the subtests of sexual experience and sexual drive and higher scores in the measures of psychological symptoms and affect. The scores of the marital adjustment measures were within the normative limits of the tests. There were no significant differences in marital adjustment and satisfaction with age, based on independent reporting by both partners.

The correlations between psychosexual, marital, and behavioral variables with the measures of sexual satisfaction are summarized in Table 4.1. *Satisfaction with the subject's own sexual function* was positively related to the subject's reported degree of subjective and physiological arousal, with coital frequency and with more liberal attitudes. It was negatively related to the subject's perceived erectile

Table 4.1. Correlation coefficients of psychosexual, behavioral and marital variables with measures of sexual satisfaction

Variables	Satisfaction with own sex function	General sexual satisfaction	Enjoyment of marital sexuality
Age	−0.18	−0.08	−0.03
Psychosexual measures (DSFI)			
Information	0.14	0.37 ***	0.26 *
Experience	0.03	0.12	0.04
Drive	0.12	0.02	0.19
Attitude	0.29 **	0.22	−0.04
Symptoms	0.17	0.27 *	0.30 **
Affect	0.12	0.20	0.43 ***
Gender role	0.07	0.26 *	0.13
Fantasy	0.00	−0.07	0.07
Body image	0.15	0.26 *	0.10
Behavioral measures			
Subjective arousal	0.26 *	0.17	0.35 **
Degree coital erections	0.53 ***	0.48 ***	0.44 ***
Coital frequency	0.45 ***	0.40 ***	0.54 ***
No. orgasms/month	0.22	0.23	0.12
Problem with erections	−0.73 ***	−0.55 ***	−0.50 ***
Marital measures			
L–W (self)	0.20	0.36 **	0.46 ***
L–W (partner)	0.22	0.22	0.35 **
DAS (self)	0.17	0.28 *	0.43 ***
DAS (partner)	0.21	0.26 *	0.35 ***

Notes:

* $p < 0.05$; ** $p < 0.01$; *** $p < 0.001$. (Reprinted with permission from Schiavi et al. 1994. Sexual satisfaction in healthy aging men, *Journal of Sex and Marital Therapy* 20, 3–13, with permission from Brunner/Mazel, Inc., New York.)

difficulties but was not associated with measures of marital adjustment. In contrast, marital adjustment, psychosexual and behavioral measures were significantly related to *general sexual satisfaction* and to *enjoyment of marital sexuality.* Of the psychosexual measures, information, symptoms, gender role, and body image correlated positively with *general sexual satisfaction,* as did behavioral measures of arousal and coitus, and most of the measures of marital adjustment. *Enjoyment of marital sexuality* correlated with psychosexual measures of sexual information, symptoms and affect, as well as with coital and marital adjustment measures.

Problems with erections were strongly and negatively associated with all three measures of sexual satisfaction. In the second phase of statistical evaluation, stepwise regression analyses were performed using psychosexual, marital behavioral measures, and age as predictor variables and the three measures of sexual satisfaction as dependent variables. This approach permitted the simultaneous evaluation of all the variables, identification of independent factors and estimation of the magnitude of the effects on the measures of sexual satisfaction. The subjects' erectile problems were the sole predictors of the degree of *satisfaction with their own sexual function*, with no other variable providing significant additional information. The presence of erectile problems was also an important negative predictor of *general sexual satisfaction*, but, in addition, sexual information and the men's marital adjustment scores were also independent contributors accounting for 45.6% of the variability in this measure. Significant independent predictors of *enjoyment of marital sexuality* were coital frequency, positive affect, subjective sexual arousal and, in a negative direction, presence of erectile problems. Marital adjustment measures, because of their intercorrelation with the other measures, did not make a significant, independent contribution beyond the variables previously mentioned. It is interesting that the presence of positive affect was more influential than erectile capacity on marital sexual enjoyment. It is also worth mentioning that age per se, when entered as an independent variable in the multiple regression analysis, was not associated with any of the sexual satisfaction variables.

The conclusions that may be drawn from this study of healthy couples are limited by its cross-sectional design, by the lack of psychometrically validated measures of sexual satisfaction and by the nature of the population investigated. However, it is important to consider these data otherwise our view of the sexuality of aging people is distorted by the focus on the medically ill or on sexually dysfuntional couples seeking psychological counseling. This study shows that, in addition to erectile capacity, psychosexual and marital determinants influence aging men's sexual satisfaction considerably. The interaction between interpersonal and marital adjustment measures and male sexuality will be discussed further in the next chapter.

Summary

The emotional responses to age-related variations in sexual function differ considerably among men. Some integrate sexual changes into their overall life with no effect on well-being while others react with considerable distress, self-doubt and impaired self-esteem. Individuals differ markedly in how they value sexuality, reflecting their personalities and their personal circumstances at the time. Sexual attitudes and knowledge, shaped by sociocultural influences and by personal experience, play an important role in the interpretation and reaction to sexual changes. How the individual appraises the effects of age on sexual function largely determines how the individual adapts and copes in later life.

Studies of the sexuality of aging have been concerned primarily with sexual performance, neglecting sexual satisfaction as an independent measure that is theoretically and clinically relevant. Several cross-sectional studies have shown that sexual satisfaction does not decline with age, despite decrements in sexual function and behavior. This observation, still awaiting prospective validation, may be caused by the parallel declines in sexual motivation and sexual activity and, possibly, to a decrease in sexual expectations. There is evidence, from healthy aging volunteers, that sexual information, affect and marital adjustment, in addition to the subjects' perception of erectile difficulties, significantly and independently contribute to sexual enjoyment and satisfaction. The observation that some couples develop successful strategies to cope with marked age-related changes in sexual function points to the need and clinical relevance of moving beyond performance measures to multivariate investigations of factors that determine sexual satisfaction in the later years.

Case studies

Case study 4.1

Mr. and Ms. A volunteered to participate in a study of sexual behavior because of his concerns about sexual function. They were 64 and 62 years of age respectively and had been married for 37 years. Mr. A had been noticing progressive difficulties in gaining and maintaining erections for four years and was only able to achieve insertion in about half of the attempts at intercourse which occurred approximately twice per month; his sexual drive was not impaired and he masturbated regularly with close-to-full erections three times per week. Because of his preoccupation with his sexual potency Mr. A had undergone a complete medical and urological evaluation with negative results.

Mr. A, an only child, was raised as a practicing Catholic within a strict and conservative family milieu. He met his wife while working for the Foreign Service in Europe and they were married after five months of courtship. The couple had an active and mutually satisfying sex life prior to the onset of the current sexual problem; they had a committed marriage and a harmonious relationship after having successfully raised four children and becoming free from economic concerns. Mr. A's consulting company, which he established following his forced retirement from a Wall Street firm when aged 60, had become a lucrative and considerably demanding enterprise. During this period marital sex became perfunctory, his sexual desire for his wife declined and, during one of his frequent trips, he initiated an affair which was fraught with considerable guilt. The realization that his erectile difficulties were not limited to his relationship with his wife but also occurred extramaritally damaged his self-esteem and exacerbated his self-criticism and the feeling that he was 'old and over the hill'. Marital sex became strained by his attempts to prove that he could achieve an erection and by his wife's efforts to reassure him about his masculinity.

Comment

Sexuality had always been an important aspect of Mr A's well-being and marital adjustment. He had experienced over several years before the onset of his sexual problems some decrease in erectile capacity which had not been noticed by his wife but was a latent source of concern for Mr. A. His unanticipated retirement had been traumatic, leading to self-doubts and diminished self-esteem. Mr. A coped by immersing himself in a new enterprise which, although successful, was a source of stress and decreased their marital intimacy. His extra-marital relation did little to enhance self-worth in this individual who was governed by rather high moral principles. Feelings of guilt and self-recrimination were associated, instead, with extramarital sexual failure reinforcing his belief that 'he was too old to function sexually'.

The recording of nocturnal erections demonstrated normal erectile capacity and all hormonal values were within the normal range for his age. Although Mr. A did not show clinical evidence of a mood disorder; psychological testing revealed an elevated depressive score, impaired body image and low sexual satisfaction in keeping with the clinical presentation.

Case study 4.2

Mr. and Mrs. B, both 67 years of age, had been married for 41 years. He was a retired salesman working part-time as a teacher. They joined the study prompted by intellectual curiosity about the nature of the research project. Mr. B was in good health, free from drugs or medications. During the preceding six months, the couple had had intercourse once a week on average. He had noticed a gradual decrease in sexual desire and 'deliberately created my own desire' by fantasizing, seeking erotic stimuli and inviting his wife to wear enticing undergarments. Sexual experiences were mutually initiated during which he gained erections rated, independently by each partner, as 7 (on a 1–10 scale; 5 sufficient for penetration with manual assistance, 10 maximum erection). Both described their sexual experiences as enjoyable, although he was somewhat disappointed by the loss of orgasmic intensity. Mr. B did not masturbate and was no longer aware of sleep-related erections. Sexuality had been an important aspect of the couple's relationship, which was not without difficulties due to an extramarital relationship that he had had about ten years previously. At the time of the interview both reported fully enjoying their life and companionship, free from monetary worries and the responsibilities of raising their family.

Nocturnal penile tumescence recordings showed a marked diminution in frequency, duration and degree of erectile episodes consistent with organic impairment of erectile capacity. An evaluation of sleep disorders revealed that he had a periodic disorder of leg movement. Hormonal assessments during sleep revealed primary testicular hyposecretion with low total plasma testosterone and elevated luteinizing hormone. As part of the study, Mr. B completed daily reports of sexual behavior prospectively over a month's period. The couple mutually initiated intercourse four times, leading to intravaginal ejaculation, rated by Mr. B as very satisfactory.

Comment

The overall pattern of abnormal physiological findings contrasted with a lack of clinical evidence of sexual dysfunction and with the couple's report of satisfying sexual relations. A phenomenological assessment suggested that, despite physiological limitations, his cognitive ability and motivation to proactively seek sexual cues to enhance his sexual arousal, the high value placed on sexuality over the span of their marital life and the supportive attitude of his wife played important compensatory roles in Mr B's age-related decline in sexual function. (Reproduced in modified form with permission, Schiavi R. C. (1992). *Psychiatric Medicine* **10**, 217–25.)

Case study 4.3

Mr. C, a 68-year-old man, had decided to retire three years ago because he found his work as a mechanical engineer physically taxing. Retirement was for him 'boring', devoid of challenging experiences and lacking in interpersonal relationships. His curiosity and desire for intellectual stimulation led him to volunteer in the research project on aging. After the couple's initial surprise at the sexual focus of the study, they were willing participants in it.

Mr. C had had limited sexual experiences prior to his marriage at the age of 28. Their sexual activity during the first 20 years of marriage had been problem free and fully satisfying, with a coital frequency of twice per week. He denied extramarital relations and having ever masturbated. At age 50 his sexual desire began to decline and about four years prior to the evaluation the couple was no longer having intercourse. Since Ms. C sexual drive was also low the couple did not view the absence of coitus as problematic. Their engaging in regular kissing and embracing while sleeping in close physical contact was a source of considerable pleasure for both. Mr. C stated that his involvement with work and her preoccupation with their children had previously interfered with their relationship. As the external demands decreased, his affection for his wife increased and the emotional and physical intimacy with his wife became an important aspect of his sexuality, even if it did not involve coitus. Mr. C was unable to explain why his desire for intercourse had disappeared. He felt sexually satisfied and did not perceive himself as having a sexual problem. A complete medical and urological evaluation conducted as part of this investigation was normal. Mr. C's assessment in the sleep laboratory showed that his nocturnal penile tumescence was significantly impaired, with a mean of two brief erectile episodes during the three study nights, all of partial tumescence. Sleep architecture, hormonal determinations and psychological testing were within the normal range.

Comment

Mr. C reported a gradual, age-related decline in coital desire and need for ejaculatory relief but did not consider himself devoid of sexual feelings. He redefined his sexuality as a physically affectionate exchange without performance pressure and considered his intimate sensual experiences with his wife as an important aspect of his self-image as a sexual being. The couple viewed the change in their sexual interaction as a natural aspect of their growing old; the correspondence, in both partners, of decreased sexual motivation and low sexual expectations contributed to their experiencing a satisfying sexual life.

References

Barlow, D. H. (1986). Causes of sexual dysfunction. The role of anxiety and cognitive interference. *Journal of Consulting and Clinical Psychology* 54, 140–8.

Beck, J. D. and Barlow, D. H. (1986). The effects of anxiety and attentional focus on sexual responding. *Behavioral Research and Therapy* 24, 9–17.

Botwinick, J. (1984a). Sexuality and sexual relations. In *Aging and Behavior*, ed. J. Botwinck, pp. 91–109. New York: Springer Publishing Co.

Botwinick, J. (1984b). Well-being. In *Aging and Behavior*, ed. J. Botwinck, pp. 77–90. New York: Springer Publishing Co.

Bultena, G. L. and Powers, E. A. (1978). Denial of aging: aging identification and reference group orientations. *Journal of Gerontology* 33, 748–54.

Byrne, D. and Schulte L. (1990). Personality dispositions as mediators of sexual responses. *Annual Review of Sexual Research* 1, 93–117.

Cameron, P. (1970). The generation gap: beliefs about sexuality and self-reported sexuality. *Developmental Psychology* 3, 272–5.

Cohen, F. and Lazarus, R. S. (1983). Coping and adaptation in health and illness. In *Handbook of Health, Health Care and the Health Professions*, ed. D. Mechanic, pp. 608–35. New York: Free Press.

Cranston-Cuebas, M. A. and Barlow, D. H. (1990). Cognitive and affective contributions to sexual functioning. *Annual Review of Sexual Research* 1, 119–61.

Creti, L. and Libman, E. (1989). Cognitions and sexual expression in the aging. *Journal of Sex and Marital Therapy* 15, 83–101.

Cutler, N. E. (1979). Age variations in the dimensionality of life satisfaction. *Journal of Gerontology* 34, 573–8.

Derogatis, L. R. and Melisaratos, N. (1979). The DSFI: a multi-dimensional measure of sexual functioning. *Journal of Sex and Marital Therapy* 5, 244–81.

Glamser, F. D. (1974). The importance of age to conservative opinions: a multivariate analysis. *Journal of Gerontology* 29, 549–54.

Kaplan, H. S. (1974). *The New Sex Therapy*. New York: Brunner/Mazel.

Kaplan, H. S. (1990). Sex, intimacy and the aging process. *Journal of the American Academy of Psychoanalysis* 18, 185–205.

Kausler, D. H. (1982). *Experimental Psychology and Human Aging*, p. 622. New York: Wiley.

Kimmel, D. and Van der Veen, F. (1974). Factors of marital adjustment. Locke's Marital Adjustment Test. *Journal of Marriage and Family* 36, 57–63.

Larson, R. (1978). Thirty years of research on the subjective well-being of older Americans. *Journal of Gerontology* 33, 109–25.

Lazarus, R. S. and DeLongis, A. (1983). Psychological stress and coping in aging. *American Psychologist* 38, 245–54.

Martin, C. E. (1981). Factors affecting sexual functioning in 60–70-year-old married males. *Archives of Sexual Behavior* 10, 399–420.

McKinlay, J. B. and Feldman, H. A. (1994). Age-related variations in sexual activity and interest in normal men: results from the Massachusetts Male Aging Study. In *Sexuality across the Life Course*, ed. A. S. Rossi, pp. 261–85. Chicago, IL: University of Chicago Press.

Palmore, E. and Kivett, V. (1977). Change in life satisfaction: a longitudinal study of persons aged 46–70. *Journal of Gerontology* 32, 311–16.

Pfeiffer, E. and Davis, G. C. (1972). Determinants of sexual behavior in middle and old age. *Journal of American Geriatrics Society* 20, 151–8.

Schiavi, R. C. (1992). Normal aging and the evaluation of sexual dysfunction. *Psychiatric Medicine* 10, 217–25.

Schiavi, R. C., Mandeli, J. and Schreiner-Engel, P. (1994). Sexual satisfaction in healthy aging men. *Journal of Sex and Marital Therapy* 20, 3–13.

Snyder, E. E. and Spreitzer, E. (1976). Attitudes of the aged toward non traditional sexual behavior. *Archives of Sexual Behavior* 5, 249–54.

Spanier, G. C. (1976). Measuring dyadic adjustment: new scale for assessing the quality of marriage and similar dyads. *Journal of Marriage and the Family* 38, 15–29.

Steinke, E. E. (1994). Knowledge and attitudes of older adults about sexuality in aging: a comparison of two studies. *Journal of Advanced Nursing* 19, 477–85.

Stimson, A., Wase, J. F. and Stimson, J. (1981). Sexuality and self-esteem among the aged. *Research on Aging* 3, 228–39.

White, C. B. (1982). Sexual interest, attitudes, knowledge, and sexual history in relation to sexual behavior in the institutionalized aged. *Archives of Sexual Behavior* 11, 11–21.

White, C. B. and Catania, J. A. (1982). Psychoeducational intervention for sexuality with the aged, family members of the aged, and people who work with the aged. *International Journal of Aging and Human Development* 15, 121–38.

5   Aging and marital sexuality

The substantial increase in life span since the beginning of the twentieth century has had notable consequences for the social relationships of older individuals. As society norms and attitudes have become less restrictive, there has been increased fluidity in the development and realignment of partnerships encompassing marriage, separation, divorce, remarriage, extramarital, and same-sex relationships. Although this range of possibilities has greatly expanded sexual options, marriage remains the most prevalent social arrangement within which normatively sanctioned sexual experiences take place. Because women have a longer life expectancy and men tend to be older when they marry, and marry more frequently, there are marked age-related gender differences in opportunities for sexual partnerships (Figure 5.1). The percentages of men married at ages 55–69, 75–79 and 85 and older are 93, 82 and 80% respectively. In contrast, the percentages of women who are married within the same age spans are 66, 40 and 18% respectively (US Bureau of the Census, 1985).

Marital status is associated with marked differences in the number of sexual partners. In a full-probability cross-sectional survey of the adult population of the United States conducted in 1989 (Smith, 1991), the widowed reported the fewest sexual partners during the preceding year (a mean of 0.21), followed by the married (0.96), the divorced (1.31), the never married (1.84) and the separated (2.41). There was a gradual decline with age in the mean number of sexual partners from 1.7 partners among individuals younger than 30 years of age to 0.35 among those older than 70. The age-related decreases in the number of partners and the frequency of intercourse remained significant even when marital status and gender were controlled for. In contrast to the popular belief that extramarital relationships are highly prevalent, faithfulness was the norm among the married. The percentage of couples who reported having had sexual partners other than their spouse in the year before this survey was 2.1% for men and 0.8% for women. The cumulative number of extramarital relationships increased with age and presumably with the duration of marriage. The number of sexual partners did not vary significantly with race, education or region of residency but there was evidence of a cohort effect, in that members of earlier cohorts had significantly fewer partners than members of more recent cohorts.

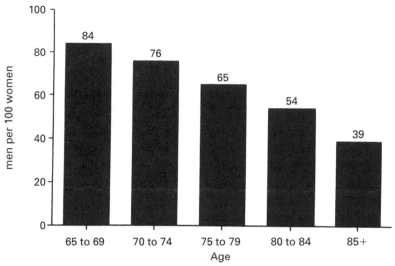

Source: U.S. Bureau of the Census, "U.S. Population Estimates, by Age, Sex, Race, and Hispanic Origin: 1989," by Frederick W. Hollman, *Current Population Reports* Series p-25, No. 1057 (March 1990).

Figure 5.1   Number of men per hundred women, by age group: 1989. (Reprinted from the *Statistical Handbook on Aging*, 1994 edn. ed. Frank L. Schick and Renee Schick. Published by the Oryx Press, 4041 N. Central Avenue, Suite 700, Phoenix, AZ 85012, USA.)

There is little evidence for the role that marital status plays in mediating the effects of age on male sexual behavior and satisfaction. This is partly caused by the narrow focus on coital frequency, with limited attention given to aging couples redefining their relationships and accommodating to the passage of time. In this chapter we review the limited information available on how marriage affects the sexuality of aging males. We consider how aging affects marriage, and explore the interaction between marital relationships and the frequency and nature of sexual expression. The variety of marital experiences associated with male sexual function and behavior is illustrated by observations from our study of healthy aging couples and by three case histories.

Marital aspects of the sexuality of aging males

Kinsey, Pomeroy and Martin (1948) devoted several chapters to marital status and sexual activity but they only studied men younger than 60. They noted that sexual intercourse within marriage provides less than 85% of total 'sexual outlets', with the proportion of orgasms derived from masturbation, nocturnal emissions and extra-marital experiences increasing with age. Men who are divorced continued to be as sexually active as when married, deriving up to 80% of their orgasms from hetero-sexual intercourse and the rest from masturbation. This contrasts markedly with the majority of women in their samples who, when widowed or divorced, ceased sexual activity. Kinsey's extensive study provides little information on marital inter-action effects on men's sexual activity.

The results of the Duke's studies (Verwoerdt, Pfeiffer and Wang, 1969; Pfeiffer, Verwoerdt and Davis, 1972) show that marital status has little effect on sexual inter-est and activity. The frequency of sexual intercourse within marriage decreased with age, with both partners attributing the decline to the man. The most frequent reasons why sexual relations stopped were the death of a spouse, an illness or the husband's inability to perform sexually. Udry, Deven and Coleman (1982), however, challenged the notion that married couples have sexual intercourse less frequently as they age because men have a diminished sexual capacity. They provide cross-cultural data suggesting that this decline is a function of the woman's age, not the man's, and that it is probably because the women become less interested in sex. Even though it is questionable whether their observations are valid for older couples, their research directed attention towards the role of the female partner.

Frank, Anderson and Rubinstein (1978), in a frequently quoted study, examined the sexual interactions of 100 couples living in stable relationships for 1–20 years, who defined their marriage as well adjusted. They found an unexpectedly high fre-quency of sexual dysfunction and sexual difficulties that were not dysfunctional in nature. Among the latter were an inability to relax, being uninterested, poor timing for the initiation of sexual activities and lack of adequate foreplay. Of note is the observation that couples were able to tolerate sexual dysfunction and difficulties without compromising the quality of their sexual interaction, providing the affective tone of their marriage was satisfactory. There was an inverse relationship between the frequency of intercourse and the sexual difficulties the husbands reported for their wives. The wives' 'sexual difficulties' emerged as a salient factor in the frequency and quality of the male sexual experience. Nowinski and LoPiccolo (1979), in a study of nondysfunctional couples, reported that for males the best predictor of sexual behavior was their estimate of their partner's level of sexual pleasure while for women it was self-reported pleasure. Bancroft (1984), in an article on gender differences in marital sexuality, refers to research showing that the decline in sexual activity in elderly couples is influenced more by the wife than by the husband. Based on the clinical presentation of couples with sexual problems, Bancroft noted that the postmenopausal decline in sexual interest, although not necessarily distressing for the wife, may have serious repercussions for the older husband, unbalancing his borderline adjustment towards coital failure. Among the several variables investigated by Marsiglio and Donnelly (1991), the partner's health status emerged as being more significantly and positively associated with the frequency of sexual relations of older married couples during the preceding month than the husband's own health.

Aging and marital satisfaction

It seems important to explore how aging influences marital adjustment, and how the nature of the marital relationship affects the frequency and quality of sexual experiences of older individuals. The majority of older men have been married for a long time, despite the current rise of divorce rates in middle and old age. Life events, such as relocation, retirement, emotional losses, as well as physical and mental disabilities, challenge the adaptive resources of individuals and couples, modifying well-established patterns of marital interaction. With the passage of time, marital roles are redefined, issues of trust and commitment come to the fore and the nature of intimacy evolves, influencing individual well-being and the quality of marital relationships.

A considerable amount of research has been carried out on marital satisfaction with inconsistent results. Marital satisfaction has been reported to decline gradually with the duration of marriage or to remain unchanged as couples grow older (Dentler and Pineo, 1960; Pineo, 1969). More recent studies suggest a curvilinear pattern, with high levels of satisfaction immediately after marriage, subsequently declining because of economic concerns, problems about raising children or coping with their adolescence and then increasing in late middle and old age as couples enjoy greater freedom and financial security (Rollins and Cannon, 1974; Anderson, Russell and Schumen, 1983). The impact of retirement on couples' well-being has been variously described as enhancing marital satisfaction (Gilford, 1984), having no demonstrable effect (Eckerdt and Vinick, 1991) or resulting in marital strain (Lee and Shehan, 1989). Chronic illness and disability appear to have more impact than retirement on marital relationships and satisfaction. Typically, the spouse is the main enabling and emotional resource of the disabled, and the single most important factor in preventing the aged from being institutionalized (Johnson, 1985). Several, although not all, reports favorably compare the degree of marital adjustment, enjoyment and companionship of long-term marriages to that of couples who have not been married as long (Stinnett, Carter and Montgomery, 1972; Peterson, 1973; Parron, 1982). Men and women perceive the quality of marital relationships differently. Husbands, at all ages, are more satisfied than wives; in addition married men report a better sense of well-being than single men (Sporakowski and Hughston, 1978; Sporakowski and Axelson, 1984; Markides, 1995).

The validity of research on marital satisfaction has been criticized on several grounds. Global measures of marital quality have been used without assessing or attempting to integrate the broad range of psychological dimensions that influence marital interactions and without controlling for the tendency of older individuals to respond in socially desirable ways. Since much of this research is cross-sectional, it is difficult to determine the extent to which the apparent increase in marital satisfaction of older couples is artifactual, as dissatisfied couples often divorce or separate and therefore are not included in the samples. Generation effects may also influence the results, with older couples who were raised in the traditional norms prevailing during the first half of the twentieth century being more committed to marriage and having a tendency to minimize marital problems when compared to younger cohorts. Cohorts who will enter old age at the beginning of the twenty-first century have been, at the forefront of the gender revolution, exposed to high rates of marital breakdown and their first marriage is likely to end in separation and/or divorce (Goldscheider, 1990).

An increasing number of longitudinal studies of marital quality have been published in recent years. Karney and Bradbury (1995) critically reviewed the methods and findings of 115 longitudinal studies as the basis for a model of marital development aimed at explaining how marriages change over time. Meta-analytical techniques were used to estimate the aggregate effect of close to 200 variables on marital quality and marital stability. As expected, education, positive behavior and employment predict positive marital outcomes, whereas neuroticism, negative behavior and an unhappy childhood predict negative marital outcomes. Although sexual satisfaction is a positive predictor of marital satisfaction for men and women, the magnitude of the correlation is not high and is based on a single prospective study. Marital satisfaction has a greater effect on marital stability than most other variables. However, a longitudinal examination of the duration of marriage shows that marriages tend to become more stable but less satisfying with the passage of time. The occurrence of stressful life events predicts decreased marital satisfaction and marital stability. An exception to this trend is the experience of becoming a parent which, similar to other stressful events, may lead to decreased marital satisfaction, but, unlike other stressors, may enhance marital stability. The appraisal of stressful events by the couples, as well as their interaction and the adaptive processes they bring to bear in response to marital difficulties and transitions are important determinants of marital stability over time. Weiss (1983) investigated the relationship between couples' intimacy and adaptation to stress throughout adult life. He found that the level of an operationally defined measure of a couple's intimacy changes significantly across the life span, with women's lowest levels occurring when their children leave home and men's when they retire. He also observed that intimacy with a spouse has consequences for adaptation to old age, helping to buffer older married individuals from the stresses that accompany the aging process.

Levenson, Carstensen and Gottman (1993) conducted a well-designed investigation on 156 couples in long-term marriages. They studied two cohorts aged 40–50 years and 60–70 years selected to represent, within each group, maritally satisfied and dissatisfied couples. Spouses completed several questionnaires and psychological inventories and then participated in a laboratory procedure to assess areas of conflict and sources of pleasure. The authors hypothesized that: (1) older married couples would report less conflict and more pleasure than middle-aged married couples, (2) children would be a source of greater conflict for middle-aged married couples, and (3) gender differences would be less evident in older couples than in middle-aged couples. All the hypotheses were supported by the data. Of particular interest is a comparative analysis of the sources of conflict and pleasure in the two age cohorts. Children were a relatively less important source of disagreement between older couples compared with middle-aged couples, while communication and recreation were the greatest sources of conflict in old age. Sexuality was ranked fifth among ten sources of potential disagreement (after communication, recreation, money, and children) with no differences in ranking position between the two age groups. Among the 16 areas of potential enjoyment, older couples derived greater enjoyment than middle-aged couples from talking about children and grandchildren, sharing activities and vacations. Dissatisfied couples, regardless of their age group, reported a wide source of conflicts including communication, sex, jealousy, children, recreation, friends, alcohol, and drugs. Although the cross-sectional study design does not permit the drawing of general conclusions, the results suggest that, in this sample of healthy, upper-middle-class individuals, there is less potential for conflict and more potential for pleasure for older married couples compared to middle-aged married couples. The results are consistent with the Baltes and Baltes (1990) model of selective optimization with compensation. As the responsibilities of raising children and work commitments decrease and the extended social networks become less important, greater value is placed by older couples on intimate emotional interactions and shared activities within the family.

Marriage and sexuality

The narrowing range of social involvement and responsibilities associated with aging, and increasing investment in the marriage has not only potential for increasing intimacy but also for conflict with still unexplored consequences for the sexual relationship between the aging couple. There is a substantial body of information from national surveys and systematic research on the association between marital adjustment and sexuality regardless of age and duration of marriage. Two surveys (Starr and Weiner, 1981; Brecher, 1984) show that there is a relationship between sexuality and marital well-being. In the Brecher study of older respondents, for example, the author found a strong association for both husbands and wives between sexual enjoyment and marital happiness. For both men and women marital well-being was positively related to satisfaction with marital sex and the ease with which sex is discussed. Although these reports are nonrepresentative, they do provide phenomenological, albeit highly selective, information on the interaction between sexual and marital satisfaction.

Edwards and Booth (1994) conducted one of the few systematic studies of changes in sexual expression and marital well-being over time in a randomly selected national sample of middle-aged married persons in the USA. More than 2000 individuals at the outset were interviewed on three occasions between 1980 and 1988 with a completion rate of 66%. While the majority of individuals reported being 'very happy' or 'pretty happy' with marital sex, men reported greater dissatisfaction during early-middle age while for women this occurred during late-middle age. Satisfaction with marital sex and interest in sex significantly declined during the course of the study, suggesting that these variables are influenced by the duration of marriage. A significant relationship was evident between sexual satisfaction and marital happiness and marital stability. Individuals in early-middle age, compared to late-middle age, had higher marital instability scores and were more likely to consider divorce when they were unhappy with their sexual relationship or had lost interest in sex. Assessment of change over the eight-year period of the investigation found a significant association between changes in sexual behavior and marital well-being. As dissatisfaction with marital sex and loss of sexual interest increased, psychological well-being and the perceived quality of the marriage decreased. However, these data do not assess the different effects of gender, and neither do they determine the causal link between marital well-being and sexuality.

While some investigators conclude that the quality of the marital relationship is an important determinant of satisfaction with sexuality within marriage, others consider that sexual satisfaction is an independent variable that influences marital adjustment. Although cause cannot be determined because of the correlational design of these studies, it is likely that both sexual and marital variables interact, in ways still to be determined, shaping the quality of the couples' overall experience. Empirical research has considered sexual satisfaction in marriage in relation to equity (Hatfield et al., 1982), communication over sexual matters (Cupach and Comstock, 1990), the meaning of life (McCann and Biaggio, 1989), partners having shared perceptions (Fields, 1983), and personality traits (Schenk, Pfrang and Rausche, 1983). The studies neglect the effects of aging and duration of marriage, and the complexity of the issues makes it difficult to relate or integrate their results. However, it may be valuable to apply some of these constructs when assessing sexual satisfaction in the later years.

Little attention has been paid to the way that perceptions of physical attractiveness affect marriage. The prevailing stereotype is that men place higher value on physical characteristics, such as body shape and weight, while women are more sensitive to psychological attributes such as truthfulness and emotional warmth. Margolin and White (1987) hypothesized that a decline in physical attractiveness, usually associated with aging, will affect the marital sexual relationship to a greater extent for men than for women. They surveyed a large, representative sample of married individuals who were asked to assess both their own and their spouse's physical aging and to identify possible problems in marriage. Nine per cent of the sample considered lack of interest in sex as a problem in the marriage, a proportion that was significantly influenced by gender, with 11% of the wives and 6% of the husbands reporting this problem. However, men reported unhappiness with the sexual aspects of their marriage significantly more often than women. Men who believed that their wife's physical appearance, but not their own, had declined were more likely to report a lack of sexual interest, sexual unhappiness and to a lesser extent problems caused by unfaithfulness. This pattern was not observed in women and was independent of the duration of marriage and relative economic status. Although the study should be repeated, the findings suggest a gender bias, in that the perceived decline in the wives' physical attractiveness associated with aging may have greater consequences for the quality of marital sexuality compared with the perceived decline in the husbands' appearance.

Male aging and sexuality; a phenomenological view

During the course of our study on aging men we systematically evaluated their marital relationship with a semistructured interview lasting two hours (Schiavi, Mandeli and Schreiner-Engel, 1994). The couples, together and separately, were allowed considerable latitude to respond to a 300-item questionnaire, and, in addition, completed two marital adjustment measures. Table 5.1 summarizes information on marital adjustment, assessed independently by both partners, using the Locke–Wallace (L–W) Test (Kimmel and Van der Veen, 1974) and the Dyadic Adjustment Scale (DAS) (Spanier, 1976). Age had no significant effect on the husband's and wives' responses, with median L–W and DAS scores all falling within the instrument's norms. The ranges of ratings are broad, suggesting that there is considerable individual variability in marital adjustment. The relationship between measures of marital adjustment and sexual satisfaction is reviewed in the previous chapter. No attempt will be made to quantify further the interactions between marriage and sex. Instead a phenomenological description of the most salient themes that characterize the relationships of these mainly middle-class, economically comfortable and well-educated couples, as they unfold over time, will be summarized. Some, but not all, of these observations concur with the results of the research previously described.

Generation effects are most evident in older couples who had a conservative

Table 5.1. Marital adjustment scores in three age groups

Marital measures*	Age group		
	45–54	55–64	65–74
Locke-Wallace test			
Self	108 (75–129)	107 (57–133)	113 (58–132)
Partner	112 (73–137)	108 (58–131)	109 (71–125)
Dyadic adjustment scale			
Self	116 (92–143)	112 (65–141)	119 (62–146)
Partner	111 (80–141)	113 (56–141)	117 (80–136)

Notes:

* Median values; range within parenthesis. (Reprinted with permission from Schiavi et al. 1994. Sexual satisfaction in healthy aging men, *Journal of Sex and Marital Therapy* 20, 3–13, with permission from Brunner/Mazel, Inc., New York.)

and religious upbringing and limited sexual activities prior to marriage. Characteristically, the men have adopted the responsibility for being the initiators and main advocates of marital sexuality, have been frustrated by their wives' sexual passivity and regret not having had greater sexual opportunities during their youth. The wives' response to the aging men's decrease in erectile capacity is an important determinant of the quality of their relationship as time progresses. Some women, sensitive to their partner's sexual insecurity and careful to encourage their self-esteem, become more active sexually to enhance their husband's arousal. Although not always sexually desirous, they are willing to accommodate to their husband's expectations; in the process they may become sexually excited and orgasmic, or feel emotionally rewarded by the intimacy of the shared experience. Other wives resent their husband's overconcern with their declining erectile function to the detriment of affection within their relationship and resist their mate's request for genital stimulation, resulting in feelings of guilt and anger and marital strain.

The retrospective assessment of the couples' interaction over the course of their marriage reveals that the frequency of sexual experiences does not plateau or decline with time; rather it fluctuates, depending on life events and marital difficulties. In general, sexual desire differs between men and women, such that husbands express a greater and more constant interest in sexual activity, and wives are more likely to feel sexually unresponsive during marital problems or when stressed. Although only two men reported ongoing extramarital experiences, several, primarily middle-aged husbands, acknowledged having had extramarital affairs, the discovery of which led to marked, and at times lasting, marital disruption. Menopause was found to be a salient marker that has a significant impact on the sexual life of many of the couples of the study. Most frequently, wives reported a decline in sexual interest associated with it, but others indicated an increase in sexual assertiveness, a response that was not always welcomed by their mates. We suspected, but were unable to confirm, that the perception of changes in sexual attractiveness influenced the husbands' sexual responses to their mates in a consistent manner.

Marital satisfaction is an encompassing concept that, in the couples of this study, appeared to rest on a number of factors that extended beyond the confines of their sexual experience. Retrospective reporting suggests a predictable pattern of change in satisfaction in keeping with age and the marital stage. During their younger years, the couples' marital satisfaction is restricted by the pressure of professional responsibilities, economic concerns, the needs of growing children, and the expectations of elderly parents. As stated by an older man, 'In my 40's I was so invested in accomplishing that I lost track of being'. As couples grow older they report less pressure, more financial security and fewer responsibilities toward older and younger generations. Marital commitment, companionship, more leisure time and the sharing of emotional rewards from children become important contributors to marital well-being. In this context sexual satisfaction is predicated on the congruence of mutual expectations, the couples' capacity to modulate their sexual demands in keeping with their mates' sexual desire and functional capacity, and the ability to communicate and compromise.

The following statement by a 71-year-old man, married 40 years previously, characterizes the experience of several older couples in the study, 'the nature of our sex is different but the satisfaction remains the same. . . . I miss the passion but feeling relaxed and sexually comfortable with my wife has become more important and it is equally enjoyable'.

Conclusion

Most aging men remain married throughout their lives or remarry soon after divorce. Characteristic of older cohorts is their conservative attitude towards sexuality, which is expressed mainly in the context of their marital relationships. Their sexual behavior is not only directly influenced by age but also by changes in the character of their interaction as it evolves over time. There is evidence of an association between the quantity and quality of sexual experiences and marital adjustment but the nature of this relationship is uncertain. Fulfilling sexuality may enhance marital well-being or, conversely, be the consequence of a satisfying marital life. Until prospective studies identify causality, it seems plausible to assume that there is a mutual relationship between sexual and marital satisfaction.

Noted in the literature, and reported by several older couples in our study, is a curvilinear pattern of marital and sexual satisfaction, with higher levels during the first years of marriage, declining during early-middle age because of professional and family pressures and economic concerns and increasing again during late-middle age. Sex, a central component of marital adjustment during early marriage, becomes less frequent and passionate, but no less significant for older couples in the context of broader, more family-focused sources of reward.

The degree of congruence of sexual needs and expectations between sexual partners and their ability to communicate and compromise are critical components for marital and sexual adjustment, and an important source of variability as exemplified by the three case studies that follow. Perceived changes in sexual interest and functional capacity associated with male aging and with female menopause can disrupt the sexual equilibrium of aging couples. The behavioral outcome depends, in great measure, on the nature of the couple's interaction and on their adaptive resources. Without a doubt, when assessing the effects of age one needs to consider the context of the relationship in which male sexuality is experienced and expressed.

Case studies

Case study 5.1

Mr. D, a 65-year-old man, was about to retire from his position as city administrator when he was interviewed. He came with his wife, aged 61, to whom he had been married for 34 years. They both described a stable and basically uneventful marriage and, together as well as separately, expressed their satisfaction with the current relationship. They were nostalgic about the romanticism of their earlier years but were also relieved at having survived their children's rebellions in adolescence and at no longer needing to carry two jobs to support the family. Frequency of intercourse had gradually decreased from four times per week in their 30's to twice per month. Sex was described as less passionate but equally satisfying for both. Mr. D stated, 'in our 40's the kids were in the next room, I used to go to bed tired and sex was brief; now sex is more relaxed and we can choose the best time for it'. When Mr. D became 50, for unclear reasons he went through a two-month period of erectile losses prior to ejaculation. He recovered his erectile function after antibiotic treatment for presumed 'prostatitis'. Five years later his wife entered the peri-menopausal phase which was associated with depression, irritability, a significant loss of sexual desire, and vaginal dryness. He had been the sexual initiator but during this period, which lasted three years, he became tentative because of his awareness of her lack of desire and fear of inflicting coital pain. He had a reactive decrease in sexual drive and would occasionally lose his erection when attempting vaginal penetration. The use of estrogen patches restored his wife's sexual drive, increased her lubrication and markedly improved the quality of their sexual lives. The couple compensated for the decrease in erectile firmness by extending the duration of foreplay and having sex in the morning when he felt more rested. Mr. D acknowledged some apprehension about sexual performance but his capacity for intercourse has remained consistently intact over the past seven years.

Comment

This vignette is prototypical of couples who report continued sexual satisfaction into later years. The character of sexual experiences evolved from lust to more affectionate and comfortable sexual experiences that, although less pressing, occur at a frequency that meet their mutual needs and expectations. Menopause can be a turning point that disrupts the marital equilibrium, particularly when it occurs at a time when men start noticing a decrease in erectile firmness. The outcome depends, at least in part, on the couples' marital stability, the value of sexuality for each partner, the ability to communicate and compromise, and their adaptive capacities. Mr. and Ms. D were able to negotiate the menopausal transition with relatively minimal disruption to the quality of their marital life. Marital, psychological, sleep, and hormonal assessments were all normal.

Case Study 5.2

Mr. E volunteered to participate in the aging study wishing to have a medical evaluation and was initially surprised by its focus on sexuality. Mr. and Ms. E, aged 74 and 64 years respectively, had been married for 42 years. Mr. E had retired from a senior administrative position ten years previously, while Ms. E continued her artistic work as a sculptor. The couple, who had had a conservative Jewish religious upbringing, were both virgins when they married after two years of courtship. They described a 'rocky' marriage due to his over-involvement at work and high sexual expectations. On several occasions she expressed her desire to separate but he refused despite continued marital upheaval. The overall relationship had markedly improved after his voluntary retirement ten years prior to the interview. They were financially secure, did not take their good health for granted, shared enjoyable leisure-time activities and their children were a continuous source of emotional satisfaction; however, their sexual interactions remained problematic. Since their first sexual attempts Ms. E had markedly less sexual desire than her husband. Usually she complied with his sexual demands and, after overcoming initial resistance, would become aroused and find the experience gratifying. As time passed she increasingly refused his advances which led to his stopping initiating sex. Eventually Ms. E felt guilty about depriving her husband and began self-stimulating to arouse sufficient desire to initiate intercourse. This pattern had altered during the preceding two years because of the joint effects of his declining erectile capacity and her loss of motivation to continue generating sexual desire by masturbation. At a follow-up session one year after the completion of the study Mr. E reported increasingly frequent coital failures and requested a referral for sex therapy evaluation.

Comment

A discrepancy in sexual desire had been a prevailing source of sexual distress and of marital problems since the beginning of this couple's relationship. When Mr. B retired and became more affectionately involved with his wife, marital satisfaction markedly improved despite the persistence of sexual difficulties. Mr. B's sustained erectile capacity into his early 70's appears to have been predicated, at least in part, by Ms. B determination to be an active, albeit reluctant, participant in their sexual experiences. The lack of active sexual involvement by his wife and the presence of an organic erectile deficit, evident in the markedly abnormal nocturnal penile tumescence (NPT) recordings (only one partial erectile episode during three study nights), are both likely determinants of his increased coital failures. Mr. E had abnormally low bioavailable testosterone levels and high luteinizing hormone levels suggestive of testicular hypofunction. It is difficult to interpret the role of hypogonadism since his sexual drive remained unimpaired.

Case study 5.3

Mr. and Ms. F, aged 64 and 61 years, had married 35 years previously and were the parents of three children no longer living at home. Mr. F described a strict Catholic upbringing and an emotionally deprived childhood, having been raised in an orphanage following his mother's physical disablement and his father's family desertion. Mr. F's determination, hard work and consistency of purpose permitted him to overcome this background, becoming a lawyer and rising to a top position in a large brokerage house. He was described by his wife as a good provider, strict, self-involved and totally invested in his career. Two years before the interview, unexpectedly, he was given a 'golden handshake' and invited to retire from the firm. He missed his loss of status, power and control; although now wealthy, could not accept remaining unoccupied and began working as an independent lawyer.

The couple's sexual life was described as uneventful and uninspiring, with a coital frequency that, over the years, had gradually decreased to about once-per- week. Two months after leaving the old firm Mr. F entered a three-month period of coital failures that remitted in response to reassurance from a urologist; however, he still had sporadic erectile difficulties. Mr. F reported, confidentially, a loss of desire for his wife whom he was finding increasingly unattractive, and stated that his erectile problems permitted his avoidance of unwelcome marital sex. His previous work in the brokerage firm had allowed escape from marital intimacy while providing psychological stimulation in the form of attractive and slim female employees that fed his fantasies when having sex with his wife. He had resisted sexual affairs because of religious reasons but acknowledged one extramarital experience seeking sexual reassurance during the period of erectile failure. When interviewed alone Ms. F stated that she had eagerly anticipated her husband's retirement expecting that it would lead to more shared activities and greater emotional intimacy; now she felt hopeless and rejected. Although committed to remain married, it was difficult for her to accept that their mutual alienation would continue in the years ahead.

Comment

This case study illustrates several interwoven themes: the husband's achievement orientation born from unhappy early experiences, his over-commitment to work seeking self-esteem and avoidance of marital intimacy, and the traumatic consequences of unwanted retirement leading to a loss of sexual desire for his wife and to erectile difficulties. Ms. F's frustrated disappointment at his increasingly distant behavior led to depressed mood and to a neglect of personal appearance, further contributing to her husband's loss in sexual interest. Characteristic of the couple's impaired communication and of Mr. F's denial, he lacked awareness that his wife was clinically depressed and in need of treatment. The low scores of marital adjustment measures in both partners corroborated the presence of severe marital maladjustment, probably aggravated by his forced retirement. His abnormally elevated interpersonal sensitivity score in the SCL-90, a self-report test of psychological symptoms, probably reflects characterological problems associated with his constricted emotional behavior. All other psychological and physiological measures were within normal limits.

References

Anderson, S. A., Rusell, C. S. and Schumen, W. R. (1983). Perceived marital quality and family-cycle categories: a further analysis. *Journal of Marriage and Family* 45, 127–39.

Baltes, P. B. and Baltes, M. M. (1990). Psychological perspectives on successful aging: the model of selective optimization with compensation. In *Successful Aging: Perspectives from the Behavioral Sciences*, ed. P. B. Baltes and M. M. Baltes, pp. 1–34. Cambridge, UK: Cambridge University Press

Bancroft, J. (1984). Interaction of psychosocial and biological factors in marital sexuality – differences between men and women. *British Journal of Guidance and Counselling* 12, 62–71.

Brecher, E. L. (1984). *Sex and Aging: A Consumers' Union Report*. Boston, MA: Little Brown.

Cupach, W. R. and Comstock, J. (1990). Satisfaction with sexual communication in marriage: links to sexual satisfaction and marital adjustment. *Journal of Social and Personal Relationship* 7, 179–86.

Dentler, R. A. and Pineo, P. C. (1960). Sexual adjustment, marital adjustment and personal growth of husbands: a panel analysis. *Marriage and Family Living* 22, 45–8.

Eckerdt, D. J. and Vinick, B. H. (1991). Marital complaints in husband-working and husband-retired couples. *Research on Aging* 13, 364–82.

Edwards, J. N. and Booth, A. (1994). Sexuality, marriage and well-being: the middle years. In *Sexuality Across the Life Course*, ed. A. S. Rossi, pp. 233–59. Chicago, IL: The University of Chicago Press.

Fields, N. S. (1983). Satisfaction in long term marriages. *Social Work* 28, 37–41.

Frank, E., Anderson, C. and Rubinstein, D. (1978). Frequency of sexual dysfunction in 'normal' couples. *New England Journal of Medicine* 299, 111–15.

Gilford, R. (1984). Contrasts in marital satisfaction throughout old age: an exchange theory analysis. *Journal of Gerontology* 39, 325–33.

Goldscheider, F. K. (1990). The aging of the gender revolution. What do we know and what do we need to know. *Research on Aging* 12, 531–45.

Hatfield, E., Greenberger, D., Traupmann, J. and Lambert, P. (1982). Equity and sexual satisfaction in recently married couples. *Journal of Sexual Research* 18, 18–32.

Johnson, C. L. (1985). The impact of illness on late-life marriages. *Journal of Marriage and the Family* 47, 165–72.

Karney, B. R. and Bradbury, T. N. (1995). The longitudinal course of marital quality and stability: a review of theory, method and research. *Psychological Bulletin* 118, 3–34.

Kimmel, D. and Van der Veen, F. (1974). Factors of marital adjustment. Locke's Marital Adjustment Test. *Journal of Marriage and the Family* 36, 57–63.

Kinsey, A. C., Pomeroy, W. B. and Martin, C. E. (1948). *Sexual Behavior in the Human Male.* Philadelphia: W. B. Saunders.

Lee, G. R. and Shehan, C. L. (1989). Retirement and marital satisfaction. *Journal of Gerontology* 44, S226–S230.

Levenson, R. W., Carstensen, L. L. and Gottman, J. M. (1993). Long-term marriage: age, gender and satisfaction. *Psychology and Aging* 8, 301–13.

Margolin, L. and White, L. (1987). The continuing role of physical attractiveness in marriage. *Journal of Marriage and Family* 49, 21–7.

Markides, K. S. (1995). Marital satisfaction. In *The Encyclopedia of Aging*, 2nd edn, ed. G. L. Maddox, pp. 601–2. New York: Springer Publishing Co.

Marsiglio, W. and Donnelly, D. (1991). Sexual relations in later life: a national study of married persons. *Journal of Gerontology* 46, S338–S344.

McCann, J. T. and Biaggio, M. K. (1989). Sexual satisfaction in marriage as a function of life meaning. *Archives of Sexual Behavior* 18, 59–72.

Nowinski, J. K. and LoPiccolo, J. (1979). Assessing sexual behavior in couples. *Journal of Sex and Marital Therapy* 5, 225–43.

Parron, E. M. (1982). Golden wedding couples: lessons in marital longevity. *Generations* 7, 14–16.

Peterson, J. (1973). Marital and family therapy involving the aged. *The Gerontologist* 13, 27–31.

Pfeiffer, E., Verwoerdt, A. and Davis, G. C. (1972). Sexual behavior in middle life. *American Journal of Psychiatry* 128, 82–7.

Pineo, P. C. (1969). Development patterns in marriage. *Family Coordinator* 18, 135–40.

Rollins, B. C. and Cannon, K. L. (1974). Marital satisfaction over the family cycle: a reevaluation. *Journal of Marriage and the Family* 36, 271–82.

Schenk, J., Pfrang, H. and Rausche, A. (1983). Personality traits versus the quality of the marital relationship as the determinant of marital sexuality. *Archives of Sexual Behavior* 12, 31–42.

Schiavi, R. C., Mandeli, J. and Schreiner-Engel, P. (1994). Sexual satisfaction in healthy aging men. *Journal of Sex and Marital Therapy* 20, 3–13.

Schick, F. L. and Schick, R. (1994). *The Statistical Handbook on Aging.* Phoenix, AZ: Oryx Press.

Smith, T. W. (1991). Adult sexual behavior in 1989: number of partners, frequency of intercourse and risk of AIDS. *Family Planning Perspectives* 23, 102–7.

Spanier, G. C. (1976). Measuring dyadic adjustment: new scale for assessing the quality of marriage and similar dyads. *Journal of Marriage and the Family* 38, 15–29.

Sporakowski, M. J. and Axelson, L. J. (1984). Long-term marriages: a critical review. *Lifestyles: A Journal of Changing Patterns* 7, 76–93.

Sporakowski, M. J. and Hughston, G. A. (1978). Prescriptions for happy marriage: adjustments and satisfactions of couples married for 50 or more years. *The Family Coordinator* 27, 311–27.

Starr, B. D. and Weiner, M. B. (1981). *The Starr–Weiner Report on Sex and Sexuality in the Mature Years.* Briarcliff Manor, NY: Stein & Day.

Stinnett, N., Carter, L. M. and Montgomery, J. E. (1972). Older persons' perception of their marriages. *Journal of Marriage and the Family* 32, 428–34.

Udry, R., Deven, F. R. and Coleman, S. J. (1982). Cross-national comparison of the relative influence of male and female age on the frequency of marital intercourse. *Biosociety of Science* **14**, 1–6.

US Bureau of the Census 1985. *Current Population Reports Series P-60. No 146.* Washington, DC: US Government Printing Office.

Verwoerdt, A., Pfeiffer, E. and Wang, H. S. (1969). Sexual behavior in senescence. II. Patterns of sexual activity and interest. *Geriatrics* **24**, 137–54.

Weiss, L. J. (1983). Intimacy and adaptation. In *Sexuality in the Later Years*, ed. R. B. Weg, pp. 147–66. New York: Academic Press.

6   Aging and homosexual relationships

The relationship between aging and the psychosocial adjustment of homosexual individuals has been neglected as a topic of research. Accurate information about the aging and adaptation of homosexuals is important, not only to correct pervasive stereotypical notions, but also for the general understanding of the social context of sexual diversity and the health-care needs of an important portion of the aging population.

Aging homosexual individuals are variously described as lonely, isolated from other homosexual males because of the over-emphasis on youth in the gay subculture, thinking of themselves as middle-aged and old before their heterosexual counterparts, unable to sustain close relationships, dysfunctional, unhappy, and lacking in self-esteem (Kelly, 1977; Berger, 1980; Pope and Schulz, 1991; McDougall, 1993). Descriptive studies, conducted mostly during the 1970s and 1980s, do not support these stereotypical beliefs. Weinberg and Williams (1975), who analyzed questionnaire data from a subsample of men aged over 45 as part of a survey of over 2000 homosexual volunteers, found that younger and older respondents did not differ on several measures of personal adjustment. Older men had more stable self-concepts and were less likely to desire psychiatric treatment. Kelly (1977) also noted that most older participants in his investigation reported satisfactory social and sexual lives. Berger (1980), in a study of 112 homosexual men aged 41–77, found that the majority of respondents lived in stable relationships, had many friends, scored within the normative range in all measures of psychological adaptation and life satisfaction and that older men, in comparison to younger homosexuals, had lower levels of depression and psychosomatic symptoms. Pope and Schulz (1991) assessed the sexual attitudes and behavior of 87 homosexual males divided into three age cohorts, 40–49, 50–59 and 60+ groups. Although there was an age-related decline in sexual interest and frequency of sexual activity, there was no change in reported enjoyment of sex from the subjects' younger years to the time of the study.

Several studies have specifically assessed some of the presumed negative characteristics of aging homosexuals. The notion that homosexual men self-perceive an earlier onset of middle and old age than do heterosexual men, labeled as accelerated aging, has been supported by some (Kelly, 1977; Friend, 1980) but not all studies (Minnigerode, 1976; Laner, 1978). Bennett and Thompson (1991), in an investigation of 478 Australian homosexual men, found that, consistent with research on male heterosexuals, the subjects perceived middle age beginning around 41 years and old age at 63 years. However, in contrast, the subjects believed that other homosexual men define middle age as beginning around 39 years and old age at 54 years. The authors concluded that the contradictory information about male homosexuality and accelerated aging may be largely dependent on the discrepancy between self-perception and the subject's belief about the perception of others, based on the youthful orientation of the gay community. Feeling 'over the hill' and devalued for not appearing youthful may be a contributing factor to the feelings of depression and isolation experienced by some individual men (Friend, 1987), but there is no evidence that homosexuals as a group are more depressed and socially isolated than their heterosexual cohort. Dorfman and collaborators (1995) surveyed 108 homosexual and heterosexual subjects ranging in age from 60 to 93. The two respondent groups did not differ significantly in depression and overall social support, measured by scales validated for use in elderly populations. There were, however, interesting group differences in the sources of support: while heterosexual subjects obtained more support from family members, gay men and lesbians derived significantly more support from friends. Homosexual individuals, having had to manage family crises caused by their sexual orientation, are more likely to have compensated for a real or imagined loss of family support in old age by developing a strong network of friends and engaging in gay community activities. The results, suggesting the importance of friendship networks for aging homosexuals, are consistent with the socioemotional selectivity theory proposed by Carstensen (1992), which is discussed in the following chapter. It should be noted that the respondents in Dorfman et al.'s study were drawn from urban areas and the findings may not be generalizable to gays from nonurban regions where there are fewer networks for gay populations.

Problems about the generalizability of results is a generic issue applicable to all studies of homosexuality and aging. A central methodological problem is the bias inherent in recruiting primarily urban-located homosexuals active in the gay community who are usually white, well-educated and of relatively high socioeconomic status, and may be invested in denying the stigma of growing older (Harry, 1986). Few studies have been able to recruit an adequate number of homosexuals older than 65. It is likely that older homosexual men who became socialized in a repressive social climate are less inclined to participate in the gay subculture, less open about their sexual orientation and less prone to volunteer for studies about homosexuality.

Aging, adaptation of homosexuals and life-styles

There are marked socialization differences in the life histories of older and younger homosexuals. Today's 70-year-old homosexual men lived through an important phase of their formative years during the post World War II and the McCarthy era, a period of social oppression and active discrimination against homosexuals. They were already in their 40s when the gay rights' movement was born, following the riots triggered by police raids on gay bars in Greenwich Village and gay organizations became established (Heil, 1989). This dramatic social change variously influenced the self-concept and emotional adjustment of aging homosexual individuals with overt consequences for the degree of concealment of their sexual identity, living patterns and participation in the gay community.

Several authors have noted the diversity of relationship patterns of older homosexual men (Kimmel, 1977, 1979; Berger, 1982; Friend, 1991). Kimmel, based on life history interviews of a small number of men aged 55–81 years, described three gay-men lifestyles: 'long-term relationships', 'previously married gay men' and 'loners or serial lovers'. A similar categorization based on a study of 112 homosexual men older than 40 was developed by Berger (1982). Men in 'long-term relationships' may or may not be monogamous and show considerable variability in traditional gender roles. 'Previously married gay men' usually develop a homosexual life-style following marital separation or divorce and some may have had repeated homosexual affairs during their marital life. The 'loners or serial lovers' are characterized by Kimmel as mostly single, living alone, having engaged in short-term homosexual affairs devoid of intimacy and often fearful that their sexual orientation would be discovered. Friend (1991), based on social construction theory, proposed a cognitive–behavioral model of identity formation which characterizes at least three distinct groups of older gay adults. Individuals described as 'stereotypic older gay people' are those who, having internalized negative ideas about their sexual orientation, are more likely to experience low self-esteem, shame and guilt, are fearful of discovery and engage in distant relationships devoid of sexual intimacy. At the other end of the continuum, 'affirmative older gay people' represent those individuals who 'have reconstructed what it means to be gay or lesbian into something positive', have a high level of self-acceptance and are open and engaged in their homosexual life-styles. In the middle range are the 'passing older gay people', married or single, who have a fragmented sense of self, compartmentalizing their lives and engaging in homosexual experiences while spending considerable energy trying to appear heterosexual. This theory predicts that successful aging will depend on the degree to which homosexual men develop effective adaptive skills, coping with a socially unaccepting environment, in the way of achieving high levels of self-acceptance as gay individuals. The linear structure of this model has been criticized for not capturing the diversity and complexity of patterns of identity development; nevertheless, it describes how the sexual identity of homosexuals develops as they age, an area devoid of theory and empirical data.

Frequently mentioned in the literature on aging and homosexuality is the concept of 'crisis competence' (Kimmel, 1978; Berger, 1982; Friend, 1991; Quam and Whitford, 1992). This notion suggests that attitudes and coping processes that had permitted successful social adaptation to homosexuality and positive self-attributions, also facilitate the management of issues and feelings associated with aging. Changes associated with potential role losses as aging progresses, due to retirement, separation or death, may also be less severe for homosexual individuals because of their greater gender role flexibility. Traditional gender role definitions involve sustaining 'appropriate', socially accepted behaviors in the face of the challenges posed by old age. A heterosexual widower, for example, may have inadequate skills that ensure autonomous living when confronted with the tasks of cooking and house cleaning. A more flexible gender role allows the older homosexual greater freedom to learn skills that are considered 'nontraditional' and are more likely to be part of women's repertoire. The notion of 'crisis competence' has been challenged, however, by Lee (1987). In a four-year longitudinal study of 47 homosexual men, 50–80 years old, Lee found that life satisfaction scores were not related to the number and intensity of life crises reported by the subjects, rather they were significantly associated with self-rated health, income, education and close relationships. Therefore, it would appear, based on this study, that homosexual and heterosexual men are more alike than dissimilar on the factors that contribute to satisfactory aging.

Sexual problems and concerns

Some of the problems experienced by aging homosexuals, such as issues of health, income and loneliness, are similar to those frequently cited by their heterosexual counterparts. Quam and Whitford (1992), for example, explored age-related concerns in a sample of 80 homosexual individuals, 41 male, aged 50–73 years living in a Midwestern metropolitan region in the USA. Forty-one percent of the sample indicated health concerns as a serious problem facing respondents. Additional problems listed included isolation (19.2%), finances (19.2%), planning and funding retirement (13.7%), and developing relationships in the future (12.3%). Health and associated emotional concerns are magnified by the destructive effects of the acquired immunodeficiency syndrome (AIDS) epidemic in the gay community. Issues of loss, bereavement and emotional needs are particularly salient for gay survivors, many of whom are alienated from their families and rely on the support of friends, and gay community programs and self-help groups. Most of these programs, however, are located in urban centers and are not easily available elsewhere. The difficulty in managing terminal illness for same-sex unmarried partners may be magnified by the interaction with hostile relatives and legal issues arising from absent or contested wills and inheritance conflicts. Availability of well-informed legal counsel is of considerable importance not only for the protection of the legal rights of the surviving partner but also for addressing discriminatory practices concerning housing, employment, or purchasing insurance (Berger and Kelly, 1996).

The negative consequences of early social stigmatization is particularly relevant to older homosexuals, not only because they are reflected in their fears of social isolation and physical violence, whether reality based or not, but also because they are frequently confirmed by their interaction with health-care professionals and institutional settings. Health-care professionals frequently ignore the sexual orientation of their patients, even when important for their adequate care. In the following chapter we discuss the repressive attitudes of long-term care institutions for the aged concerning sexual expression. Nursing homes' failure to recognize the affective and sexual needs of their residents is particularly obvious in the case of homosexual patients, who may not disclose their sexual orientation for fear of ostracism or find that visits by same-sex partners are discouraged and opportunity for intimacy not available.

Sexual and intimacy problems

There is almost no information on the patterns of sexual adjustment among homosexual men in the community. Most of the available knowledge is derived from gay couples or individuals who have sought treatment because of sexual difficulties. By and large, the sexual dysfunctions for which gay men seek help do not differ greatly from those of heterosexual men (McWhirter and Mattison, 1980; Paff, 1985). They include low sexual desire, sexual desire discrepancies, erectile dysfunction, premature ejaculation, and delayed ejaculation. A distinct problem among homosexual men is aversion to penetrate or be penetrated anally and, possibly, a higher prevalence of delayed ejaculation. The age of homosexual men seeking treatment usually ranges from their 20s to early 50s and, apart from an age-related decrease in sexual interest and erectile capacity, there are no objective data on the effect of aging on their sexual function.

Coleman and collaborators (1988, 1992) thoughtfully discuss the particular challenges that confront homosexual individuals in the development of a positive sexual adaptation and life-style which, when disrupted, result in sexual and intimacy dysfunctions. Among the psychological determinants of specific relevance to being a homosexual are disturbances in the formation of their identity as a homosexual, discordant sex roles, and internalized homophobia. The stigma attached to homosexuality, fear of social disapproval and issues raised by the AIDS epidemic all conspire to generate confusion over sexual orientation and to disrupt the development of an integrated homosexual identity, self-confidence and self-esteem. Conflict and dysphoria concerning sexual orientation have been identified as common factors associated with sexual dysfunction in homosexual individuals (McWhirter and Mattison, 1980). Rigid adherence to stereotypical male roles may create problems in homosexual relationships that call for more fluid life-styles, freer from the traditional 'masculine' and 'feminine' dichotomy. Sexual maladjustment may occur when an individual's sexual behavior is not compatible with his perceived masculine gender role, such as being passive or receptive during sexual intercourse. Individual problems in the development of an integrated homosexual identity and lack of congruence between sexual orientation, sexual role and behavior may, according to Coleman, Rosser and Strapko (1992), be the consequence of internalized homophobic attitudes prevalent in present society. These attitudes, in addition to avoidance of interpersonal intimacy and sexual dysfunction, contribute to maladaptive behaviors such as drug abuse and sexual compulsivity. The AIDS epidemic is an important social determinant of internalized homophobia and lack of self-acceptance. The community misperception of AIDS as a problem for homosexuals has led to further stigmatization and, at the individual level, to disruptive anxiety, somatic preoccupation, sex-orientation dysphoria, loss of sexual desire, erectile difficulties or sexual avoidance (Quadland and Shattls, 1987). Yet, for many, it has reinforced, instead, the value of sustaining relationships, becoming sexually responsible, abstaining from anonymous sex, and increasing community involvement to provide as well as receive emotional and practical support.

Case study 6.1

Mr. G, a 67-year-old divorced man sought treatment because of his inability to ejaculate anally with his 42-year-old lover. He could ejaculate following vigorous manual stimulation by his companion but the pressure to reach orgasm triggered intense frontal headaches and Mr. G was concerned that it may lead to a stroke. He had suffered from essential hypertension, controlled with diet alone, but was otherwise healthy and on no drugs or medication. Mr. G's partner was invited but was unwilling to participate in evaluation or treatment.

The patient was brought up in Brooklyn, New York, in the context of a recently immigrated, traditional, lower-middle-class Eastern European family. At the age of 17, following an uneventful childhood and early adolescence, he began an active period of homosexual experimentation, resulting in considerable parental upheaval and in his decision to enlist in the Army. During his Army days and following his discharge he engaged in several long-term homosexual affairs that were not free from conflict. He felt 'different', 'socially isolated', 'diminished' by his homosexuality, sad at no longer relating to his family and began to question his sexual orientation. The manufacturing company he had established following his

Army discharge was flourishing and, by the age of 43, he felt economically secure and able to seek psychoanalytical help. He began heterosexual experimentation, fraught initially with considerable anxiety and fear of erectile failure, and three years after treatment onset met the woman he eventually married. Mr. G experienced his wife-to-be as 'good company', intellectually stimulating and physically attractive, and was able to have sexual relations without difficulty. She was a successful antique dealer, and through her he entered a socially sophisticated world that fulfilled his narcissistic aspirations. Several years into his marriage he felt increasingly neglected and resentful of her full devotion to her antique gallery, and began experiencing erectile difficulties and a reactivation of his sexual attraction to men leading, eventually, to separation and divorce. Soon after his divorce the patient met a young art designer with whom he had been living for 15 years at the time of the initial interview. He was attracted by his lover's handsomeness and felt proud to be with him among his friends. The relationship was characterized by Mr. G's ambivalent feelings about his own sexual orientation and doubts about his lover's motivation and commitment. Although the patient denied that the age difference was a negative factor, there were frequent arguments due to life-style preferences and his lover's feeling that Mr. G was too possessive and did not allow enough 'space' to pursue interests of his own. The patient, responding to his lover's expressed fears of economical insecurity, had included him in his will, but, despite this, he continued to request further monetary assurances. The event that precipitated the patient's orgasmic dysfunction was the discovery of lice in the partner's pubis in the face of his continuing denial of extrarelationship experiences. Despite this upheaval, the patient decided to continue the relationship providing that his partner entered psychotherapy. Mr. G's own therapy focused on issues of trust, commitment and self-esteem, was helpful in relieving his depressive mood but did not ameliorate his sexual dysfunction. At the time the patient decided to terminate treatment, Mr. G had been diagnosed as HIV positive and his lover was engaged in a battle with Mr. G's family concerning the will.

Comment

This case history illustrates several issues previously discussed, including conflict over homosexual identity, family alienation, problems of intimacy and self-esteem and the onset of HIV-related legal difficulties in a couple divergent in age. The patient's conflict concerning sexual orientation interacted with his narcissistic personality and with the couple's difficulties around issues of power and control. Particularly striking was Mr. G's onset of orgasmic dysfunction in relation to a serious crisis that threatened his trust and commitment. A follow-up session revealed that Mr. G had ended the relationship with his lover, was no longer sexually active, felt lonely but not depressed, participated in an HIV-support group and was devoting most of his energies to a newly discovered artistic vocation.

References

Bennett, K. C. and Thompson, N. L. (1991). Accelerated aging and male homosexuality: Australian evidence in a continuing debate. *Journal of Homosexuality* 21, 65–75.

Berger, R. M. (1980). Psychological adaptation of the older homosexual male. *Journal of Homosexuality* 5, 161–75.

Berger, R. M. (1982). The unseen minority: older gays and lesbians. *Social Work* 27, 236–41.

Berger, R. M. and Kelly, J. J. (1996). Gay men and lesbian grown older. In *Textbook of Homosexuality and Mental Health*, ed. R. P. Cagaj and T. S. Stein, pp. 305–16, Washington DC: American Psychiatric Press.

Carstensen, L. L. (1992). Social and emotional patterns in adulthood: support for the socioemotional selectivity theory. *Psychology and Aging* 7, 331–8.

Coleman, E. and Reece, R. (1988). Treating low sexual desire among gay men. In *Sexual Desire Disorders*, ed. S. R. Leiblum and R. C. Rosen, pp. 413–45, New York: The Guilford Press.

Coleman, E., Rosser, B. R. S. and Strapko, N. (1992). Sexual intimacy dysfunction among homosexual men and women. *Psychiatric Medicine* 10, 257–71.

Dorfman, R., Walters, K., Burke, P., Hardin, L., Karanik, T., Raphael, J. and Silverstein, E. (1995). Old, sad and alone: the myth of the aging homosexual. *Journal of Gerontological Social Work* 24, 29–44.

Friend, R. A. (1980). GAYing: adjustment and the older gay male. *Alternative Lifestyles* 3, 231–48.

Friend, R. A. (1987). The individual and social psychology of aging: clinical implications for lesbian and gay men. *Journal of Homosexuality* 14, 307–31.

Friend, R. A. (1991). Older lesbian and gay people: a theory of successful aging. *Journal of Homosexuality* 20, 99–118.

Harry, J. (1986). Sampling gay men. *Journal of Sex Research* 22, 21–34.

Heil, B. S. (1989). Homosexuality: a social phenomenon. In *Human Sexuality. The Societal and Interpersonal Context*, ed. K. McKinney and S. Sprecher, pp. 321–49. Norwood, NJ: Ablex Publishing Corporation.

Kelly, J. (1977). The aging homosexual: myth and reality. *Gerontologist* 17, 328–32.

Kimmel, D. C. (1977). Psychotherapy and the older gay man. *Psychotherapy: Theory, Research and Practice* 14, 386–93.

Kimmel, D. C. (1978). Adult development and aging: a gay perspective. *Journal of Social Issues* 34, 113–30.

Kimmel, D. C. (1979). Life-history interviews of gay aging men. *International Journal of Aging and Human Development* 10, 239–48.

Laner, M. R. (1978). Growing older male: heterosexual and homosexual. *The Gerontologist* 18, 496–501.

Lee, J. A. (1987). What can homosexual aging studies contribute to theories of aging? *Journal of Homosexuality* 13, 43–69.

McDougall, G. J. (1993). Therapeutic issues with gay and lesbian elders. *Clinical Gerontologist* 14, 45–57.

McWhirter, D. P. and Mattison, A. M. (1980). Treatment of sexual dysfunction in homosexual male couples. In *Principles and Practice of Sex Therapy*, ed. S. R. Leiblum and L. A. Pervin, pp. 321–45, New York: The Guilford Press.

Minnegerode, F. A. (1976). Age status labeling in homosexual men. *Journal of Homosexuality* 1, 273–6.

Paff, B. A. (1985). Sexual dysfunction in gay men requesting treatment. *Journal of Sex and Marital Therapy* 11, 3–18.

Pope, M. and Schulz, R. (1991). Sexual attitudes and behavior in midlife and aging homosexual males. *Journal of Homosexuality* 20, 169–77.

Quadland, M. C. and Shattls, W. D. (1987). AIDS, sexuality and sexual control. *Journal of Homosexuality* 14, 269–90.

Quam, J. K. and Whitford, G. S. (1992). Adaptation and age-related expectations of older gay and lesbian adults. *The Gerontologist* 32, 367–74.

Weinberg, M. S. and Williams, C. J. (1975). *Male Homosexuals: their Problems and Adaptations*, pp. 206–7. New York: Penguin Books.

7   The social context

Sexuality evolves throughout our lives, and is shaped by social conventions that give meaning and significance to life events and influence individual responses in keeping with the values and expectations prevailing at that time. According to life-span developmental theory (Baltes, 1987), people move through identifiable phases or periods requiring adaptation to personal or environmental changes that alter social roles, personal identity, and expectations. Individual adaptation to life events is not just a passive phenomenon, but a dynamic process that is influenced by the social context in which adult transitions take place. Socialization processes, with their implied expectations, norms, and values, help shape the sexual thoughts, interest, and activities of older individuals. The aged may incorporate these normative sanctions and perceive them not only as external constraints but also as a reflection of their personal values and preferences.

Social attitudes toward aging and sexuality

Cultural stereotypes about the sexuality of aging people are embedded in general negative attitudes towards the aged. Several authors have written about negative beliefs that prevail in Western societies concerning the aged (Hendricks and Hendricks, 1977; Rogers, 1979; Hultsch and Deutsch, 1981). Butler (1969) coined the term 'ageism' to indicate prejudicial attitudes toward older people, as well as discriminatory practices against this social group. Sexuality is popularly viewed as a youth-oriented activity. Prevailing social stigmas are that sexual interest and activity among the aged is inappropriate, that elderly people are either uninterested or unable to engage in sex and that they are physically unattractive and therefore sexually undesirable (Riportella-Muller, 1989). Traditionally, the mass media has both reflected and contributed to these myths by portraying sexual expression of older men and women as, 'humorous, ridiculous, repugnant, appropriate for patronizing response or extraordinarily exceptional' (Robinson, 1983).

Society's attitudes towards sexuality have evolved considerably in recent years. The strict Victorian sexual standards that prevailed when today's elderly were growing up differs markedly from the social and sexual climate that influenced the development of presently middle-aged individuals. Dramatic social movements in the USA in the 1960s and 1970s involving gender and race had significant impact on gender roles and sexual relations. During this period the problems of the elderly came to the nation's attention and government policies on aging began to be developed. However, the degree to which these social changes influenced cultural attitudes towards the sexuality of aging people is unclear. Arluke, Levin and Suchwalko (1984) investigated romantic and sexual advice in books for the elderly published prior to and after 1970 as a reflection of cultural changes over a 30-year period. The results suggest less negative attitudes towards the sexual activity of elderly people since the 1970s, but they provide little support for older people's dating and remarrying. Although the aged presently enjoy more sexual freedom, the cultural myth that aging men are asexual or sexually inappropriate still persists (Hall, Selby and Vanaclay, 1982). This stereotype coexists with contemporaneous emphasis on sexual proficiency as an essential component of sexual identity and male self-esteem. It is in this social context that what has been termed the 'midlife crisis' or 'male menopause' may be considered.

The midlife crisis

The terms midlife crisis, male menopause, andropause, and male climacteric refer to an elusive constellation of hormonal changes, psychological symptoms, and behavioral problems in middle-aged men. Sexual difficulties, depression, irritability, insomnia, marital problems, and hypochondriac complaints have been viewed as a syndrome ascribed to androgen deficiency analogous to the changes reported during female menopause. Age-related decreases in testosterone production and spermatogenesis in men have been documented (see Chapter 3). These changes are gradual, moderate and highly variable across individuals, in marked contrast to the generally abrupt decline in estrogen levels and irreversible anovulation during the female menopause (McKinlay, Longcope and Gray, 1989; Vermeulen, 1993). Despite the lack of evidence of a relationship between hormonal changes, psychological symptoms, and sexual difficulties in middle-aged men, popular literature on 'the male climacteric' continues to grow. There is an increased professional interest in the use of androgen replacement for the treatment of the 'low-testosterone male-menopausal syndrome' (Morley et al., 1997).

Featherstone and Hepworth (1985) suggest that the persistence and popular appeal of the notion of a male menopause and midlife crisis reflects, in part, middle-aged men's experience of sexual anxiety about, and/or dissatisfaction with, their sex life as it occurs in the current cultural context. They draw attention to two pervasive social forces: the emergence of a sexualized life-style extending into late middle-age, and changes in the social status of men. Erotic images pervade everyday life and help change expectations and reinforce the stereotype of male performative sex, a source of anxiety when sexual capacity begins to decrease. Sexological research has contributed valuable clinical information but, 'the result has not been an uncomplicated demythologization of sex, as some would have hoped, but the creation of a stimulating mixture of science, stereotypes and fantasies which constitutes the most persistent and persuasive images of our contemporary sexualized consumer culture.' (Featherstone and Hepworth, 1985). According to these authors, the term consumer culture refers to the impact of mass consumption on everyday life, which is reinforced through the mass media with the promotion of images of slim and attractive bodies, and proficient sexual behavior. Psychological distress and anxiety over masculinity, sexual identity, and sexual expression during men's transition into middle-age are viewed as the result of conflicting forces stemming from the youthful, sexualized life-style that characterizes cultural expectations and the changes in sexual role and balance of power between the sexes in contemporary Western societies. The term 'male menopause', while not physiologically valid, expresses and gives meaning to a constellation of events and experiences involving the aging process, sexual identity and cultural influences as men confront middle-age.

Late adulthood

The considerable popular and professional attention attracted by the midlife transition and 'male menopause' contrasts with the lack of a systematic examination of the psychosocial aspects of older men's sexuality. Critical 'turning points' occurring at a later stage of life, such as retirement, illness, widowerhood and institutionalization, can have profound consequences on sexual identity, sexual expression, and gender role expectations. Work provides a major source of men's identity, social status and self-esteem. Thus, retirement is, potentially, a crisis point for the individual, challenging his sense of masculinity, as defined by society, and impinging on patterns of interpersonal behavior and intimate relationships (Gradman, 1994). Simon (1996) discusses getting older in terms of necessary losses – loss of prestige and status due to retirement, loss of sexual competency, loss of friends and spouses and threatened or real loss of health and financial security. These significant life changes threatens men's social roles, and sense of autonomy and control. Kaas (1981), borrowing from Kuypers and Bengtson's social breakdown syndrome (1973), proposed the concept of the Geriatric Sexuality Breakdown Syndrome to analyze the relationship between sexuality of the aging and the social environment. According to this model, a decline in sexual capacity, in the context of diminished social roles and uncertain identity, renders the aged susceptible to a 'negative breakdown cycle'. The breakdown is characterized by increased dependency on prevailing social cues regarding appropriate behavior, since frames of reference based on past experiences are no longer available. The social context ignores the sexuality of the aged or overtly conveys the belief that sex is wrong, sinful or inappropriate. These negative stereotypes are incorporated by the aged, to the extent that their self-esteem is compromised and they are more susceptible to negative sexual prejudices and myths. The elderly learn to disavow sexual feelings or desire as a result of guilt or shame, leading to sexual withdrawal and enhanced sensitivity to negative labeling and stigmatization. Although this model takes into account the interactions between society, aging and sexuality, there is limited empirical evidence to validate it. In fact, more recent gerontology contributions, not directly focused on sexuality, have challenged some of its assumptions.

A broader sociopsychological perspective of aging

The notion that the elderly are the subject of widespread negative stereotyping is not a generally accepted conclusion. While several authors agree that negative perceptions towards older people are common in our culture (Butler, 1969; Levin and Levin, 1980; Palmore, 1982), others such as Lutsky (1980), Green (1981) and Schonfield (1982) believe that there is little or no firm scientific evidence for negative stereotypes of the aged. Crockett and Press (1981), based on a critical review of this literature, draw a distinction between general attitudes towards the elderly as a group and the perception of specific elderly individuals. The data do not support the existence of global negative stereotypes, although they do show that unfavorable beliefs about the nature of old age often outnumber favorable ones. The findings suggest that perceptions of the aged are not simply shaped by general attitudes but by the interaction between such attitudes and the characteristics of the particular individual. They postulate that perceivers differentiate between subcategories of the elderly, and have different attitudes towards them. These subcategories are composed of elements such as physical characteristics, traits, interests, and abilities. The evaluation of an older individual would depend on the subcategory to which the person is assigned based on the match between the person's observed characteristics and the qualities that are prototypical for the various subcategories.

How do individuals adjust or manage their own aging? Two influential theories that addressed this question were the previously alluded social breakdown theory of Kuypers and Bengtson (1973) and the disengagement theory (Cumming and Henry, 1961). The social breakdown theory posits that the elderly, who lack clear role definitions and reference groups, internalize society's pejorative labels leading to a self-reinforced negative cycle. The disengagement theory proposes that the aged and society mutually withdraw from each other, and that this decrease in social interaction is psychologically adaptive for the elderly and advantageous for society. Both theories have been criticized for their sparse scientific evidence and for being time bound. They have been replaced by more positive conceptualizations in which the aged actively adapt their interaction with society, with emphasis on role change rather than role loss.

Frequently noted in recent studies is a positive sense of self-worth and self-esteem among the aged (Brown, 1990) and satisfaction with their social relationships (Herzog and Rodgers, 1981; Field and Minkler, 1988). Maintaining personal worth or developing a new basis for self-esteem are dynamic social processes that are negotiated as roles change and new ones acquired. Of particular importance in this process is the interaction of the aged with their mates, families, and significant others. Carstensen (1991, 1992) challenged the inference that reduced social interaction in old age indicates a loss of emotional social experience and reduced social competence. She proposed a model, termed socioemotional selectivity theory, in which older people proactively manage reductions in social interaction to maximize emotional ties and intimate relationships and to minimize social and emotional risks. The theory predicts that, relative to younger people, older people are less invested in emotionally meaningless social interactions and make, instead, social choices based on the potential for emotional gains. Lang and Carstensen (1994) conducted a cross-sectional study of 156 community-dwelling and institutionalized people, aged 70–104 years, stratified by age and sex. They hypothesized that the number of intimate emotional relationships would not differ with age and that, when family members were not available to occupy the 'inner circle', such roles would be filled by people outside the family. Furthermore, they expected that fewer emotional partners would be needed if nuclear family members were available. The results supported their predictions. Although the overall social network size was negatively related to age, and the social network of very old people was nearly half that of old people, the actual number of very close relationships was the same for both age groups. Reductions in social relationships were limited to social partners who were less close. Those subjects with spouses or children placed them in the innermost circle and placed other relatives and friends in the middle circle. Those without nuclear family placed other kin in the inner circle, suggesting an adaptive process by which social partners other than nuclear family members ensure intimacy even in very old age. These results are in keeping with the Baltes and Baltes (1990) model of selective optimization with compensation described in Chapter 1. Consistent with the concept of selection, older people managed emotional resources so that the most valuable and rewarding relationships were maintained and the less significant ones abandoned. There was also evidence in this study that the old people were proactively involved in social interactions that compensated for emotional and physical losses. They were also engaged in strategies that met their practical needs while optimizing the emotional value of close relationships.

The institutionalized aged

One consequence of the extended life-span is that more elderly people spend a significant portion of their life in institutional facilities. It has been estimated that 5% of people older than 65 are in extended care facilities and that during the course of their lives 30% of men spend some time in nursing homes (Cohen, Tell and Wallack, 1986). The sexuality of the institutionally aged has been ignored or severely restricted and too little research attention has been devoted to it. Wasow and Loeb (1979) and White (1982) found that although most institutionalized residents were sexually inactive, a significant proportion acknowledged having sexual thoughts and feelings. Mulligan and Palguta (1991), in a survey of male nursing home residents, also observed the persistence of sexual interest, reported as strong by 61% of those who had a potential sexual partner. Although only one-fifth of residents continued to have intercourse, 90% engaged in hugging, caressing, and kissing. Of note is the observation that, despite their limited sexual activity, most subjects were relatively satisfied sexually. Conflicting attitudes concerning the sexual behaviors of institutionalized residents among health-care professionals have been found, and many find themselves unprepared to respond in a constructive rather than in a punitive manner (Kaas, 1978; Szasz, 1983; Brown, 1989). Traditionally, institutional rules concerning sexual expression, whether they involve hugging and petting behaviors, masturbation or overnight conjugal visits, have been repressive. Privacy was restricted, sexes were frequently separated and no provisions were made even for married residents to share a room. In the USA, these policies may be changing partly in response to federal statutes concerning the older person's rights (Patients' Rights Section, 1980). However, administrative changes in response to federal regulations have been implemented slowly. Equally important for effective change is the development of training programs addressing the sexual attitudes and required knowledge and skills of health-care providers responsible for the needs of institutionalized aged individuals (Glass, Mustian and Carter, 1986; Hillman and Stricker, 1994).

Conclusion

What is the relevance of current sociopsychological perspectives of aging to our views on the sexuality of older men? Few are the studies that have incorporated sexual role and behavior dimensions into modern social theories of aging. The marked social changes in sexual attitudes and behavior that have occurred over the last 30 years limit the validity of cross-sectional research involving age cohorts with dissimilar social backgrounds, values, and experiences. The majority of social studies on aging have investigated white, well-educated populations and the relationship between the sexuality of older men and variables such as ethnicity and socioeconomic class remain to be explored. Its relevance is exemplified by a study of the sexual function and behavior of older men of lower socioeconomic status who attended a Veterans Administration Geriatric Clinic (Cogen and Steinman, 1990) in the USA. Fifty-nine per cent of men reported significant or total loss of erectile capacity but, in contrast to data from surveys of more economically advantaged groups, few of the men in their study engaged in alternative sexual practices such as mutual masturbation or oral sex. A significant proportion of subjects, when unable to have intercourse, ceased to be sexually active altogether.

Current theories suggest that the interaction between the aged and society is gradually changing and that older persons are not necessarily passive recipients of negative sexual prejudices. Influenced by more sexual information, their peers and changes in family structure, the aged are becoming increasingly proactive in the development of intimate relationships, shaping their sense of sexual worth and identity. However, while the social stereotype of the asexual older man may be gradually diminishing, it is being replaced by the expectation of undiminished capacity for sexual performance as age progresses. Sociocultural approaches to the sexuality of the aged should rise above an exclusive focus on sexual intercourse to consider other forms of sexual expression, the meaning of sexuality in later life and issues of intimacy, pleasure, and satisfaction. There is increasing fluidity in the patterns of sexual interaction as cultural norms change with time and over a lifetime. We are living longer, gender roles are evolving, and social variations in sexual expression are becoming increasingly heterogeneous, be it heterosexual, homosexual, bisexual or celibate.

References

Arluke, A., Levin, J. and Suchwalko, J. (1984). Sexuality and romance in advice books for the elderly. *The Gerontologist* 24, 415–18.

Baltes, P. B. (1987). Theoretical propositions of life-span developmental psychology: on the dynamics between growth and decline. *Developmental Psychology* 23, 611–26.

Baltes, P. B. and Baltes, M. M. (1990). Psychological perspectives on successful aging: the model of selective optimization with compensation. In *Successful Aging: Perspectives from the Behavioral Sciences*, eds. P. B. Baltes and M. M. Baltes, pp. 1–34. Cambridge, UK: Cambridge University Press.

Brown, A. S. (1990). A social psychology of aging. In *The Social Processes of Aging and Old Age*, ed. A. S. Brown, pp. 40–53. Englewood, NJ: Prentice Hall.

Brown, L. (1989). Is there sexual freedom for our aging population in long term care institutions. *Journal of Gerontological Social Work* 13, 75–93.

Butler, R. N. (1969). Age-ism: another form of bigotry. *The Gerontologist* 9, 243–6.

Carstensen, L. L. (1991). Socioemotional selectivity theory: social activity in life-span context. *Annual Review of Gerontology and Geriatrics* 11, 195–217.

Carstensen, L. L. (1992). Social and emotional patterns in adulthood: support for the socioemotional selectivity theory. *Psychology and Aging* 7, 331–8.

Cogen, R. and Steinman, W. (1990). Sexual function and practice in elderly men of lower socioeconomic status. *Journal of Family Practice* 31, 162–6.

Cohen, M. A., Tell, E. J. and Wallack, S. S. (1986). The lifetime risks and costs of nursing home use among the elderly. *Medical Care* 24, 1161–72.

Crockett, W. H. and Press, A. N. (1981). Perceptions of aging and the elderly. In *The Dynamics of Aging*, eds. F. Berghorn and D. Schafer, pp. 217–41. Boulder, CO: Westview.

Cumming, E. and Henry, W. (1961). *Growing Old: the Process of Disengagement*. New York: Basic Books.

Featherstone, M. and Hepworth, M. (1985). The male menopause: lifestyle and sexuality. *Maturitas* 7, 235–46.

Field, D. and Minkler, M. (1988). Continuity and change in social support between young-old and old-old or very-old age. *Journal of Gerontology: Psychological Sciences* 43, P100–6.

Glass, J. C., Mustian, R. D. and Carter, L. R. (1986). Knowledge and attitudes of health care providers toward sexuality in the institutionalized elderly. *Educational Gerontology* 12, 465–75.

Gradman, T. J. (1994). Masculine identity from work to retirement. In *Older Men's Lives*, ed. E. H. Thompson, pp. 215–32. Thousand Oaks, CA: Sage.

Green, S. K. (1981). Attitudes and perceptions about the elderly: current and future perspectives. *International Journal of Aging Human Development* 13, 99–119.

Hall, A., Selby, J. and Vanclay, F. M. (1982). Sexual ageism. *Australian Journal of Ageing* 1, 29–34.

Hendricks, J. and Hendricks, C. D. (1977). *Aging in Mass Society: Myths and Realities*. Cambridge, MA: Winthrop Publishers.

Herzog, R. A. and Rogers, W. L. (1981). Age and satisfaction: data from several large surveys. *Research on Aging* 3, 142–65.

Hillman, J. L. and Stricker, G. (1994). A linkage of knowledge and attitudes toward elderly sexuality: not necessarily a uniform relationship. *The Gerontologist* 34, 256–60.

Hultsch, D. F. and Deutsch, F. (1981). *Adult Development and Aging: A Life-span Perspective*. New York: McGraw and Hill.

Kaas, M. J. (1978). Sexual expression of the elderly in nursing homes. *The Gerontologist* 18, 372–8.

Kaas, M. J. (1981). Geriatric sexuality breakdown syndrome. *International Journal of Aging Human Development* 13, 71–7.

Kuypers, J. and Bengtson, V. L. (1973). Social breakdown and competence: a model of normal aging. *Human Development* 16, 181–201.

Lang, F. R. and Carstensen, L. L. (1994). Close emotional relationships in late life: further support for proactive aging in the social domain. *Psychology and Aging* 9, 315–24.

Levin, J. and Levin, W. C. (1980). *Ageism: Prejudice and Discrimination Against the Elderly*. Belmont, CA: Wadsworth. Publishing Co.

Lutsky, N. S. (1980). Attitudes toward old age and elderly persons. In *Annual Review of Gerontology and Geriatrics*, vol. 1, ed. C. Eisdorfer, pp. 287–336. New York: Springer.

McKinlay, J. B., Longcope, C. and Gray, A. (1989). The questionable physiologic and epidemiologic basis for a male climacteric syndrome: preliminary results from the Massachusetts Male Aging Study. *Maturitas* 1, 103–15.

Morley, J. E., Kaiser, F. E., Sih, R., Hajjar, R. and Perry, III H. M. (1997). Testosterone and frailty. *Clinics in Geriatric Medicine* 13, 685–95.

Mulligan, T. and Palguta, R. F. (1991). Sexual interest, activity and satisfaction among male nursing home residents. *Archives of Sexual Behavior* 20, 199–204.

Palmore, E. B. (1982). Attitudes toward the aged: what we know and need to know. *Research on Aging* 4, 333–48.

Patients' Rights Section (1980). Marital Privacy, 405 1121 (K 14). In *Federal Regulations Guidelines for Directors of Nursing*, eds. M. L. Kander and K. May. Owings Mill, MD: National Law Publishing.

Riportella-Muller, R. (1989). Sexuality in the elderly: a review. In *Human Sexuality. The Societal and Interpersonal Context*, eds. K. McKinney and S. Sprecher, pp. 210–36. Norwood, NJ: Ablex Publishing Co.

Robinson, P. K. (1983). The sociological perspective. In *Sexuality in the Later Years*, ed. R. B. Weg, pp. 81–103. San Diego: Academic Press.

Rogers, D. (1979). *The Adult Years: An Introduction to Aging*. Englewood Cliffs NJ: Prentice Hall Inc.

Schonfield, D. (1982). Who is stereotyping whom and why. *The Gerontologist* 22, 267–72.

Simon, J. (1996). Getting older. *Psychiatric Annals* 26, 41–4.

Szasz, G. (1983). Sexual incidents in an extended care unit for aged men. *Journal of the American Geriatrics Society* 31, 407–11.

Vermeulen, A. (1993). Environment, human reproduction, menopause and andropause. *Environmental Health Perspectives Supplements* 101 [Suppl 2], 91–100.

Wasow, M. and Loeb, M. B. (1979). Sexuality in nursing homes. *Journal of the American Geriatrics Society* 27, 73–9.

White, C. B. (1982). Sexual interest, attitudes, knowledge, and sexual history in relation to sexual behavior in the institutionalized aged. *Archives of Sexual Behavior* 11, 11–21.

8   The nature and prevalence of sexual disorders in the aged

The nosological system for sexual disorders incorporated in the *Diagnostic and Statistical Manual of Mental Disorders* (DSM-IV) (American Psychiatric Association, 1994) characterizes sexual dysfunction as disturbances in sexual response defined to include four phases: desire, excitement, orgasm, and resolution. This classification, psychophysiologically based and oriented towards sexual performance, does not fully encompass the experiences and problems of the aging male. Aging is mostly neglected in DSM-IV as an associated feature of sexual dysfunction and its subjective aspects, which become more salient as age progresses. However, a significant improvement in the DSM-IV edition should be recognized. The diagnostic criteria for sexual dysfunction now require that the disturbance causes marked distress or interpersonal difficulties (Table 8.1). Consequently, age-related declines in a man's sexual function may not be categorized as dysfunctional unless they are problematic for the individual or his partner.

Sexual problems and concerns, not classifiable as dysfunctional according to DSM-IV diagnostic categories, are highly prevalent in the aging population. Their importance as a source of dissatisfaction and as a determinant of help-seeking behavior has been frequently ignored. The large body of data on sexual problems in the aging male is remarkable for its almost exclusive focus on erectile disorders. Regrettably, the health-care delivery system in the Western world tends to focus on the functional decrements in erectile capacity with limited attention given to underlying individual and interpersonal difficulties. In this chapter we shall summarize information from selected surveys, representative samples of the community at large and clinical populations. Among the latter we shall describe our clinical experience over a 17-year span at the Human Sexuality Program at Mount Sinai Medical Center. Finally, three case examples will illustrate frequently noted sexual problems in aging patients.

Sexual concerns and sexual difficulties

Sexual concerns are a universal phenomenon, 'are we doing it too frequently or not frequently enough?', 'are we doing it in the right way?', 'are we enjoying it as much as others?'. Behind these questions is a quest for reassurance about the normality of individual experience. The frequent inclusion of articles on sexual behavior in

Table 8.1. Diagnostic criteria for male sexual dysfunctions (DSM-IV)

Criterion A

Hypoactive sexual desire disorder
Persistently or recurrently deficient (or absent) sexual fantasies and desire for sexual activity.
The judgment of deficiency or absence is made by the clinician, taking into account factors that
affect sexual functioning such as age and the context of the person's life.

Male erectile disorder
Persistent or recurrent inability to attain, or to maintain until completion of the sexual activity,
an adequate erection.

Male orgasmic disorder
Persistent or recurrent delay in, or absence of, orgasm following a normal sexual excitement
phase during sexual activity that the clinician, taking into account the person's age, judges to be
adequate in focus, intensity, and duration.

Premature ejaculation
Persistent or recurrent ejaculation with minimal sexual stimulation before, on, or shortly after
penetration and before the person wishes it. The clinician must take into account factors that
affect the duration of the excitement phase, such as age, novelty of the sexual partner or
situation, and recent frequency of sexual activity.

Dyspareunia
Recurrent or persistent genital pain associated with sexual intercourse.

Criterion B (applies to all dysfunctions)
The disturbance causes marked distress or interpersonal difficulty.

Criterion C (applies to all dysfunctions)
The sexual dysfunction is not better accounted for by another Axis I disorder (except another
sexual dysfunction) and is not due exclusively to the direct physiological effects of a substance
(e.g., a drug of abuse, a medication) or a general medical condition.

Notes:
Taken from *Diagnostic and Statistical Manual of Mental Disorders (DSM-IV)*, 4th edn. (1994).
Washington, DC: American Psychiatric Association.

the popular press is not only stimulated by the readers' natural curiosity but also by
their sexual worries. Prevalent concerns reported by older volunteers in our study
of healthy aging centered around the unpredictability of erectile function,
decreased penile rigidity, body image, loss of sexual attractiveness, sexual boredom,
and distress about their partner's loss of sexual interest.

The dividing line between sexual concerns and sexual difficulties is not of easy
demarcation. Frank, Anderson and Rubinstein (1978), in a study described in

Chapter 5, analyzed the responses to a self-report questionnaire of predominantly white, well-educated couples who believed, 'their marriages were working reasonably well'. The investigators not only inquired about sexual dysfunctions but also about sexual difficulties, which included problems not dependent on sexual performance, such as an inability to relax, lack of interest in sex, too little foreplay before intercourse and the partner choosing inconvenient times for sex. Half of the men and 77% of the women acknowledged sexual difficulties that were not dysfunctional in nature. Sexual dysfunctions were reported by 50% of men (mainly premature ejaculation but also erectile difficulties) and by two-thirds of the women (mainly arousal and orgasm dysfunctions). Sexual dissatisfaction was more closely related to the occurrence of sexual difficulties than to the existence of sexual dysfunction. While recognizing the problem of generalizing from this selected sample, the authors conclude that, 'it is not the quality of sexual performance but the affective tone of the marriage that determines how most couples perceived the quality of their sexual relations'. This conclusion is congruent with the data reported in preceding chapters on the factors that sustain sexual satisfaction in older men.

Sexual dysfunctions

Several nonrandom studies of sexual behavior in older men have shown age-related increases in the prevalence of male erectile disorders. Kinsey, Pomeroy and Martin (1948), for example, reported that the percentage of men with impotence remained less than 7% until 60 years of age. Subsequently, the percentages gradually increased to 25%, 55%, and 75% at ages 70, 75, and 80 respectively. No information was provided on male orgasmic disorders in the small sample of older men included in their survey. In the Duke Study of Aging which included 261 men at the beginning of the study, 29% of men gave loss of potency as the reason for stopping intercourse and 15% loss of interest. There was general agreement between spouses that cessation of intercourse was due to the husbands' illnesses or inability to perform sexually (Pfeiffer, Vewoerdt and Wang, 1968). The proportion of men who had partial or total erectile dysfunction in the Baltimore Longitudinal Study of Aging increased from 7% in the 20–30 age group to 57% at ages 70–79. Seventy-five per cent of the less sexually active men, 46% of the moderately active and 19% of the most active subjects reported significant erectile problems. In addition 21% of the least active as compared to 8% of the most active men reported long-term premature ejaculation (Martin, 1981). Martin attributed the age-related increase in erectile problems and the decrease sexual activity to a loss of sexual motivation. The wide differences in population characteristics, lack of systematic focus on sexual dysfunction, unclear definitions of 'impotence', and the confounding of problems of sexual desire with those of arousal do not allow the prevalence of sexual disorders in older men to be estimated from these data.

Representative studies from the community

Diokno, Brown and Herzog (1990) conducted, as described in Chapter 2, a probability sample survey of noninstitutionalized individuals aged 60 years and older living in a Michigan county. As part of the clinical assessment carried out by trained interviewers, medical and psychosexual information was obtained from a total of 1956 individuals. The proportion of married men who were sexually active decreased from 87% at ages 60–64 to 50% at ages 75–79. Forty per cent of all the men in the sample reported having difficulties getting or maintaining erections; the prevalence increased significantly from 28% to 62% between ages 60–64 and 75–79 respectively. Impotence was reported by 38% of the married respondents and, among those, 40% indicated that they did not have any erection at all and 26% rated their erections between 1 and 50% of a full erection. A history of myocardial infarction, urinary incontinence, and sedative use were associated with a higher prevalence of erectile problems. The study did not provide information on orgasmic dysfunction but indicated that 1.4% of men suffered from dyspareunia.

The Massachusetts Male Aging Study is presently the most definite source of epidemiological data on the prevalence of erectile dysfunction in noninstitutionalized aging men (Feldman et al., 1994). As mentioned in Chapter 2, the study was carried out between 1987 and 1989 on a random sample of men 40–70 years of age living in selected towns around Boston. The response rate was 53% and included primarily white and well-educated volunteers in keeping with the population composition of the region. Because of the study's importance, we shall expand on methodological aspects relevant to the assessment of erectile capacity (see Chapter 2 for additional information on this study). A nine-item self-administered sexual questionnaire was completed by 1290 respondents. The following multiple-choice questions related to potency were asked:

1   In an average week, how often do you usually have sexual intercourse or activity?
2   During an average 24-hour day, how often do you have a full hard erection?
3   During the last six months have you ever had trouble getting an erection before intercourse begins?
4   During the last six months have you ever had trouble keeping an erection once intercourse has begun?
5   How frequently do you awaken from sleep with a full erection?
6   How satisfied are you with your sex life?
7   How satisfied are you with your sexual relationship with your present partner or partners?
8   How satisfied do you think your partner(s) is (are) with your sexual relationship?
9   Has the frequency of your sexual activity with a partner been: (a) as much as you desire? (b) less than you desire? (c) more than you desire?

In addition, the respondents were asked to characterize themselves as non-impotent, minimally impotent, moderately impotent or completely impotent. Finally a discriminant formula combining all the sexual responses was generated to estimate the probability of each subject having nil, minimal, moderate or complete impotence.

The mean prevalence of erectile difficulties in the entire sample of men was 52%; 9.6% were rated as completely impotent, 25% as moderately impotent, and 17.2% as minimally impotent. Age was the variable more strongly associated with impotence; between ages 40 and 70 the prevalence of complete impotence increased from 5.1% to 15% and the probability of moderate impotence doubled from 17 to 34%. It should be noted, however, that 33% of the 70-year-old respondents did not have erectile difficulties. Several medical conditions and life-style factors were significantly related to a higher probability of impotence following adjustment for age effects. They include hypertension, heart disease, diabetes, ulcer, arthritis, certain medicaments, cigarette smoking, and indices of anger and depression. The significance of these conditions for the pathogenesis of erectile failure will be discussed further in the next chapters.

The Massachusetts Male Aging study is unique for permitting generalization of findings to a well-defined, free-living population of men, encompassing a wide range of psychosocial, life-style, medical and hormonal characteristics, and obtaining well-defined information on erectile function. There was also evidence of age-related increases in male orgasmic problems and genital pain during intercourse but the questions were not couched in a manner that permits assessment of the prevalence of orgasmic disorders or dyspareunia in this sample.

Sexual problems in medical clinics

The high prevalence of erectile disorders in community studies, and their association with aging and disease, underlies the importance of considering sexual dysfunction in clinical populations. Among the 1180 patients from a Veterans Administration's Medical Clinic surveyed by Slag et al. (1983), 401 men (34%) acknowledged having erectile difficulties and among those 180 (45%) agreed to be examined for their problem. Impotent patients were significantly older than non-dysfunctional men (66.9 versus 56.5 years) and had a greater prevalence of medical illnesses. The majority of the sexually dysfunctional patients reported a gradual onset of erectile difficulties in the presence of adequate libido. Among the patients with erectile dysfunction who received a full medical examination, medical illness was considered the likely cause in 55%, medication in 25%, psychological factors in 14% and unknown cause in 7%. Of note is the observation that, before the investigators conducted their systematic inquiry, only 6 of 401 men had been identified as having an erectile dysfunction.

The role of aging and chronic disease in sexual dysfunction was also explored by a questionnaire which was distributed to all 347 patients from a VA geriatric ambulatory care clinic (Mulligan et al., 1988). The respondents (65% response rate) were divided into a 'young-old' group aged 65–75 years and a 'old-old' group aged over 75. They were compared to an 'old-young' group of less than 65 years from a general medical clinic. Lack of libido was reported by 30% of 'old-young', 31% of 'young-old', and 47% of 'old-old'. Erectile dysfunction was noted in 26% of 'old-young', 27% of 'young-old' and 50% of 'old-old', a difference that was significant. A stepwise logistic regression analysis identified age, self-reported poor health status, diabetes and urinary incontinence as predictor risk factors for sexual dysfunction.

Increasing awareness of the association between erectile impotence and chronic illness fostered the establishment, beginning in the middle 1970s, of medically based, impotence-evaluation units and the development of diagnostic methods for assessing erectile dysfunction. These clinics are aimed at a comprehensive evaluation of patients with erectile problems with particular emphasis on medical and pharmacological causes. Most of the referred patients tend to be in their middle 50s or older and to suffer from coexisting medical conditions. The nature and extent of the psychosexual assessment have varied considerably, as have the ancillary diagnostic procedures employed. The diagnostic results have ranged from 30% of patients classified as having organic sexual dysfunctions (Shrom, Lief and Wein, 1979) to 85% in other reports (Davis et al., 1985). Interpretation of the pathogenic significance of medical findings for erectile impotence has also varied depending on the specialty or research orientation of the clinic, be it focused on vascular (Lue et al., 1989) or hormonal (Kaiser et al., 1988) mechanisms.

To summarize, community- and clinical-based studies demonstrate a significant age-related increase in erectile disorders but provide little information on the prevalence of hypoactive sexual desire, or orgasmic and sexual pain disorders in older men. The high frequency of medical illness and drug effects associated with erectile problems in the aged, which will be discussed in detail in the following chapters, have led some authors to state that impotence has, primarily, an organic basis. Neglected in this conclusion is recognition of a bias that favors referral of organically disturbed patients to medically based diagnostic clinics. Evidence of selection bias in referral patterns was demonstrated in a study of two sexual dysfunction clinics in the departments of urology and psychiatry in the same institution (Segraves et al., 1981). Evaluation by both centers of the same patients, who self-referred or were initially referred to either one of the two clinics, demonstrated clear differences in the nature of patient groups. Organic forms of impotence predominated in patients initially referred to the urologically based clinic, while psychogenic impotence was the most common final diagnosis of patients first evaluated in the psychiatry clinic. This distinction emphasizes the importance of considering referral patterns and the nature and orientation of the clinic when interpreting diagnostic findings.

Sexual dysfunction clinics

The 1970s were characterized by the rapid development of sex therapy clinics based on the pioneering work of Masters and Johnson (1970), Kaplan (1974), and Lief (1981). These clinics reflected increasing public recognition of the prevalence of sexual problems and the availability of treatment for these conditions. The most frequent male dysfunctions evaluated in these units were premature ejaculation in younger patients and erectile dysfunction in older patient groups. A psychological orientation towards diagnosis and treatment predominated but also included some medical evaluation and laboratory testing to rule out organic pathology. Although the clinical characteristics of sexually dysfunctional men seeking sex therapy have been described frequently, there are almost no reports specifically focused on the aging male. One exception is an article by Wise, Rabins and Gahnsley (1984), who reviewed the records of all patients older than 50 evaluated from 1972 to 1981 in the sexual behaviors clinic of the department of psychiatry at the Johns Hopkins Hospital. The evaluation included psychosexual and psychiatric assessments and determination of organic factors based on history, physical examination, and laboratory testing. During the study period, 150 (5.8%) of the 2550 patients evaluated were men over 50 years of age. They were predominantly white, of middle socioeconomic class and were self-referred or had been referred, mainly by non-psychiatric physicians. Seventy per cent of these patients had an erectile dysfunction, and among those 22% were judged to have an organic dysfunction, 21% a psychogenic dysfunction and 27% had uncertain etiology. Desire-phase disorders and premature ejaculation were each diagnosed in 7% of patients. A high proportion of male patients (63%) received a concurrent psychiatric diagnosis, mainly depression, anxiety or personality disorder. A psychogenic cause for the sexual dysfunction was more frequently found among the self-referred patients than among those referred by medical practitioners. Among the medical conditions associated with sexual dysfunction, chronic cardiovascular diseases, diabetes, and postsurgical states were the most prevalent.

We conducted a chart review of patients evaluated in a multidisciplinary diagnostic and treatment program at the department of psychiatry, Mount Sinai Medical Center. Out of over 2500 individuals and couples seen between 1974 and 1991, 1775 were men and among them 236 (13.3% of the male sample) were aged 60 years and over. Referral sources were mainly general practitioners and medical specialists, some requesting specialized nocturnal penile tumescence (NPT) diagnostic testing, the remainder were community organizations and self-referrals. More than half of the older patients were married or had a stable sexual partner, but, despite our encouragement, they usually came alone for the initial evaluation. The psychosexual evaluation consisted of sessions, lasting from one to several hours, to gather systematic data on the nature and development of the sexual problem, the quality of interpersonal relations, medical, drug-intake and psychiatric history, and relevant developmental information. The interaction between the sexual problem and marital adjustment was explored in detail and, if available, the partner was interviewed alone during the second session. Recent medical records were reviewed and referrals to medical specialists carried out to acquire or complement available medical data. In addition to routine laboratory indices and hormonal assessments, ancillary (noninvasive) diagnostic testing was carried out, when necessary, to clarify the sexual diagnosis. This testing included NPT assessments in our sleep laboratory, penile responses to visual erotic stimulation, and Doppler recordings of penile blood pressure. These approaches are discussed in detail in Chapter 13.

Table 8.2 summarizes demographic and diagnostic information about this sample of older men. They were, mainly, in their middle 60s, white, well-educated and economically comfortable. A significant proportion among them were divorced, separated or widowers struggling with the vicissitudes of new relationships. Following chart review, the patients were classified according to DSM-IV diagnostic criteria. In keeping with the referral pattern, most of them met criteria for erectile disorder; the prevalence of patients diagnosed as having another dysfunction in isolation was remarkably low. Hypoactive sexual desire was, in 14% of patients, associated with erectile disorders; in some men it was causally related to the erectile difficulties, in others it was the consequence of repeated erectile failures and in most it was not possible to determine the primary dysfunction. Premature ejaculation usually occurred in association with erectile dysfunction and, as others have reported of the aged, it was frequently reactive to erectile problems. In almost all patients the sexual dysfunction developed after a period of normal sexual functioning.

In keeping with modern views about the etiology of sexual dysfunction (to be discussed in detail in Chapter 13), we approached our assessment of psychological, interpersonal and medical determinants as independent and not mutually exclusive causative factors. The degree of psychological and relationship impairment was rated on a three-point scale, based on a priori operational definitions. The significance of medical disorders and drug intake was determined in relation to the onset and maintenance of the sexual dysfunction. As may be seen in Table 8.3, the majority of patients suffered from chronic illness or were taking medications with potentially deleterious consequences for sexual function. An attempt was made to classify men with erectile disorders ($n=134$), into one of four diagnostic subtypes as defined in DSM-IV (Table 8.4): (1) due to psychological factors; (2) due to combined factors; (3) due to a general medical condition and (4) substance-induced sexual dysfunction. Table 8.5 summarizes this information: psychological factors

Table 8.2. Male patients 60 years of age and older evaluated between 1974 and 1991 (*n*=236)

Men's age (years):							
Mean: 65.7			Median: 66			Range: 60–84	
Marital status:							
Single:	10	4%					
Married:	135	57%					
Separated:	11	5%					
Divorced:	37	16%					
Widowed:	38	16%					
No information:	5	2%					
Partners' age (years):							
Mean: 60.2			Median: 60			Range: 33–79	
Duration of marriage (years):							
Mean: 29.8			Median: 34			Range: 1–50	
Occupation:							
Skilled:	35	15%					
Semi-professional	49	21%					
Professional:	55	23%					
Retired	70	30%					
No infornation	27	11%					
Psychosexual evaluation:							
Men alone:	169	72%					
Couples:	67	28%					
Psychosexual diagnosis:							
Hypoactive sexual desire disorder (HSDD):			8	3%			
Erectile disorder (ED):			155	66%			
Premature ejaculation (PE):			5	2%			
Male orgasmic disorder (MOD):			5	2%			
Other:			2	1%			
Double dysfunctions							
HSDD–ED:			34	14%			
ED–PE:			27	11%			
Characteristics of the dysfunction:							
Global:	119	50%	Progressive:	106	45%		
Situational:	83	35%	Intermittent:	101	43%		
No information:	34	14%	No information:	29	12%		

Table 8.3. Male patients with sexual problems 60 years of age and older. Causal factors and disposition

Psychological determinants			Relationship determinants		
None–Mild	27	11%	None-Mild	55	30%
Moderate	50	21%	Moderate	20	11%
Severe	113	48%	Severe	73	39%
No information	46	20%	No information	38	20%
Medical disorders*					
Cardiac/hypertension	93	39%	Postsurgical	31	13%
Neurological	14	6%	Musculoskeletal	7	3%
Hormonal	11	5%	Pulmonary	4	2%
Diabetes/metabolic	48	20%	Other	14	6%
Urologic	16	7%	None	60	25%
Gastrointestinal	7	3%	No information	9	4%
Drug Intake*					
Cardiovascular/antihypertensives	79	33%	Hypnotics	12	5%
Hypoglycemic agents	28	12%	Drugs of abuse	8	4%
Hormonal	12	5%	Anticholinergics	5	2%
Antidepressants	18	8%	Other medications	15	6%
Anticonvulsants	7	3%	None	80	34%
H_2 blockers	7	3%	No information	15	6%
Disposition					
Sexual counseling/sex therapy	70	30%			
Psychotherapy/psychopharmacology	22	9%			
Marital therapy	4	2%			
Medical treatment	47	20%			
Surgical approaches	16	7%			
No treatment	37	16%			
Evaluation not completed	12	5%			
No information	28	12%			

Note:

* Patients may receive multiple diagnoses or be listed under more than one medication.

Table 8.4. Male erectile disorders. DSM-IV diagnostic subtypes

Due to psychological factors
This subtype applies when psychological factors are judged to have the major role in the onset, severity, exacerbation, or maintenance of the sexual dysfunction, and general medical conditions and substances play no role in the etiology of the sexual dysfunction.

Due to combined factors
This subtype applies when: (1) psychological factors are judged to have a role in the onset, severity, exacerbation, or maintenance of the sexual dysfunction, and (2) a general medical condition or substance is also judged to contribute but is not sufficient to account for the sexual dysfunction.

Due to a general medical condition
Presence of a clinically significant sexual dysfunction that is judged to be due exclusively to the direct physiological effect of a general medical condition.

Substance-induced sexual dysfunction
Presence of a clinically significant sexual dysfunction that is fully explained by substance use, occurs during or within a month of substance use, and is judged to be due exclusively to the direct physiological effect of the substance.

Note:
Taken from *Diagnostic and Statistical Manual of Mental Disorders (DSM-IV)*, 4th edn. (1994). Washington, DC: American Psychiatric Association.

were judged to have a major etiological role in 33% of patients (see Case studies 8.1 and 8.2), and a contributory role in association with a medical condition or substance use in 38% of men (see Case study 8.3). In 29% of patients the erectile problem was judged to be caused exclusively by a medical disorder or to be fully explained by substance use. There were no differences among subtypes in demographic characteristics; as expected, the duration of the erectile disorder was significantly less when substance induced. The findings of this chart review should be interpreted with caution, however, in view of its retrospective nature, which was not conducted 'blind'. It lacks inter-rated reliability data for diagnostic categorization and, at the time of the initial evaluation, the more recently developed physiological testing procedures were unavailable.

Case studies

Case study 8.1
Mr. H, a 70-year-old jeweler, requested an evaluation for his erectile difficulties which had begun after his wife's death from uterine cancer two years before. For most of their 35 years

Table 8.5. Men with erectile disorders aged 60 years and older. DSM-IV diagnostic subtypes (*n* = 134)

	Due to psychological factors	Due to combined factors	Due to medical conditions	Substance induced
Number of patients (%)	44 (33%)	51 (38%)	27 (20%)	12 (9%)
Age: median (range)	66 (60–75)	65 (60–84)	66 (60–80)	64 (61–72)
Marital Status(%)				
Single	4.5	0	11.5	0
Married	48	60	58	75
Separated/divorced	30	28	8	17
Widowed	18	12	23	8
Duration of marriage [median years (range)]	35 (4–48)	35 (2–49)	40 (1–45)	29 (5–50)
Duration of dysfunction percentage of patients				
less than 2 years	49	41	23	67
2–5 years	19	10	12	8
more than 5 years	32	49	65	25

of marriage they had been sexually active and problem free; during the last year of her terminal illness he had limited his sexual activities to masturbation. Although he thought he was prepared for it, his wife's death came as a 'shock'; his children were far away and he felt lonely and in need of companionship. After several brief 'affairs' which were devoid of erectile difficulties, he renewed a relationship that had predated his marriage. As he became emotionally involved, and began having fantasies of living together, he found himself losing his erection when he attempted intercourse. Although the patient denied feelings of depression, discussion of his wife's final illness evoked a considerable emotional abreaction during the session.

A full medical and urological evaluation, hormonal tests, and penile vascular assessments provided negative results.

Comment

This vignette illustrates several features of common clinical occurrence in what has been labeled 'the widower's syndrome'. They include a committed marital relationship broken by the wife's terminal illness and the premature resumption of sexual activity while the widower is still in the process of grieving. Not uncommonly, as in this case, men are not fully aware of or deny their underlying emotional disarray and reinforce the problem by misguided attempts at 'forcing their erections'.

Case study 8.2

Mr. and Ms. I were referred by his cardiologist for evaluation of his sudden loss of sexual desire. The cardiologist had initially thought that the sexual problem was due to treatment with beta-blockers but the sexual problem had persisted following discontinuation of the antihypertensive medication. Mr. and Ms. I were 61 and 55 years of age respectively, had been married for 20 years and were the parents of three children no longer living at home. The loss of sexual desire had begun suddenly when he became 60 years old, an event he found very traumatic. Despite being a Dean of a Graduate School and having achieved considerable professional recognition, he felt 'at the end of the line', without having fulfilled the expectations he had set for himself. He resented his wife for his having had to relinquish a potentially successful political career in order to accept an administrative position that provided financial security for his family. After losing his sexual desire, he continued to engage in intercourse with his wife out of a sense of obligation, but began having episodes of erectile failure which were associated with anxiety, self-blame and sexual avoidance. The sexual history revealed that on one occasion, at the time of his 50th birthday, Mr. I had encountered similar sexual difficulties which had resolved spontaneously.

A central theme during the evaluation was Mr. I's regret at not having being with his father during the last days of life, his inability to mourn his death, and the sense that whatever unspoken expectations his father had had for him concerning a political career, he would never be able to meet them. Psychotherapy, in the past, had been helpful in allowing him to gain some insight into the sources of his guilt and distress. To his surprise the psychological conflict became reactivated once again around his 60th birthday.

Comment

Mr. I met criteria for hypoactive sexual desire disorder as the primary dysfunction and erectile disorder as the secondary dysfunction. It seemed obvious that the genesis of the sexual problem was psychological. Although the patient was dysphoric, he did not have an affective disorder that could explain the dramatic loss of sexual drive. Mr. I was not inclined to reenter psychotherapy to examine still unresolved dynamic issues; unfortunately, the attempt at sex therapy with his wife was severely compromised by his initiating an extramarital experience primarily motivated by the need to enhance his self-esteem.

Case study 8.3

Mr. and Ms. J, aged 65 and 59 respectively, were referred by his internist for evaluation of their sexual problems. They had been married for 38 years and for most of their married life had engaged in intercourse once to twice per week. Erectile problems had begun progressively ten years before and, at the time of the interview, he was only infrequently able to effect insertion with manual assistance. Mr. J's sexual desire persisted, although somewhat diminished; he occasionally masturbated with a partial erection and was no longer aware of full nocturnal erections.

Ms. J was a reluctant participant during the evaluation. She described a submissive but resentful attitude during the early stages of marriage caused by her husband's limited concern for her inhibitions, and felt that the situation was now reversed with her husband dependent on her to sustain his masculinity. Regrettably, her sexual desire was low and was particularly lessened towards her mate because of his increasing obesity. Their sexual pattern involved very limited foreplay and struggling attempts at achieving vaginal penetration. Mr. J resented her passivity and was 'turned off' by the impression that she engaged in sex 'as a favor' to him. Contributing to the marital tension and to his dysphoria was the loss of most of their savings following an ill-conceived investment after his retirement from a civil service position two years earlier.

Mr. J had had a mild heart infarct five years previously and was treated with antihypertensive medication. Treatment discontinuation did not improve sexual functioning. Intracavernosal testing with prostaglandin resulted in functional erections but the patient refused continued treatment with penile injections. He was studied in the Sleep Laboratory on three nights. On each of these nights he slept for over seven hours, had normal sleep stages and normal percentages of rapid eye movement (REM) sleep. He had a mean of three erectile episodes per night with circumference increases of up to 27mm. Unfortunately it was not feasible to assess the degree of penile rigidity by direct observation. The patient was given a special tape measure and instructed to measure the circumference of his penis in the flaccid and erect state at home, attempting to obtain maximum tumescence by any means he chose. A week later he reported that by self-stimulation he had attained several erections amounting to 30mm and that, although not full, they would have been more than adequate for intercourse. He had not had erections of this magnitude for a long time.

Comment

This clinical case characterizes the multiplicity of factors that frequently operate in concert with age-related decreases in penile rigidity leading to erectile dysfunction. Among the more obvious contributing determinants are possible underlying vascular pathology, power and control marital issues, his wife's unwilling participation in their sexual experiences, and his low self-esteem and mild depression following his business failure. The recording of NPT demonstrated that his erectile potential was superior than his sexual function with his wife. It is of note that this patient, as with others, after being told the results of our findings, was able to attain adequate erections by self-stimulation at home. Mutual recriminations dominated an attempt at marital/sex therapy and prevented its implementation.

Conclusion

Erectile difficulties are commonly noted among noninstitutionalized older men and are the most frequent reason for seeking sexual help. Sexual dissatisfaction and the call-for-help are not only dependent on decreased penile rigidity, but also on issues rooted in personal history, and the partner's attitude and emotional reaction to the change. Desire and orgastic difficulties are not frequently noted among the aged, but this may be artifactual, because of the focus on erectile function prevailing in most surveys. Men with loss of sexual desire may not be motivated to seek help unless pressured by their partners, as was the case for most of the older men with hypoactive sexual desire disorder evaluated in our clinic.

Data on the prevalence of erectile disorders among aging men varies considerably, according to the population screened, the definition of 'impotence', and the setting in which the study is conducted. Erectile problems in older men are frequently associated with medical disorders and drug intake but their prevalence and the significance of this relationship much depends on referral patterns and the orientation of the clinician. Central to diagnostic conclusions and therapeutic recommendations is the conceptualization about etiology. The tendency to interpret an association as having causal significance or to view causation as dichotomous (either organic or psychogenic) frequently leads to inaccurate or unbalanced views about the nature of sexual problems in the aged. The multidimensional approach to sexual problems, frequently advocated but seldom implemented, demands a comprehensive assessment of both psychological and organic dimensions as well as their interaction. It is important to keep this perspective in mind as we approach the next chapters on medical illness and pharmacological agents to balance their etiological focus on the sexual disorders of older men.

References

American Psychiatric Association (1994). *Diagnostic and Statistic Manual of Mental Disorders*, 4th edn. Washington, DC: American Psychiatric Association.

Davis, S. S., Viosca, S. P., Guralnik, M., Windsor, C., Buttigliery, M. W., Baker, J. D., Mehta, A. J. and Korenman, S. G. (1985). Evaluation of impotence in older men. *Western Journal of Medicine* 142, 499–505.

Diokno, A. C., Brown, M. B. and Herzog, A. R. (1990). Sexual function in the elderly. *Archives of Internal Medicine* 150, 197–200.

Feldman, H. A., Goldstein, I., Hatzichristou, D. G., Krane, R. J. and McKinlay, J. B. (1994). Impotence and its medical and psychosocial correlates: results of the Massachusetts Male Aging Study. *Journal of Urology* 151, 54–61.

Frank, E., Anderson, C. and Rubinstein, D. (1978). Frequency of sexual dysfunction in 'normal' couples. *New England Journal of Medicine* 299, 111–15.

Kaiser, F. E., Viosca, S. P., Morley, J. E., Mooradian, A. D., Davis, S. S. and Korenman, S. G. (1988). Impotence and aging: clinical and hormonal factors. *Journal of American Geriatrics Society* 36, 511–19.

Kaplan, H. S. (1974). *The New Sex Therapy*. New York: Brunner/Mazel.

Kinsey, A. C., Pomeroy, W. B. and Martin, C. E. (1948). *Sexual Behavior in the Human Male*. Philadelphia: W. B. Saunders Co.

Lief, H. (1981). *Sexual Problems in Medical Practice*. Monroe, WI: American Medical Association.

Lue, T. F., Mueller, S. C., Jow, Y. R. and Hwang, T. I.-S. (1989). Functional evaluation of penile arteries with Duplex ultrasound in vasodilator-induced erection. *Urologic Clinics of North America* 16, 799–807.

Martin, C. E. (1981). Factors affecting sexual functioning in 60-79 year-old married males. *Archives of Sexual Behavior* **10**, 399–420.

Masters, W. H. and Johnson, V. E. (1970). *Human Sexual Inadequacy.* Boston, MA: Little Brown.

Mulligan, T., Retchin, S. M., Chinchilli, V. M. and Bettinger, C. B. (1988). The role of aging and chronic disease in sexual dysfunction. *Journal of American Geriatrics Society* **36**, 520–4.

Pfeiffer, E., Verwoerdt, A. and Wang, H. S. (1968). Sexual behavior in aged men and women. *Archives of General Psychiatry* **19**, 753–8.

Segraves, R. T., Schoenberg, H. W., Zarins, C. K., Camic, P. and Knopf, J. (1981). Characteristics of erectile dysfunction as a function of medical care system entry point. *Psychosomatic Medicine* **43**, 227–34.

Shrom, S. H., Lief, H. I. and Wein, A. J. (1979). Clinical profile of experience with 130 consecutive cases of impotent men. *Urology* **13**, 511–15.

Slag, M. F., Morley, J. E., Elson, M. K., Trence, D. L., Nelson, C. J., Nelson, A. E., Kinlaw, W. B., Beyer, S., Nuttall, F. Q. and Shafer, R. B. (1983). Impotence in medical clinic outpatients. *Journal of the American Medical Association* **249**, 1736–40.

Wise, T. N., Rabins, P. V. and Gahnsley, J. (1984). The older patient with a sexual dysfunction. *Journal of Sex and Marital Therapy* **10**, 117–21.

9   Impact of medical illnesses on sexuality

Community surveys and studies of patients in medical and sex therapy clinics, summarized in Chapter 8, make abundantly clear the high prevalence of medical illnesses associated with erectile disorders in aging men. Any illness that is accompanied by weakness, fever, pain, malaise, and limited mobility is likely to have a generalized, nonspecific effect on sexual function. Medical disorders may also have direct actions by interfering with vascular, neural, and endocrine processes that mediate the sexual response. Their sexual effects are frequently multifactorial, involving physiological mechanisms interacting with psychological processes. Aging contributes significantly to the nature of this interaction; a person's age not only influences the probability of being affected by a specific illness but also determines their biobehavioral response to the medical problem (Mulligan, 1989). The effect of illnesses on individual sexual responses is also influenced by factors such as prior experiences of, and attitudes to, sex, coping styles, personality characteristics, and the nature of ongoing relationships. Regretfully, little empirical, systematic data on these critically important aspects are available for determining the effect of illness on sexual satisfaction.

A wide range of chronic organic conditions are associated with male sexual disorders (Table 9.1). The following is a discussion of the most prevalent diseases and surgical interventions that affect the sexual life of aging men. Coping and adaptive responses, as well as diagnostic and management issues will be considered in subsequent chapters.

Cardiovascular disease

Coronary artery disease, cerebrovascular lesions, peripheral arterial insufficiency and hypertension are frequently associated with sexual problems in the aged. The underlying pathophysiology is atherosclerosis, an age-related degenerative condition of the vascular tree that limits the blood supply to the tissues. The specific processes that contribute to sexual difficulties are complex, depending on the anatomical localization and degree of vascular pathology, the rate of progression of the disease, and the psychological and interpersonal factors that shape individual reactions to the organic insult.

Table 9.1. Chronic diseases and surgery associated with sexual dysfunction

Cardiovascular	Angina pectoris
	Myocardial infarction
	Hypertension
	Peripheral vascular insufficiency (atherosclerosis)
	Vascular surgery (aortoiliac/aortofemoral bypass)
Endocrine	Primary hypogonadism
	Hypogonadotrophic hypogonadism
	Hyperprolactinemia
	Thyroid disorders
	Addison's disease
	Cushing's syndrome
	Postsurgical: gonadectomy
Metabolic	Diabetes mellitus
	Chronic renal insufficiency
	Chronic hepatic insufficiency
Neurological	
Central	Temporal lobe pathology
	Multiple sclerosis
	Parkinson's disease
	Amyotrophic lateral sclerosis
	Cerebrovascular lesions (stroke)
	Sleep disorders (apnea)
	Alzheimer's disease
	Tumors and traumatic lesions (brain and spinal cord)
Peripheral	
Degenerative	Diabetic neuropathy
	Alcoholic neuropathy
Postsurgical	Transurethal surgeries
	Radical prostatectomy
	Abdominoperineal resection
	Bilateral lumbar sympathectomy
Anatomical	Peyronies' disease
	Postsurgical (genital tumors)
Other systemic conditions	Chronic obstructive pulmonary disease
	Arthritis
	Obesity

Patients who have coronary artery disease may experience angina because of myocardial ischemia during intercourse. The associated discomfort frequently interferes with sexual function and enjoyment. The pathogenesis of transient ischemia during sexual activity, similar to exercise-induced ischemia, involves an increased heart rate and enhanced demand for myocardial oxygen (Drory et al., 1995). A recent study of patients with ischemic heart disease who underwent coronary angiography (Greenstein et al., 1997) demonstrated a significant correlation between the number of coronary vessels affected and the degree of erectile impairment.

Numerous studies have reported a diminished frequency and quality of sexual activity, loss of sexual drive and sexual disorders in 10–70% of patients after myocardial infarction (Papadopoulos, 1989a). In addition to erectile dysfunction, premature ejaculation and orgasmic difficulties have been noted (Mehta and Krop, 1979). Resumption of sexual activity following a myocardial infarction has been found to vary from 2 weeks to 12 months with an average of 11 weeks (Papadopoulos, 1978). Among the factors implicated in the sexual consequences of myocardial infarction are angina, shortness of breath, fatigue, palpitations, medication effects, depression, and the patient's and partner's fear of cardiac complications during intercourse (Trelawny-Ross and Russell, 1987; Rosal et al., 1994). Methodological issues that contribute to the wide range of findings include lack of consideration of age effects and the level of sexual function prior to infarction. Retrospective evaluation shows that in two-thirds of patients the sexual problems had preceded the occurrence of the infarct (Wabrek and Burchell, 1980). In addition, Dhabuwala, Kumar and Pierce (1986) showed no differences in the prevalence of sexual problems between men with myocardial infarction and a control group matched for age, smoking history, and hypertension.

Fear and anxiety over resumption of sexual activity are a frequent source of sexual difficulties after a heart attack (Case study 9.1). A recent, well-designed study which estimated, in a large sample of patients with coronary heart disease, the risks of myocardial infarction triggered by sexual activity provides some reassurance in this regard (Muller et al. 1996). The absolute risk of sexual activity triggering a myocardial infarction is extremely low (one chance per million in a healthy individual) and is not increased in patients with prior coronary disease. Regular exercise further decreases the patient's risks of triggering an ischemic episode. Physiological investigation show that mean maximal heart rate and systolic blood pressure during intercourse do not differ between cardiac patients and normal subjects (Hellerstein and Friedman, 1970). The equivalent maximum oxygen cost during intercourse at orgasm in normal subjects has been calculated at six calories per minute, which is below the maximum capacity of average patients who have recuperated from myocardial infarction. Larson et al. (1980) compared the heart rates and blood pressure responses to sexual activity and stair climbing in healthy volunteers and those with coronary artery disease whose mean age was 50 years. The results supported the clinical use of ten minutes of rapid walking followed by climbing two flights of stair in ten seconds as a physiological test of readiness to resume activity after myocardial infarction. The occurrence of dysrhythmias during coitus may require further medical evaluation, including stress testing and ambulatory Holter (electrocardiogram, ECG) recording during sexual activity (Tardif, 1989).

Coronary artery bypass graft surgery is a frequently employed procedure aimed at relieving angina, improving the quality of life and diminishing mortality risk for cardiac patients. Numerous articles have assessed quality of life in coronary bypass patients but few have focused on sexual activity. There is considerable variability in sexual adjustment following surgery both within and across studies. Overall, the percentage of previously sexually active patients who resume sexual activity after bypass surgery appears to be higher than after myocardial infarction and more patients increase rather than decrease the frequency of sexual activity after surgery (Papadopoulos, 1989b).

The literature on sexual behavior after stroke reports decrements in sexual desire and sexual activity and increased erectile difficulties (Boldrini, Basaglia and Calanca, 1991; Angeleri et al., 1993). There is no agreement as to whether the site of the lesion, right or left hemisphere, has a differential impact on sexual function. The psychological factors that influence the sexual consequences of cerebrovascular lesions include depression, problems of self-esteem and body image, fear that sexual activity may precipitate death, and marital difficulties. In addition muscle weakness, sensory impairment, loss of sphincter control and speech limitations also contribute to sexual problems and dissatisfaction (Binder, 1984). Patients with stroke frequently suffer from associated medical conditions such as peripheral vascular disease, hypertension and previous myocardial infarction, all of which may independently affect sexual function.

Peripheral vascular disease caused by atherosclerosis is an important pathological determinant of erectile dysfunction in the aged. Atherosclerotic degeneration of the vascular supply to the penis decreases arterial inflow to the erectile tissues and impairs penile rigidity (see Chapter 3 for vasculogenic erectile mechanisms). Michal (1982) documented by angiography the presence of arterial stenosis or occlusion in 89% of men with erectile dysfunction aged 35 and over. Virag, Bouilly and Frydman (1985), in a study of 220 impotent men, related the presence of organic impotence to four arterial risk factors: hypertension, hyperlipidemia, tobacco, and diabetes. An elevated risk of myocardial infarction and stroke in impotent men was predicted by abnormal penile-brachial indices, suggesting the existence of generalized arterial disease (Morley et al., 1988). Furthermore, low penile-brachial indices predict abnormal ECG responses to exercise stress (Kaiser et al., 1989). These studies, mostly conducted on older patients, suggest that vascular pathology contributes significantly to age-related erectile disorders. It should be noted, however, that the coexistence of vascular lesions and sexual problems does not demonstrate pathogenesis. Few vascular studies of men with erectile disorders have included matched controls or have followed prospectively the sexual functioning of patients at risk of vascular disease.

Hypertension

Hypertension is highly prevalent among the aged and a major cause of morbidity and mortality associated with peripheral vascular disease, myocardial infarction, and stroke. While there is considerable information on the sexual consequences of antihypertension treatment, few data on sexual disorders in unmedicated patients are available. Bulpitt, Dollery and Carne (1976) found, in response to a questionnaire, that 17% of newly diagnosed untreated hypertensive men reported erectile problems compared to 6.9% of normotensive controls. In addition there was a 7.3% prevalence of 'ejaculatory incompetence' among the untreated hypertensives in comparison to none among the normal subjects. In another study (Bauer et al., 1978), 20% of untreated hypertensive men (n=75) reported erectile dysfunction, a figure that was double the prevalence in normotensive controls (n=126). However, these differences are not compelling, as the authors did not consider the effects of age and comorbidity. The results of the Massachusetts Male Aging Study (Feldman et al., 1994) demonstrate that hypertension, heart disease, and diabetes are significantly associated with erectile dysfunction after adjustment for age, but the results are confounded by medication effects. Karacan and collaborators (1989) measured penile blood flow during a nocturnal penile tumescence (NPT) study of three groups of middle-aged men: nonmedicated hypertensive patients with and without erectile dysfunction, and normotensive controls free of erectile difficulties. Hypertensive patients with erectile problems had reduced NPT and abnormal penile pulsatile blood flow, indicating hemodynamic impairment. Furthermore, penile blood flow during rapid eye movement (REM) sleep differed significantly among the three groups: normotensive controls had the highest amplitudes, patients without erectile problems had lower values and patients with erectile dysfunction had the lowest blood flow measures. The investigators concluded that penile blood flow measures may help to identify hypertensive men at risk of developing vasculogenic impotence. The pathogenesis of erectile dysfunction in older, nonmedicated, hypertensive patients probably involves hemodynamic factors associated with generalized arterial disease as they impinge on erectile mechanisms. Despite clinical impressions, there are no data on the role of psychological factors in the sexual dysfunction of hypertensive men in the absence of comorbid conditions.

Diabetes mellitus

Diabetes mellitus is among the most frequent systemic disorders associated with sexual dysfunction in the aged. Several surveys of diabetic men have reported a prevalence of erectile impotence ranging from 27 to 59%; there is a consistent relationship between age and erectile problems which parallels but is markedly higher than the prevalence of erectile disorders in the general population (Schiavi and Hogan, 1979; McCulloch et al., 1980). Increased comorbidity as age progresses contributes to the higher frequency of erectile difficulties in older diabetic individuals, but there are few controlled investigations that have considered the effects of age, current illnesses, and medication. We found that, compared to age-matched healthy controls, diabetic men, screened for nondiabetic pathology, show extensive behavioral decrements in sexual desire, arousal, activity, and satisfaction. In addition, diabetic patients reported decreased penile sensitivity and a range of ejaculatory and orgasmic difficulties (Schiavi et al., 1993). The validity of these differences was confirmed by independently assessing the sexual partners. Typically, there is a gradual impairment of erectile capacity with a loss of spontaneous and early morning erections, and an increasing inability to achieve masturbatory erections and intercourse (Case study 9.2). There are frequent exceptions to this characteristic clinical picture, however. Erectile difficulties may begin abruptly because of metabolic decompensation or psychological factors; conversely, some impotent diabetic patients may occasionally have full erections during sleep or exceptional sexual stimulation. There is little evidence that the type of diabetes (insulin-dependent versus noninsulin-dependent diabetes) is an important determinant of differences in sexual function when age is considered. The effect of blood sugar control on the development of sexual problems is uncertain. Jensen (1981) observed that sexual dysfunction is unrelated to diabetes regulation; in contrast, in a prospective study McCulloch et al. (1984) found that erectile impotence is associated with poor control of blood sugar. While we found no differences between insulin-dependent and noninsulin-dependent diabetic patients in prevalence of sexual problems, there were significant relationships between the lack of metabolic control, complications of diabetes, and impaired NPT (Schiavi et al., 1993). The duration of the disease and type of antidiabetic medication do not appear to be significantly related to the occurrence of sexual problems.

Neurological, vascular, and metabolic factors and their interactions have been implicated in the pathogenesis of diabetic erectile impotence. The association between diabetic neuropathy, reflected in peripheral sensory motor abnormalities and autonomic nervous dysfunction, and erectile problems has been repeatedly reported in the literature (Buvat et al., 1985b; Jensen, 1986). Bemelmans et al. (1994) conducted a neurophysiological study of somatic and autonomic sensory nerves in diabetic men with and without erectile disorders, compared with impotent nondiabetic patients. Impotent diabetic men suffered more from more severe peripheral and autonomic neuropathy, an effect related to age. Intracavernosal pharmacological testing of the same patients suggested that angiopathy was of secondary importance. There are no methods, however, that directly assess the competence of autonomic nervous function in the mediation of penile erections. Cardiovascular reflexes, evaluated as an indirect and nonspecific test of penile autonomic neuropathy, suggest that diabetic-related *and* age-related abnormalities are associated with erectile dysfunction (Nisen et al., 1993).

NPT recording has been frequently employed as a physiological test of neurovascular competence in men with erectile problems (Schiavi, 1988). Impotent diabetic men have significantly less NPT during REM sleep than psychogenically impotent and normal control individuals (see Chapter 13 for the diagnostic significance of NPT testing). The markedly impaired NPT activity in diabetic men with symptomatic neuropathy or retinopathy, noted in our age-matched controlled study (Schiavi et al., 1993), supports the notion that peripheral neurovascular pathology participates in the pathogenesis of diabetic erectile dysfunction. However, sexually nondysfunctional diabetic men also had significant NPT abnormalities. Diabetic men with no coital failure may have subclinically impaired erectile function which, although not enough to interfere with penetration, is reflected in NPT measures. Abnormalities in sleep architecture and REM sleep (Nofzinger et al., 1992; Schiavi et al., 1993) suggest, in addition, central nervous system involvement. There is growing evidence that central autonomic dysregulation may be associated with deficient metabolic control of glucose (Vinik and Mitchell, 1988; Cryer, 1992). The possibility that a central autonomic dysfunction, reflected by abnormal REM activity, may also contribute to the erectile problems of diabetic men deserves further investigation.

Atherosclerotic vascular degeneration also contributes to diabetic impotence in the aged. Diabetes is frequently associated with hypertension (The National High Blood Pressure Education Program Working Group, 1994), and both strongly predispose to atherosclerotic cardiovascular disease which can restrict vascular flow into the hypogastric–penile arterial tree (Newman and Marcus, 1985). Hyperglycemia increases endothelial production of collagen which may cause smooth muscle atrophy and lipid deposition within the corpora cavernosa. Diabetes may also enhance age-related decreases in the compliance of the fibroelastic trabecular structure within the smooth muscle of the corpora cavernosa, leading to unrestricted penile blood outflow and impaired erectile rigidity

(Carrier et al., 1993). Decreased neurogenic and endothelium-dependent relaxation of penile smooth muscle occurs in isolated smooth muscle from the corpora cavernosa of impotent diabetic patients (Saenz de Tejada et al., 1989). Neurotransmitter alterations are also suggested, by reduced noradrenaline and vasoactive intestinal polypeptide (VIP) levels in penile tissue from diabetic patients and by the decreased responsiveness of the cavernous smooth muscle to vasoactive agents such as acetylcholine (Lincoln et al., 1987). These data, mostly derived from in vitro research, indicate the possible mediating molecular mechanisms within the corpora, but their physiological significance to the pathogenesis of diabetic erectile dysfunction and its relationship with aging remain to be determined.

Little is known about the factors that influence the rate of development and the extent of neurovascular impairment, but in many diabetic patients the progression of change may span several years. During this time the increased vulnerability to sexual failure frequently leads to performance concerns, anxiety, and marital dissatisfaction. The clinical information in support of these observations is substantial but impressionistic, and there are few controlled studies of the psychology of sexual dysfunction in diabetes (Bancroft and Gutierrez, 1996). We psychologically assessed married, male diabetic patients, whose average age was 53, who were free from the confounding effects of other illnesses and medication, and compared them to an age-matched group of healthy individuals (Schiavi et al., 1995). In diabetic men, problems of sexual desire and arousal coexisted with alterations of psychological dimensions such as sexual attitudes and body image, but they did not significantly affect the overall quality of marital adjustment as perceived by the patients and their partners. In contrast to some reports (Lustman et al., 1986; Popkin et al., 1988), there was no evidence that psychological distress or psychiatric disorders, including depression, are associated with diabetes or with its effect on sexual function.

Parkinson's disease

The onset of Parkinson's disease (PD), a chronic progressive condition of the central nervous system, generally occurs during late middle age and is frequently associated with sexual difficulties. Erectile dysfunction has been reported to occur in 60–86%, and low sexual desire in 44% of PD patients, respectively (Brown et al., 1990; Koller et al., 1990). Ejaculatory disturbances, both premature ejaculation and the inability to ejaculate, have also been noted but the nature of their relationship with the neurological disorder is less certain.

The pathogenesis of sexual problems in PD is not fully understood. Possible mediating mechanisms include autonomic dysfunction, muscle rigidity, depression, and marital difficulties. Singer, Weiner and Sanchez-Ramos (1992) evaluated clinical evidence of autonomic dysfunction in 48 men with PD (mean age 66 years), in comparison with 32 healthy males without PD (mean age 70.4 years). Erectile problems were identified in 64.4% of patients, a prevalence that was significantly higher than the value of 37.5% in the control group, but there were no group differences in sexual drive or ejaculatory disturbances. Autonomic dysfunctions more prevalent in parkinsonian patients in this study were orthostatic dizziness, sensation of incomplete bladder emptiness, urgency and constipation. However, there was no direct evidence of a link between autonomic dysfunction and erectile insufficiency.

Lipe et al. (1990) compared the sexual function of 41 married men with PD with that of 29 married men with arthritis. The prevalence of sexual dysfunctions did not differ between parkinsonian and arthritic patients but it was significantly associated, in both groups, with increased age, severity of illness and depression. These findings suggest that the sexual difficulties of parkinsonian men may not be solely due to direct CNS effects, but may also reflect associated motor impairment and psychological influences. Depression is of common clinical occurrence in parkinsonian patients (Lees, 1990) and may contribute to decreased sexual drive and erectile difficulties. However, empirical evidence that a mood disorder is causally related to their sexual dysfunction is less than compelling. PD symptoms can seriously compromise marital adjustment and impair sexual satisfaction (Brown et al., 1990; Singer, Weiner and Ackerman, 1990). They may place increased demands on the healthy sexual partner, affect sexual attractiveness, impair verbal communication, and restrict sexual interactions. Brown et al. (1990) found that the impact of the disease on marital satisfaction was greater when it was the male rather than the female who suffered from PD. The cross-sectional design of these studies does not permit assessment of the causal link between marital discord and sexual dysfunction. In summary, clinical evidence implicates several interrelated factors but not a single one has emerged from systematic research as playing a central role in the pathogenesis of sexual problems in PD.

Sleep disorders

There is considerable evidence that aging is associated with a higher prevalence of sleep disturbance (Coleman et al., 1981). Sleep-disordered breathing abnormalities, mainly frequent apneic and hypoapneic episodes, are commonly observed in older individuals (Mosko, Dickel and Ashurst, 1988). Guilleminault et al. (1977) and Schmidt and Wise (1981) noted an association between sleep apnea and erectile impotence and speculated that abnormal CNS activity may cause the erectile problems of patients with sleep disorders. We (Schiavi et al., 1991) also found, in a sample of carefully selected healthy married volunteers, significant age-related increases in sleep-disordered breathing. However, there was no evidence that sleep disorders are involved in decreases in sexual function with aging or in the pathogenesis of erectile impotence in nondiseased individuals. Most of the patients evaluated for sleep disturbances by Guilleminault were obese, on medication, clinically depressed or hypertensive, all factors that may have contributed to their sexual difficulties. The possibility that sleep disorders are more closely associated with disturbances in sexual function in seniors unselected for health status deserves further study.

Endocrine disorders

The prevalence of endocrine disorders in men with erectile dysfunction ranges up to 35%, depending on selection bias, the characteristics of clinical groups and diagnostic criteria (Sparks, White and Connolly, 1980; Slag et al., 1983; Davis et al., 1985). An increased prevalence has been noted in those attending specialized endocrine clinics and in older patient groups. The most common hormonal problem in aged men is hypogonadism. The primary pathology may be testicular, inducing a compensatory increase in pituitary luteinizing hormone (LH) secretion (primary hypogonadism); alternatively, it may be a hypothalamic pituitary defect, resulting in decreased LH secretion (secondary hypogonadism). The end result is a decrease in bioavailable testosterone (bT), with the consequent decline in sexual drive, secondary erectile difficulties and impaired ejaculatory capacity.

We have previously reviewed data (see Chapter 3) showing that aging is associated with alterations in hypogonadal–pituitary–gonadal mechanisms, but there is no evidence that, in healthy aging subjects, lower circulating testosterone, total or bioavailable, contributes to erectile dysfunction (Schiavi, 1996). In clinical samples of older men, diagnostic conclusions on the relationship between hypogonadal conditions and erectile problems are limited by uncertain criteria for distinguishing normal from pathological declines in circulating testosterone and by a lack of control groups. Korenman and collaborators (1990) studied 267 impotent men, aged 50 years and older, referred consecutively to a sexual dysfunction clinic, a comparison group of healthy potent subjects over the age of 50, and younger normal controls. They measured testosterone, bT, LH, and prolactin levels in all groups. Both older groups had markedly diminished mean testosterone and bT levels compared to the younger controls. Forty-eight per cent of the nondysfunctional older men and 39% of the impotent patients were hypogonadal as defined by a mean bT of 2.5 standard deviations below the mean levels of the young group. Ninety per cent of the hypogonadal subjects did not have a compensatory LH increase and many of them had an impaired response to gonadotrophin releasing hormone (GnRH) stimulation, suggesting hypothalamic–pituitary dysfunction.

There were no significant differences in circulating bT between the older potent and impotent hypogonadal men, supporting the notion that secondary hypogonadism and impotence are two common, overlapping but independent conditions. The observation that the older control group met endocrine criteria for hypogonadism but had normal sexual function suggests that the central hormonal threshold for sexual activation is relatively low.

Overall, it appears that the prevalence of hypogonadal conditions in unselected clinical samples of sexually dysfunctional men increases with age, and that the decrease in bT has to be substantial to be reflected in sexual function abnormalities. Most clinical studies have centered on erectile impotence to the neglect of sexual desire, thought to be a more sensitive indicator of the central effects of testosterone's action. It should also be noted that abnormal decreases in circulating androgens may impact on sexual function and behavior indirectly, through effects on general physical well-being and mood. The use of androgen treatment for the restoration of sexual function in older men will be discussed in Chapter 14.

Hyperprolactinemic conditions and thyroid disease are relatively infrequent endocrinopathies associated with sexual dysfunction in older men. Hyperprolactinemia caused by hypothalamic–pituitary tumors, medication, or chronic renal failure may impair sexual drive and erectile capacity (Buvat et al., 1985a; Leonard, Nickel and Morales, 1989). These patients usually, but not always, secrete less gonadotrophin and testosterone. Testosterone administration to those with hyperprolactinemia does not normalize sexual function. It has been suggested that a decrease in central dopaminergic activity is involved in the sexual effects of elevated prolactin levels (Drago, 1984). Administration of bromocryptine, a dopaminergic agonist, decreases prolactin levels and may restore sexual drive and erectile function before the normalization of testosterone levels.

Hypothyroidism is relatively common but difficult to diagnose in the elderly (Finucane and Anderson, 1995). It may be associated with decreased testosterone secretion and elevated serum prolactin levels (Zonszein, 1995). Low sexual drive and erectile dysfunction are not successfully treated with testosterone alone and require the thyroid disorder to be corrected. Hyperthyroidism, on the other hand, causes the estradiol production rate, and plasma testosterone and estradiol levels to rise, because of elevated sex-hormone-binding globulin levels. However, the bT is low and gonadotropin secretion may be partially suppressed. The significance of abnormal pituitary–gonadal function in the pathogenesis of sexual dysfunction in patients with thyroid disease remains to be determined.

Chronic renal and hepatic failure can impair sexual desire and sexual arousal in many ways, including the nonspecific consequences of a chronic, debilitating disease, as well as specific endocrine mechanisms. A progressive decline in renal function is a frequent but not inevitable consequence of growing old. In chronic renal insufficiency serum testosterone is usually decreased and prolactin is commonly elevated. Administration of bromocryptine to men on hemodialysis decreases prolactin levels and restores sexual interest (Bommer et al., 1979). Vascular insufficiency and uremic neuropathy may also contribute to impaired sexual arousal in chronic renal failure. Psychological factors, such as the patient's helplessness, dependency, and despair, the partner's response to the demands of the dialysis procedure and the provision of chronic care, are important in influencing the sexual outcome of the disease (Berkman, Katz and Weissman, 1982).

Low sexual desire and erectile difficulties are commonly observed in patients with hepatic insufficiency. Cornely et al. (1984) reported a 70% prevalence of erectile dysfunction in men with alcoholic liver disease, compared to 25% in patients with nonalcoholic liver cirrhosis. We assessed the sexual function of 75 men with nonalcoholic liver disease categorized on the basis of illness severity according to standard diagnostic criteria (Zifroni, Schiavi and Schaffer, 1991). There was a significant relationship between the severity of the hepatic disorder, the reduction of total and free testosterone levels, and sexual dysfunction. Diminished sexual desire and erectile difficulties were reported by 33% and 67% of patients, respectively, with most severe liver disease. Despite the lessening of sexual function with the progression of liver failure, most men reported enjoying satisfying sexual relations with their partners.

Chronic obstructive pulmonary disease (COPD)

Chronic obstructive pulmonary disease, which includes chronic bronchitis and emphysema, is characterized by a slow and insidious development of chronic cough, expectoration, shortness of breath and fatigue. The disease process usually spans many years and is a major cause of disability that increases with age. Dyspnea, caused by airway obstruction and shortness of breath after minimal exertion, can severely compromise sexual function and satisfaction. Prevalence studies of sexual dysfunction in patients with lung disease are few, mainly anecdotal, and frequently confounded by the association with cardiovascular disease, hypertension, and medications. Fletcher and Martin (1982) found a 30% rate of erectile impotence and a frequent lack of sexual desire in a small sample of men with COPD, aged 46–69, selected to exclude comorbid conditions that could affect sexual function. The pathogenesis of sexual problems in COPD patients is, like most other chronic conditions, multidimensional and includes fear and anxiety associated with physical exertion and depression. The degree of erectile impairment in COPD patients correlates with the severity of hypoxemia and the dysfunction is reversed in some patients with oxygen therapy (Fletcher and Martin, 1982; Aasebo et al., 1993). The degree of testosterone reduction appears to be related to the severity of hypoxemia.

Restoration of sexual function following long-term oxygen therapy is associated with significant increases in testosterone and with a decline in sex-hormone-binding globulin compared to nonresponders (Semple et al, 1980; Aasebo et al., 1993).

Arthritis

Arthritis is a major source of discomfort and disability in the aged. Among the numerous arthritic conditions, osteoarthritis and rheumatoid arthritis are the most common in the older adult. The occurrence, in arthritic patients, of sexual difficulties caused by pain, fatigue and restriction of movement has been assumed but seldom systematically explored. Uncontrolled studies of arthritic patients note impaired sexual interest, function, and satisfaction (Ferguson and Figley, 1979). Blake and collaborators (1988) assessed, by interview, the sexual function of 169 arthritic patients compared to 130 paired-matched controls recruited from the community; 37% of the sample were males whose mean age was 58 years. The prevalence of sexual dysfunction was notably high in both groups but only erectile impotence was reported significantly more frequently by the arthritic men than the comparison group (62% of patients versus 40% of controls). Older age, comorbidity, especially hypertension, and medications, mainly methotrexate, were significantly associated with the increased erectile difficulties of arthritic men. Depressed mood, measured by a self-report instrument, was more frequent among patients than controls; it was related to fatigue, decreased sexual drive and feelings of physical unattractiveness, but was not associated with impotence. Marital unhappiness, assessed by a validated scale, was not associated with arthritis but was related to reported sexual dysfunction and sexual dissatisfaction. In another report, based on the same study (Blake et al., 1987), patients differed from controls in their greater loss of sexual satisfaction over time. As expected, joint symptoms and fatigue impaired the sexual adjustment of patients significantly more than their matched peers. Similar results were noted by Kraimaat et al. (1996), who found that physical disability, pain and depression contributed to the impaired sexual adjustment of married patients with rheumatoid arthritis.

Surgical comorbidity

Prostate disease, mainly benign hyperplasia and malignancy, occurs commonly in aging men. It is frequently diagnosed as caused by urethral narrowing or obstruction, with consequent urinary frequency, dribbling, nocturia, and retention with overflow. Prostate carcinoma, infrequent before the age of 50, is the second most common malignancy present in possibly 90% of men in their eighth decade. Sexual dysfunction is a well-known complication of prostatic surgery. However, prevalence data vary considerably and are limited by insufficient information about sexual functioning prior to surgery, reliance on subjective reports, and failure to consider the confounding effects of age, cardiovascular disease, diabetes, and medication.

Transurethral prostatectomy (TURP), the most common procedure for patients with benign prostatic hyperplasia, has been reported to result in rates of erectile impotence of 5–40% (Padma-Nathan, 1995). Retrograde ejaculation, caused by damage to the internal bladder sphincter, may occur in up to 80% of patients after TURP. Hanbury and Sethia (1995) interviewed 268 patients about their sexual function prior to and three months after TURP. Preoperatively, 56% of patients were fully potent, 17% could only achieve partial erections and 27% were impotent. Seventeen per cent of men without prior erectile problems began having erectile difficulties after surgery, and 37% who were partially potent before the operation became impotent postoperatively. In addition to the increased risk of erectile impotence in men whose sexual function is already compromised prior to TURP, the authors found that it is significantly elevated if the prostatic capsule is damaged during the operation. The cause of erectile problems after TURP remains uncertain. Research using objective measures of erectile capacity, such as NPT recordings, have provided conflicting information (So et al., 1982; Tscholl et al., 1995). There is increasing evidence that damage to the adjacent neurovascular bundles that surround the prostate caused by electrocautery at surgery may be a significant factor for some patients (Padma-Nathan, 1995). Contributing to erectile difficulties after surgery are pre-existing, age-related, risk factors, apprehension and the emotional reaction of uninformed patients to the lack of ejaculation at orgasm.

Radical prostatectomy is commonly performed in patients with prostatic cancer. Fowler et al. (1993), in a national survey of more than 1000 Medicare patients in the USA, reported that 89% men were impotent after radical prostatectomy. Murphy et al. (1994), in a survey of 2122 patients from 484 institutions, found that impotence following radical prostatectomy occurred in 56.6% of men who were potent preoperatively. Since neither study provided information on specific surgical techniques, it is not possible to relate the type of intervention to the sexual outcome. In recent years, improved understanding of the anatomy of the prostatic nerve plexus that mediates erections has made it possible to develop nerve-sparing radical approaches with significant improvement of postoperative erectile function. Overall, Walsh, Partin and Epstein (1994) report that 68% of 503 patients who were potent preoperatively remained potent 18 months after nerve-sparing radical prostatectomy. Younger age, less invasive pathology and preservation of the adjacent neurovascular bundles correlated with the return of erectile capacity. Sexual function was maintained in almost all men younger than 50, in 75% of men 50–60 years old, in 58% of men 60–70 years old and in 25% of patients older than 70. The vulnerability to erectile failure was particularly evident in older men when the extent of the lesion necessitated unilateral excision of a neurovascular bundle. Geary et al. (1995) also found that aging effects and the number of neurovascular bundles spared were the most important factors related to the degree of maintenance of erectile function. However, they raised a note of caution against over-optimistic expectations about the sexual outcomes of nerve-sparing radical prostatectomy. The overall potency rate following bilateral nerve-sparing prostatectomy in their series was not higher than 32%. Fewer than half of the patients who retained potency were satisfied with their erections or continued to engage in intercourse for at least once a month. It is of note that, in a study of treatment management for patients with localized prostatic cancer, some men were willing to choose a treatment they were less likely to survive in order to maintain sexual potency. This choice was not influenced by age, sexual interest, intercourse frequency or even erectile capacity (Singer et al., 1991).

Radiation therapy is reserved for patients with poor prognosis because the cancer has extended beyond the prostatic capsule. These patients tend to be older, with higher rates of erectile failure and suffer frequently from other chronic medical disorders. The incidence of sexual problems occurring for the first time after radiotherapy has been estimated at approximately 25%, with more severe erectile difficulties noted in patients with borderline function prior to treatment. Administration of moderate radiation doses, as an adjuvant treatment, after nerve-sparing prostatectomy had no significant effect on recovery of potency, based on subjective reporting one year after surgery (Formenti et al., 1996). Damage to vascular erectile mechanisms and impaired gonadal function have been considered as pathogenically responsible for postradiation sexual problems, but the data remain inconclusive (Schover, 1993). Preliminary results suggest that cryosurgical ablation of the prostate and interstitial radiotherapy also have significant adverse effects on sexual function (Chaikin et al., 1996). There is a need for prospective studies that consider contributing factors such as survival concerns, disturbances in body image, anger, depression, and loss of a sense of personal control over bodily functions in the assessment of the sexual consequences of genitourinary pathology and surgery (Ofman, 1995).

Rectal cancer is diagnosed in more than 45000 persons annually in the USA (Harnsberger, Vernava and Longo, 1994). Abdominoperineal resection, the standard treatment for rectal adenocarcinoma, has been reported to induce erectile and ejaculatory problems in 69% of patients (Petrelli et al., 1993). The high prevalence of sexual disorders is caused by damage to hypogastric nerves and the pelvic autonomic plexus that runs near the rectum and pelvic wall. Technical improvements, including nerve-sparing surgery, particularly when carried out on patients younger than 50 years, have significantly improved sexual function morbidity after abdominoperineal resections (Masui et al., 1996). Abdominal stomas for the collection of urine and feces, required for some patients following surgery, can markedly affect sexual function and satisfaction. Loss of self-esteem, problems with body integrity and autonomy, fear of loss of fecal control, and concerns about the partner's reaction are determining factors in the effect of this surgery on sexuality.

Conclusion

Comments on the sexual life of the chronically ill has been relegated for many years to tangential statements or brief footnotes. During the last three decades remarkable changes have occurred, as evidenced by the extensive, and yet highly selective, literature reviewed in this chapter. Interpretation of this wealth of information, mostly derived from clinical observations, is limited by several generic, mainly methodological, issues. Age emerges as an important and frequently neglected factor that influences the nature and extent of sexual responses to chronic illness. The high prevalence of comorbid disorders and medication intake in the aged makes it difficult to ascertain the specific effect of a particular illness or medical intervention on sexual behavior. The scarcity of longitudinal studies necessitates reliance on retrospective reporting about premorbid sexual function, an approach that raises questions about the validity of the results. Few investigations have considered the sexual partner when gathering relevant information or have included age-matched control groups. The encompassing focus of most studies has been on erectile function, while other sexual dimensions and the interactive effects of psychological and interpersonal factors on sexual satisfaction have been neglected. Despite the above reservations, the data underline the importance of sexuality for the well-being and quality of life of the aged, including those who face chronic, invalidating, conditions. It reflects as well as reinforces the relevance of considering sexual function and satisfaction as part of the evaluation and management of older men with chronic medical disorders.

Case studies

Case study 9.1

Mr. and Ms. K, aged 63 and 60 respectively, had been married for over 30 years. They had a stable, mutually caring relationship and felt in an economically secure position, enjoying their work as high school teachers. The couple, who described themselves as sexually conservative, had routinely engaged in rather predictable, problem-free, intercourse usually on Fridays. During the past four to five years he had noticed increasing erectile difficulties, culminating in almost absent erections during the preceding year. Mr. and Ms. K continued to relate sensually with each other on a weekly basis with mutual caressing and genital stimulation, in response to which he could experience orgasm with a flaccid penis. Ms. K did not feel comfortable and refused his wish to begin experimenting with oral–genital stimulation. He initially denied being anxious about his inability to achieve an erection or being too concerned by issues of performance; this denial was challenged by his wife who noticed that he appeared apprehensive on the few occasions he attempted penetration and was irritable and despondent when he was unable to do so. There was no clinical evidence of depression during the evaluation. Past medical history revealed myocardial infarction ten years previously and a second coronary episode one year ago. Of interest was the presence of right lower extremity claudication for over two years, with oscillometric examination confirming virtually absent pulses in the right lower extremity; fundoscopic examination revealed marked arteriosclerotic retinal degeneration. The remainder of the physical examination was unremarkable with no anomalies of the genitalia, prostate or deep sacral reflexes. Assessment of NPT during two nights in the sleep laboratory showed markedly diminished nocturnal erections in duration, frequency, and degree. Intracavernosal papaverine testing only induced partial erections, consistent with a vasculogenic erectile disorder. Mr. K was being medicated with digoxin, quinidine, a diuretic and, occasionally, diazepam.

Comments

The clinical and laboratory results provided strong evidence that Mr. K's erectile disorder had an organic basis in generalized atherosclerotic disease. Mr. K eventually acknowledged his fear that physical exertion during sexual activity would trigger another cardiac episode. The couple decided to continue engaging in noncoital sexual experiences, as they had evolved on their own during the past five years and refused therapeutic sexual intervention.

Case study 9.2

Mr. L, a 63-year-old divorced man, was referred by his diabetologist for a sleep (NPT) evaluation of erectile capacity prior to considering penile prosthetic implantation. He had a five-year history of progressive erectile difficulties. His sexual desire was not impaired but the erectile problems were global and pervasive; he rated his erections during attempts at masturbation and upon early morning awakenings as 5 at best, on a 1–10 scale (10 maximum erections). Occasionally, he was able to achieve vaginal insertion with a woman friend but found himself, for the first time in his life, ejaculating prematurely. Mr. L felt that his sexual difficulties were responsible for the break of a long-term relation with a woman he had hoped to marry and was apprehensive that the same might occur with his new sexual partner. He denied ever having experienced coital failures prior to his current problems.

Mr. L had been diagnosed as suffering from late-onset diabetes about six years before. He was taking an oral hypoglycemic agent but metabolic control was inconsistent. There was no evidence of diabetic complications other than his erectile insufficiency. He had had a mild ischemic heart episode requiring hospitalization two years before, from which he had recovered fully and did not need cardiovascular medication. The results of recording two night's sleep were highly abnormal in that only minimal tumescence was noted during the first night and no erectile episodes occurred during the second one despite significant REM activity.

Comments

The NPT assessment was consistent with the clinical impression that Mr. L suffered from an organic erectile disorder caused by diabetes mellitus. The development of premature ejaculation in late life is not infrequent in men who anxiously engage in penile stimulation attempting to achieve vaginal insertion. Mr. L was advised to involve his partner in the decision to have a penile prosthetic implant, particularly since the couple had decided to move In together. The partner was 'turned off' by the notion of a penile implant since, for her, the quality of their relationship and sex play was more important than vaginal insertion. The couple engaged successfully in sexual counseling to enhance the sexual/erotic aspects of their interactions, de-emphasizing coital expectations.

References

Aasebo, V., Gylmes, A., Bremnes, R. M., Aakvaag, A. and Slordol, T. (1993). Reversal of sexual impotence in male patients with chronic obstructive pulmonary disease and hypoxemia with long term oxygen therapy. *Journal of Steroid Biochemistry and Molecular Biology* 46, 799–803.

Angeleri, F., Angeleri, V. A., Foschi, N., Giaquinto, S. and Nolfe, G. (1993). The influence of depression, social activity and family stress on functional outcome after stroke. *Stroke* 24, 1478–83.

Bancroft, J. and Gutierrez, P. (1996). Erectile dysfunction in men with and without diabetes mellitus: a comparative study. *Diabetes Medicine* 13, 84–9.

Bauer, G. E., Hunyor, S. N., Baker, J. and Marshall, P. (1978). Side effects of antihypertensive treatment: a placebo-controlled study. *Clinical Science and Molecular Medicine* [Suppl. 4] 55, 341s.

Bemelmans, B. L. H., Meuleman, E. J. H., Doesburg, W. H., Notermans, S. L. H. and Debruyne, F. M. J. (1994). Erectile dysfunction in diabetic men: the neurological factor revisited. *Journal of Urology* 151, 884–9.

Berkman, A. H., Katz, L. A. and Weissman, R. (1982). Sexuality and the life style of home dialysis patients. *Archives of Physical Medicine and Rehabilitation* 63, 272–5.

Binder, L. M. (1984). Emotional problems after stroke. *Stroke* 15, 174–7.

Blake, D. J., Maisiak, R., Alarcon, G. S., Holley, H. L. and Brown, S. (1987). Sexual quality-of-life of patients with arthritis compared to arthritis-free controls. *Journal of Rheumatology* 14, 570–6.

Blake, D. J., Maisiak, R., Kaplan, A., Alarcon, G. S. and Brown, S. (1988). Sexual dysfunction among patients with arthritis. *Clinical Rheumatology* 7, 50–60.

Boldrini, P., Basaglia, N. and Calanca, M. C. (1991). Sexual changes in hemiparetic patients. *Archives of Physical Medicine and Rehabilitation* 72, 202–7.

Bommer, J., Ritz, E., del Pezo, E. and Bommer, G. (1979). Improved sexual function in male hemodialysis patients on bromocriptine. *Lancet* 2, 496–7.

Brown, R. G., Jahanshahi, M., Quinn, N. and Marsden, D. (1990). Sexual function in patients with Parkinson's disease and their partners. *Journal of Neurology, Neurosurgery and Psychiatry* 53, 480–6.

Bulpitt, C. J., Dollery, C. T. and Carne, S. (1976). Change in symptoms of hypertensive patients after referral to hospital clinic. *British Heart Journal* 38, 121–8.

Buvat, J., Lemaire, A., Buvat-Herbaut, M., Fourlinnie, J. C., Racadot, A. and Fossati, P. (1985a). Hyperprolactinemia and sexual function in men. *Hormone Research* 22, 196–203.

Buvat, J., Lemaire, A., Buvat-Herbaut, M., Guieu, J. D., Bailleul, J. P. and Fossati, P. (1985b). Comparative investigations in 26 impotent and 26 nonimpotent diabetic patients. *Journal of Urology* 133, 34–8.

Carrier, S., Brock, G., Kour, N. W. and Lue, T. F. (1993). Pathophysiology of erectile function. *Urology* 42, 468–81.

Chaikin, D. C., Broderick, G. A., Malloy, T. R., Malkowicz, S. B., Whittington, R. and Wein, A. J. (1996). Erectile dysfunction following minimally invasive treatments for prostatic cancer. *Urology* 48, 100–4.

Coleman, R. M., Miles, L. E., Guilleminault, C. C., Zarcone, V. P., van der Hoed, J. and Dement, W. C. (1981). Sleep-wake disorders in the elderly: a polysomnographic analysis. *Journal of the American Geriatrics Society* 29, 289–96.

Cornely, C. M., Schade, R. R., Van Thiel, D. H., Gavaler, J. S. (1984). Chronic advanced liver disease and impotence: cause or effect. *Hepatology* 4, 1227–30.

Cryer, P. E. (1992). Iatrogenic hypoglycemia as a cause of hypoglycemia in associated autonomic failure in IDDM. A vicious cycle. *Diabetes* 41, 255–60.

Davis, S. S., Viosca, S. P., Guralnik, M., Windsor, C., Bottiglieri, M. W., Baker, D. J., Mehta, A. J. and Korenman, S. G. (1985). Evaluation of impotence in older men. *Western Journal of Medicine* 12, 499–505.

Dhabuwala, C. B., Kumar, A. and Pierce, J. M. (1986). Myocardial infarction and its influence on male sexual function. *Archives of Sexual Behavior* 15, 499–504.

Drago, E. (1984). Prolactin and sexual behavior: a review. *Neuroscience and Behavioral Review* 8, 433–9.

Drory, Y., Shapira, I., Fisman, E. Z. and Pines, A. (1995). Myocardial ischemia during sexual activity in patients with coronary artery disease. *American Journal of Cardiology* 75, 835–7.

Feldman, H. A., Goldstein, I., Hatzichristou, D. G., Krane, R. J. and McKinlay, J. B. (1994). Impotence and its medical and psychological correlates: results of the Massachusetts Male Aging Study. *Journal of Urology* 151, 54–61.

Ferguson, K. and Figley, B. (1979). Sexuality and rheumatic disease: a prospective study. *Sex and Disability* 2, 130–8.

Finucane, P. and Anderson, C. (1995). Thyroid disease in older patients. *Drug Therapy* 6, 268–77.

Fletcher, E. C. and Martin, R. J. (1982). Sexual dysfunction and erectile impotence in chronic obstructive pulmonary disease. *Chest* 81, 413–21.

Formenti, S. C., Lieskowsky, G., Simoneau, A. R., Skinner, D., Groshen, S., Chen, S.-C. and Petrovich, Z. (1996). Impact of moderate dose of postoperative radiation on urinary continence and potency in patients with prostate cancer treated with nerve sparing prostatectomy. *Journal of Urology* 155, 616–19.

Fowler, F. J., Barry, M. J., Lu Yao, G., Roman, A., Wasson, J. and Wennberg, J. E. (1993). Patient reported complications and follow-up treatment after radical prostatectomy. *Urology* 42, 622–9.

Geary, E. S., Dendinger, T. E., Freiha, F. S. and Stamey, T. A. (1995). Nerve sparing radical prostatectomy: a different view. *Journal of Urology* 154, 145–9.

Greenstein, A., Chen, J., Miller, H., Matzkin, H., Villa, Y. and Braf, Z. (1997). Does severity of ischemic coronary disease correlate with erectile function? *International Journal of Impotence research* 9, 123–6.

Guilleminault, C., Eldridge, F. L., Simmons, F. B. and Dement, W. C. (1977). Sleep apnea syndrome due to upper airway obstruction. A review of 25 cases. *Archives of Internal Medicine* 137, 296–300.

Hanbury, D. C. and Sethia, K. K. (1995). Erectile dysfunction following transurethral prostatectomy. *British Journal of Urology* 75, 13.

Harnsberger, J. R., Vernava, A. M. III and Longo, W. E. (1994). Radical abdominopelvic lymphadenectomy: historic perspective and current role in the surgical management of rectal cancer. *Diseases of the Colon and Rectum* 37, 73–87.

Hellerstein, H. K. and Friedman, E. H. (1970). Sexual activity and the postcoronary patient. *Archives of Internal Medicine* 125, 987–99.

Jensen, S. B. (1981). Diabetic sexual dysfunction; a comparative study of 160 insulin treated diabetic men and women and an age-matched control group. *Archives of Sexual Behavior* 10, 493–504.

Jensen, S. B. (1986). Sexual dysfunction and diabetes mellitus: a six-year follow up study. *Archives of Sexual Behavior* 15, 271–84.

Kaiser, F. E., Udhoji, V., Viosca, S., Morley, J. E. and Korenman, S. G. (1989). Cardiovascular stress tests in patients with vascular impotence. *Clinical Research* 37, 89A.

Karacan, I., Salis, P. J., Hirshkowitz, M., Borreson, R. E., Narter, E. and Williams, R. L. (1989). Erectile dysfunction in hypotensive men: sleep erections, penile blood flow and musculovascular events. *Journal of Urology* 142, 56–61.

Koller, W. C., Vetere-Overfield, B., Willamson, A., Busenbark, K. Nash, J. and Parish, D. (1990). Sexual dysfunction in Parkinson's disease. *Clinical Neuropharmacology* 13, 461–3.

Korenman, S. G., Morley, J. E., Mooradian, A. D., Davis, S. S., Kaiser, F. E., Silver, A. J., Viosca, S. P. and Garza, D. (1990). Secondary hypogonadism in older men: its relation to impotence. *Journal of Clinical Endocrinology and Metabolism* 71, 963–9.

Kraimaat, F. W., Bakker, A. H., Janssen, E. and Bijlsma, J. W. (1996). Intrusiveness of rheumatoid arthritis on sexuality in male and female patients living with a spouse. *Arthritis Care Research* 9, 120–5.

Larson, J. L., McNaughton, M. W., Kennedy, J. W. and Mansfield, L. W. (1980). Heart rate and blood pressure responses to sexual activity and stair-climbing test. *Heart Lung* 9, 1025–30.

Lees, A. D. (1990). The behavioral neurology of Parkinson's disease. In *Parkinson's Disease*, ed. G. M. Stern, pp. 389–413. Baltimore, MD: Johns Hopkins.

Leonard, M. P., Nickel, C. J. and Morales, A. (1989). Hyperprolactinemia and impotence: why, when and how to investigate. *Journal of Urology* 142, 992–4.

Lincoln, J., Crowe, R., Blacklay, P. F., Pryor, J. P., Lumley, J. S. P. and Burnstock, G. (1987).

Changes in VIPergic, cholinergic and adrenergic innervation of human penile tissue in diabetic and nondiabetic impotent males. *Journal of Urology* 137, 1053–9.

Lipe, H., Longstreth, W. T. Jr., Bird, T. D. and Linde, M. (1990). Sexual function in married men with Parkinson's disease compared to married men with arthritis. *Neurology* 40, 1347–9.

Lustman, P. J., Griffith, L. S., Clouse, R. E. and Cryer, P. E. (1986). Psychiatric illness in diabetic mellitus. Relationship to symptoms and glucose control. *Journal of Nervous and Mental Disease* 174, 736–42.

Masui, H., Ike, H., Yamasuchi, S., Oki, S. and Shimada, H. (1996). Male sexual function after autonomic nerve-preserving operation for rectal cancer. *Diseases of the Colon and Rectum* 39, 1140–5.

McCulloch, D. K., Campbell, I. W., Wu, F. C., Prescott, R. J. and Clarke, B. F. (1980). The prevalence of diabetic impotence. *Diabetologia* 18, 279–83.

McCulloch, D. K., Young, R. J., Prescott, R. J., Campbell, I. W. and Clarke, B. F. (1984). The natural history of impotence in diabetic men. *Diabetologia* 26, 437–40.

Mehta, J. and Krop, H. (1979). The effect of myocardial infarction on sexual functioning. *Sexuality and Disability* 2, 115–21.

Michal, V. (1982). Arterial disease as a cause of impotence. *Clinics of Endocrinology and Metabolism* 11, 725–48.

Morley, J. E., Korenman, S. G., Kaiser, F. E., Mooradian, A. D. and Viosca, S. P. (1988). Relationship of penile brachial pressure index to myocardial infarction and cerebrovascular accidents in older males. *American Journal of Medicine* 84, 445–8.

Mosko, S. S., Dickel, M. J. and Ashurst, J. (1988). Sleep apnea and sleep-related periodic leg movements in the elderly. *Sleep* 11, 340–8.

Muller, J. E., Mittleman, M. A., Maclure, M., Sherwood, J. B., Tofler, G. H. for the determinants of Myocardial Infarction Onset Study investigators. (1996). Triggering myocardial infarction by sexual activity. *Journal of the American Medical Association* 275, 1405–9.

Mulligan, T. (1989). Why aged men become impotent. *Archives of Internal Medicine* 149, 1365–6.

Murphy, G. P., Mettlin, C., Menck, H., Winchester, D. P. and Davidson, A. M. (1994). National patterns of prostate cancer treatment by radical prostatectomy: results of a survey by the American College of Surgeons commission on cancer. *Journal of Urology* 152, 1817–19.

Newman, H. F. and Marcus, H. (1985). Erectile dysfunction in diabetes and hypertension. *Urology* 26, 135–7.

Nisen, H. O., Larsen, A., Lindstrom, B. L., Ruutu, M. L., Virtanen, J. M. and Alfthan, O. J. (1993). Cardiovascular reflexes in the neurological evaluation of impotence. *British Journal of Urology* 71, 199–203.

Nofzinger, E. A., Reynolds, C. F. III, Jennings, J. R., Thase, M. E., Frank, E., Yeager, A. and Kupfer, D. J. (1992). Results of nocturnal penile tumescence studies are abnormal in sexually functional diabetic men. *Archives of Internal Medicine* 152, 114–18.

Ofman, U. S. (1995). Preservation of function in genitourinary cancers: psychosexual and psychosocial issues. *Cancer Investigation* 13, 125–31.

Padma-Nathan, H. (1995). Editorial: erectile dysfunction. *Journal of Urology* 153, 1494–5.

Papadopoulos, C. (1978). A survey of sexual activity after myocardial infarction. *Cardiovascular Medicine* 3, 821–6.

Papadopoulos, C. (1989a). Coronary artery disease and sexuality. *In Sexual Aspects of Cardiovascular Disease*, Chapter 1, pp. 1–22. New York: Praeger.

Papadopoulos, C. (1989b). Quality of life and sexual activity after cardiac surgery. In *Sexual Aspects of Cardiovascular Disease*, Chapter 3, pp. 31–44, New York: Praeger.

Petrelli, N. J., Nagel, S., Rodrigues-Bigas, M., Piedmonte, M. and Herrera, L. (1993). Morbidity and mortality following abdominal perineal resection for rectal adenocarcinoma. *The American Surgeon* 59, 400–4.

Popkin, M. R., Callies, A. L., Lewtz, R. D., Colon, E. A. and Sutherland, P. E. (1988). Prevalence of major depression, simple phobia and other psychiatric disorders in patients with long standing type I diabetes mellitus. *Archives of General Psychiatry* 45, 64–8.

Rosal, M. C., Downing, J., Littman, A. B. and Attern, D. K. (1994). Sexual functioning post-myocardial infarction: effects of beta-blockers, psychological status and safety information. *Journal of Psychosomatic Research* 38, 655–67.

Saenz de Tejada, I., Goldstein, I., Azadzoi, K., Krane, R. J. and Cohen, R. A. (1989). Impaired neurogenic and endothelium-mediated relaxation of penile smooth muscle from diabetic men with impotence. *New England Journal of Medicine* 320, 1025–30.

Schiavi, R. C. (1988). Nocturnal penile tumescence in the evaluation of erectile disorders: a critical review. *Journal of Sex and Marital Therapy* 14, 83–96.

Schiavi, R. C. (1996). Androgens and sexual function in men. In *Androgens and the Aging Male*, ed. B. Oddens and A. Vermeulen, pp. 111–25. New York: The Parthenon Publishing Group.

Schiavi, R. C. and Hogan, B. (1979). Sexual problems in diabetes mellitus: psychological aspects. *Diabetes Care* 2, 9–17.

Schiavi, R. C., Mandeli, J., Schreiner-Engel, P. and Chamers, A. (1991). Aging, sleep disorders and male sexual function. *Biological Psychiatry* 30, 15–24.

Schiavi, R. C., Stimmel, B. B., Mandeli, J. and Rayfield, E. J. (1993). Diabetes mellitus and male sexual function: a control study. *Diabetologia* 36, 745–51.

Schiavi, R. C., Stimmel, B. B., Mandeli, J., Schreiner-Engel, P. and Ghizzani, A. (1995). Diabetes, psychological function and male sexuality. *Journal of Psychosomatic Research* 39, 305–14.

Schmidt, H. S. and Wise, H. A. (1981). Significance of impaired penile tumescence and associated polysomnographic abnormalities in the impotent patient. *Journal of Urology* 126, 348–51.

Schover, L. R. (1993). Sexual rehabilitation after treatment for prostate cancer. *Cancer [Supplement]* 71, 1024–30.

Semple, P. D., Beastall, G. H., Watson, W. S. and Hume, R. (1980). Serum testosterone depression associated with hypoxia in respiratory failure. *Clinical Science* 58, 105–6.

Singer, C., Weiner, W. J. and Ackerman, M. (1990). Sexual dysfunction in early Parkinson's disease. *Neurology* 40, [Suppl. 1] 221.

Singer, C., Weiner, W. J. and Sanchez-Ramos, J. R. (1992). Autonomic dysfunction in men with Parkinson's disease. *European Neurology* 32, 134–40.

Singer, P. A., Tasch, E. S., Stocking, C., Rubin, S., Siegler, M. and Weichselbaum, R. (1991). Sex or survival? Trade offs between quality and quantity of life. *Journal of Clinical Oncology* 9, 328–34.

Slag, M. F., Morley, J., Elson, M. K., Trence, D. L., Nelson, C. J., Nelson, A. E., Kinlaw, W. B., Beyer,

S., Nutall, F. Q. and Shafer, R. B. (1983). Impotence in medical clinic outpatients. *Journal of the American Medical Association* **249**, 1736–40.

So, E. P., Ho, P. C., Bodenstab, W. and Parsons, C. L. (1982). Erectile impotence associated with transurethral prostatectomy. *Urology* **19**, 259–62.

Sparks, R. F., White, R. A. and Connolly, P. B. (1980). Impotence is not always psychogenic: newer insights into hypothalamic–pituitary–gonadal dysfunction. *Journal of the American Medical Association* **243**, 750–5.

Tardif, G. S. (1989). Sexual activity after myocardial infarction. *Archives of Physical Medicine and Rehabilitation* **70**, 763–6.

The National High Blood Pressure Education Program Working Group. (1994). National high blood pressure education program group report on hypertension in diabetics. *Hypertension* **23**, 145–58.

Trelawny-Ross, C. and Russell, O. (1987). Social and psychological response to myocardial infarction: multiple determinants of outcome at six months. *Journal of Psychosomatic Research* **31**, 125–30.

Tscholl, R., Largo, M., Poppinghaus, E., Recker, F. and Subotic, B. (1995). Incidence of erectile impotence secondary to transurethral resection of benign prostatic hyperplasia, assessed by preoperative and postoperative snap gauge tests. *Journal of Urology* **153**, 1491–3.

Vinik, K. A. and Mitchell, B. (1988). Clinical aspects of diabetic neuropathies. *Diabetes and Metabolism* **4**, 223–53.

Virag, R., Bouilly, P. and Frydman, D. (1985). Is impotence an arterial disorder? A study of arterial risk factors in 440 impotent patients. *The Lancet* i, 181–4.

Wabrek, A. J. and Burchell, R. C. (1980). Male sexual dysfunction associated with coronary heart disease. *Archives of Sexual Behavior* **9**, 69–75.

Walsh, P. C., Partin, A. W. and Epstein, J. I. (1994). Cancer control and quality of life following anatomical radical retropubic prostatectomy: results at 10 years. *Journal of Urology* **152**, 1831–6.

Zifroni, A., Schiavi, R. C. and Schaffner, F. (1991). Sexual function and testosterone levels in men with non-alcoholic liver disease. *Hepatology* **14**, 479–82.

Zonszein, J. (1995). Diagnosis and management of endocrine disorders of erectile dysfunction. *Urologic Clinics of North America* **22**, 789–802.

10   Psychopathology and sexuality in aging

The distinction between the natural changes of aging and the clinical symptoms of disease is particularly relevant when considering mental changes in late life. Clinical and research advances in geriatric psychiatry document that cognitive impairment and depressed mood, for example, are not intrinsic characteristics of growing old but that they can be indicative of mental illness. Epidemiological investigations applied to psychiatric problems have shown that mood disorders, dementia, schizophrenia, and alcohol-related disorders account for why the aged use psychiatric services so much (Blazer, 1995). The prevalence of depression has been estimated at between 2% and 4% in representative samples of noninstitutionalized individuals older than 65. The rates reach 15% and even higher when subclinical depressions are included in the sampling of older age groups (Gatz, Kasl-Godley and Karel, 1996). Depression and dementia are very prevalent among elderly patients in psychiatric units and nursing homes (Anthony and Aboraya, 1992; Gurland, 1996). Depression, as a nosological entity or as a psychiatric symptom, commonly occurs during primary medical care and ambulatory medical settings. The association between affective disorders and physical illness is manifested in a wide range of medical problems including stroke, Parkinson's disease, arthritis, endocrine disorders and renal and hepatic failure, as noted in Chapter 9. Among US community residents 65 years and older, the rate of dementia is estimated as 4.5%, with Alzheimer's disease and multi-infarct disorders accounting for the majority of cases of dementia. The prevalence of dementia rises rapidly with age, reaching 20% in patients older than 80. Alcohol abuse and dependency are also frequently detected among older men in psychiatric services and hospital and outpatient medical clinics. Surveys of the drinking behavior of the elderly have reported prevalences of 6% in Veterans Administration (VA) medical wards and 21% in psychiatric outpatients (Atkinson, Ganzini and Bernstein, 1992). Late-onset schizophrenia is uncommon, but since the life-time prevalence of this disorder is close to 1% and tends to be chronic, a significant number of older schizophrenic patients are found in health-care facilities.

The relationship between psychopathology and sexual dysfunction, as evaluated in sex therapy clinics, is unclear (Schiavi et al., 1992). Some studies indicate that sexual dysfunctions are associated with a higher prevalence of psychiatric diagnosis, and elevated levels of psychological distress, neuroticism and hostility (Eysenck, 1971; Fagan et al., 1988a). Conversely, other studies have found no conclusive evidence of a relationship between sexual dysfunction and psychological disorders (Maurice and Guze, 1970). Demographic heterogeneity and differences in clinical populations, nosological criteria, study design, and assessment techniques have contributed to the discrepant findings.

Depression

Clinically, difficulties in sexual functioning and intimate relationships are mentioned in the *Diagnostic and Statistical Manual of Mental Disorders* (DSM-IV, 4th edn. American Psychiatric Association) as one of the associated descriptive features that characterize major depressive episodes. Declines in sexual desire, arousal and behavior have been noted in depressed patients but, frequently, these findings are difficult to interpret because antidepressant medication adversely affects sexual function. (Segraves, 1992). Empirically, data on the association between depression and sexual disorders are derived from three sources: epidemiological research, surveys of depressed patients, and the psychiatric assessment of sexually dysfunctional individuals. The Massachusetts Male Aging Study assessed the relationship between depression, measured by a self-report scale, and sexual activity in 1290 older men from the general community (McKinlay and Feldman, 1994). Multivariate regression analysis demonstrated that depression strongly predicts sexual difficulties and impaired sexual satisfaction. In a further analysis, the investigators (Feldman et al., 1994) assessed the determinants of self-rated erectile impotence in this population. After adjustment for age, depression emerged as one of the factors directly correlated with a higher probability of erectile dysfunction. At the highest degree of depression, measured by the self-report scale, the age-adjusted probability of complete erectile impotence was above 40%.

There are few controlled investigations of sexual function in nonmedicated depressed patients. Mathew and Weinman (1982) observed that, compared with age- and sex-matched controls, drug-free depressed patients had significantly decreased *and* significantly increased sexual drive, but no differences in erectile or orgasmic difficulties. Howell et al. (1987) reported that nonmedicated depressed patients 21–58 years of age, compared to healthy controls, had significantly less sexual interest and satisfaction but no less sexual activity measured by a validated self-report questionnaire and a prospective daily activity log. In a related study, impaired nocturnal penile tumescence (NPT) was recorded in about one-third of patients during major depressive episodes (Thase et al., 1988). The same research group conducted a controlled, prospective investigation of 40 nonmedicated patients during a major depressive episode and after early remission in response to cognitive behavioral therapy. They included self-report and behavioral measures of sexual function as well as NPT recordings (Nofzinger et al., 1993). When depressed, patients' sexual satisfaction decreased and then improved after behavioral treatment, but their sexual drive, activity and interest were unaffected. Contrary to expectations, NPT abnormalities did not normalize after recovery from depression and restoration of sexual satisfaction. The observation that a subgroup of chronically more symptomatic depressed men, who did not remit following cognitive behavioral therapy, had shown elevated sexual interest and activity prior to treatment suggests that depressive disorders are heterogeneous with regards to sexual function. This investigation underlines the value of prospective multidisciplinary assessments that discriminate among sexual desire, activity, and satisfaction. It challenges the notion that sexual behavior is necessarily impaired in depression and emphasizes instead the relevance of the patients' cognitive appraisal of sexual function. It should be noted, however, that this study did not provide data on changes in coital frequency or in erotically induced erectile responses during and after recovery from depression. Also, relatively young patients were studied, and the effects of age were not considered. The stability of impaired NPT measures despite the change in mood following cognitive therapy, an important finding of diagnostic relevance (see Chapter 13), raises unanswered questions about the biological significance of sleep erections in mood disorders. Although older patients were included in some studies, the results were not categorized by age; therefore, conclusions that apply specifically to the aged cannot be drawn. It should be kept in mind that sadness, demoralization and despair, not uncommon affective reactions in chronically ill older individuals, are not necessarily diagnostic of a mood disorder.

Several reports provide information on mood disorders or depressive symptoms in patients with sexual dysfunction. Derogatis, Meyer and King (1981), in a study of 137 men with erectile dysfunction and 62 men with premature ejaculation evaluated in a sexual dysfunction clinic, found that 8% in both groups were diagnosed as having an affective mood disorder. A profile of the patients' symptoms was drawn up by a validated psychological text. The results confirmed that patients with erectile disorders had more symptoms of depression than the normal population. Schreiner-Engel and Schiavi (1986) studied couples in which one partner was diagnosed as having a sexual desire disorder. Although patients were not depressed at the time of evaluation, 73% of the men with inhibited sexual desire met criteria for a life-time history of affective disorder and 55% had had episodes of major depression, rates that were significantly higher than those of a matched normal control group. Furthermore, in 88% of the men with prior affective disorders, the inhibited sexual desire had developed at the same time as or after the onset of the initial depressive episode.

There is limited information on the prevalence of psychiatric disorders in older men evaluated in sexual dysfunction clinics. Wise, Rabins and Gahnsley (1984) conducted a chart review of patients seen in a Sexual Behaviors Clinic between 1972 and 1981. There were 150 men older than 50 (5.8% of all patients evaluated during the study period), most of them seeking consultation for erectile difficulties. Concurrent psychiatric pathology was found in 63% of patients, with depression, anxiety reactions, and personality disorders accounting for 77% of the psychiatric diagnoses. No relationship between psychiatric diagnosis and the nature of the sexual dysfunction was evident. Subsequently, Fagan et al. (1987) evaluated the erectile dysfunction of 50- to 70-year-old men over a one-year period in the same clinic. They found that depressive affect and anxiety symptoms, assessed by the Brief Symptom Inventory (Derogatis and Melisaratos, 1983), were significantly higher in patients with psychogenic or mixed erectile dysfunctions than in patients with erectile problems attributed to organic causes alone. In the Mount Sinai Sexuality Clinic, 17% of 236 patients aged 60 years and over, who were evaluated mainly for erectile difficulties, demonstrated clinically significant symptoms of depression (see Case study 10.1).

In summary, there is a distinct association between depression and male sexual difficulties, primarily evident as problems of sexual desire and arousal. Empirical evidence suggests that depression may have differential effects on sexual interest, activity, and satisfaction. However, there are almost no data on the nature of the relationship between mood disorders and sexual function in older patients. The deleterious effect of chronic mental illness in general, and depression in particular, on sexuality needs to take into account psychological and relationship issues, the effect of chronic physical illness, and the disruptive effects of hospitalization and pharmacological treatment. It remains unclear how much putative central neurobiological abnormalities in depression contribute to the associated sexual dysfunction.

Dementia

Dementia is characterized by a global impairment of memory, cognitive function, and personality. It may develop insidiously and become apparent by subtle behavioral changes, disturbed mood, and interpersonal difficulties. Eventually the degree of cognitive disturbance and memory deficits severely compromises the individual's social and occupational adjustment.

Despite the high prevalence of Alzheimer's disease, the most common form of dementia, and despite the concerns expressed by spouses and care-givers, there is limited empirical information about the impact of this disorder on sexual function and marital relationships. Zeiss et al. (1990) evaluated 55 male Alzheimer patients, whose mean age was 70, and found that in 52% of these men the reported onset of erectile dysfunction occurred at the same time as the cognitive symptoms started. Comparisons between patients with and without erectile dysfunction showed no differences in the degree of cognitive impairment, age, level of depression, medical problems or medications. Although a matched control group was not included in this study, and mediating mechanisms are uncertain, the results show that erectile problems commonly occur among patients with Alzheimer's disease.

Changes in functional capacity and sexual expression can be extremely distressing to spouses who become particularly vulnerable given the care-taking role they must assume (Wright, 1991). Duffy (1995) interviewed, with the help of a specifically designed questionnaire, 38 care-giver spouses of Alzheimer's patients over a one-year period, to assess the impact of the disease and its progression on the couples' pattern of sexual behavior. The patients were categorized by their mates as moderately impaired, requiring assistance with common activities of daily living. Most of the healthy spouses acknowledged that their sexual relationships had changed since the onset of the disease, but there were a few reports of behaviors characterized as bizarre or inappropriately expressed outside the marital relationship. Common sources of distress generated by their mates' behavior were awkward sequencing of sexual activity, requests for activities outside the couple's sexual repertoire and lack of regard for the sexual satisfaction of the healthy partner. The healthy spouses were troubled by the change in the perceived nature of the marital relationship, and their own loss of sexual desire as the disease progressed and they found themselves adopting the role of care-giver, nurse or mother.

Haddad and Benbow (1993) considered the wide range of sexual problems associated with dementia. They categorized them into problems involving an established partner, problems involving a new partner and problems independent of a sexual partner. Among the problems in established relationships are loss of sexual interest, increased sexual demands, inadequate sexual advances or disrupted sex play by the demented patient, loss of sexual attraction by the care-giving spouse, and marital strain or loss of intimacy resulting from the patient's cognitive and behavioral deterioration (see Case study 10.2). Issues of competency arise when a demented patient attempts to initiate a relationship with a new sexual partner, a not too infrequent occurrence in institutional settings such as elderly people's homes. Although this behavior may be disturbing to health-care providers and family alike, it raises concerns about individual's rights as well as the difficult task of determining the capacity of the patient to make informed judgments regarding new relationships. As Collopy (1988) has emphasized, competency is often context specific and not even the diagnosis of dementia precludes the patient's capacity to reach competent decisions in specific areas. Problems in determining the competency of demented patients to engage in intimate relationships has prompted the development of guidelines to assist the health-care professional. They are based on evaluating the patient's awareness of the nature of the relationship, the patient's ability to avoid exploitation and his/her awareness of potential risks (Lichtenberg and Strzepek, 1990). Among the problems independent of a sexual partner are sexual acting out, such as masturbation in public, inappropriate sexual talk and false sexual allegations. However, the data do not support the hypothesis that sexual disinhibition is a common manifestation of Alzheimer's disease (Burns, Jacoby and Levy, 1990; Bozzola, Gorelick and Freels, 1992).

Sexual behaviors occur not infrequently in geriatric residential facilities, but the concerns expressed by care-givers of demented patients may not fully correspond to the patients' sexual behavior. Zeiss, Davies and Tinklenberg (1996) conducted an observational study of 40 institutionalized demented male patients between 60 and 98 years of age. Inappropriate and ambiguous sexual behaviors were coded on nine separate occasions during the day. Inappropriate behaviors such as rubbing genitals were uncommon and only briefly noted in 18% of patients. Ambiguous behaviors, such as appearing not fully dressed in public, occurred in less than 4% of the 1800 time segments coded. There was no evidence of sexually aggressive behaviors toward staff or other patients. The same degree of concern, knowledge and skill necessitated to manage other symptoms of Alzheimer's disease is required for addressing inappropriate or ambiguous sexual manifestations when they occur. Health-care professionals, frequently, are as unprepared as family care-givers to respond to sexual expressions in a sensitive and constructive manner. Training in sexual matters relevant to demented patients may greatly assist professional care-givers to assist family members as well as the patients themselves in this often ignored aspect of Alzheimer's disease.

Alcohol-related disorders

Alcohol abuse in late life has been slow to gain attention as a significant clinical problem. Social influences, subtle or atypical symptoms and the greater prominence of associated chronic medical conditions have conspired to make substance abuse an under-recognized and under-reported problem in the aged (Gambert, 1997). Among substance-use disorders in the elderly, alcohol abuse is the most prevalent, with men being two to six times more likely than women to have documented alcohol problems. Cross-sectional community surveys of problem drinking among men 60 years of age and older show the prevalence to range from 1 to 12%. Alcohol use and abuse appear to decline with age, but data from two longitudinal studies suggest that the decrease may reflect a cohort, rather than an age effect (Atkinson, Ganzini and Bernstein, 1992; Ganzini and Atkinson, 1996).

Sexual disorders in chronic alcoholic men are reported frequently, with prevalence estimates from 8% to 58%. Although no studies have specifically focused on the aged, some have included older men in their samples (Schiavi, 1990). Whalley (1978) compared the sexual behavior of 50 hospitalized alcoholic men with a matched sample from the general population. Erectile impotence was mentioned significantly more by alcoholics (54%) than by controls (28%), but a considerable number of patients were interviewed while under psychotropic medication. Jensen (1979) compared 30 outpatient, married, alcoholic men with an age-matched control group from a general practitioner's clinic. Sixty-three per cent of the alcoholic men and 10% of the control group reported sexual dysfunctions, mainly disorders of sexual desire and arousal. Half of the alcoholic men claimed that their sexual problem began after they started drug treatment for their addiction (disulfiram). There are few studies on the prevalence of alcoholism among sexually dysfunctional patients. Fagan et al. (1988b) studied 145 consecutive patients with sexual problems at the Sexual Consultation Unit of the Johns Hopkins Hospital. Twenty-nine per cent of these patients scored within the probable alcoholism range in a widely used instrument for identifying alcoholic patients. However, only six of these patients had been diagnosed as having alcoholism by routine clinical evaluation procedures. The authors conclude that, 'alcoholism largely grows undetected among patients who present with sexual problems'.

The organic processes that mediate the chronic effect of alcohol on sexual behavior are likely to include neural and hormonal mechanisms. Neurochemical investigation has revealed that ethanol has complex effects on central mechanisms involving monoamines, choline and γ-amino-butyric acid (GABA) mechanisms and also on neuromodulator receptor–effector coupling systems. It is tempting, but would be highly speculative, to relate these neurobiological processes to the changes in sexual drive and sexual arousability observed in alcoholic individuals. Of more obvious relevance to aging men is the deleterious action of chronic alcohol intake on the peripheral neurological and autonomic processes that subserve erectile function. Considerable information has accumulated on the deleterious effect of alcohol on testicular, endocrine and hepatic physiology (Van Thiel et al., 1980; Bannister and Lowosky, 1987). Low plasma androgen levels and high estrogen and prolactin levels have been noted repeatedly in sexually dysfunctional alcoholic men. However, the relationship between alcohol-induced hormonal alterations and their impaired sexual drive and arousal has not been systematically examined. One exception is a prospective study, by Van Thiel, Gavaler and Sanghvi (1982), of 60 abstinent chronic alcoholic men with sexual desire or erectile problems. Twenty-five per cent of them experienced a spontaneous recovery of sexual function, which was predicted by their lack of testicular atrophy and their normal gonadotrophic responses to luteinizing hormone releasing hormone (LH-RH) or clomiphene.

Treatment with high doses of nonaromatizable androgen restored sexual potency in some of the men who had not recovered spontaneously.

Organic pathology and psychological factors interact in the development of sexual disorders in chronic alcoholic men, but too few studies have empirically investigated the effect of aging on this relationship. With some frequency, the pattern of addiction evolves following efforts to cope, using alcohol, with depression, bereavement, sexual anxiety, feelings of inadequacy, personality problems, and marital difficulties (Konovsky and Wilsnack, 1982; Bedi and Halikas, 1985; O'Farrell et al., 1997). Concerns about sexual performance, poor self-esteem, guilt, shame, and marital problems may also be the consequence of alcohol abuse, and contribute to sustain the addiction. However, most frequently, the reciprocal interaction between drug intake and psychological factors is so closely interwoven that it is difficult to identify the nature of this relation (Case study 10.3).

The empirical evidence of an association between alcohol dependency and sexual disorders is limited by varied or imprecise characterization of alcohol status at the time of the assessment, the confounding effects of physical illness or medication, lack of validation of subject's reports by sexual partners, and lack of objective measures of erectile capacity. Several studies have shown that alcoholics experience loss of sexual desire and erectile or ejaculatory problems during the alcohol-abuse phase, but there is little behavioral information on the sexual consequences of chronic alcoholism after abstinence. Decreased erectile episodes during sleep were observed three weeks after detoxification (Snyder and Karacan, 1981), but little is known about the long-term effects of alcohol dependence on nocturnal penile tumescence in alcoholic patients who abstain from drink.

We conducted a study (Schiavi et al., 1995) to assess sexual function, marital adjustment, sleep-related erections and pituitary–gonadal activity in abstinent, chronic alcoholic men aged 28–59 years, living in stable sexual relationships. Contrary to expectation, alcoholic men selected to minimize the confounding effects of unrelated physical illnesses or medications did not differ from a matched nonalcoholic control group in the prevalence of sexual dysfunction following sobriety, despite the significant marital dissatisfaction reported by their sexual partners. Furthermore, there were no differences in the two groups in nocturnal penile tumescence and in pituitary–gonadal function during sleep. That most of the subjects of this study did not suffer from sexual disorder may be explained by the paucity of clinical and biochemical signs of liver failure and by the lack of gonadal changes, as reflected in their normal testosterone secretion during sobriety. Age-related changes in hepatic or testicular function, possibly associated with concurrent medical illness or drug effects, are likely to play a more important role in older men, rendering them more vulnerable to the long-lasting effects of alcohol on sexual behavior.

Schizophrenia

There is a considerable lack of clarity about the effect of schizophrenia on sexual function. The sexual behavior and functioning of schizophrenic patients have been variously reported as increased, decreased, impaired, or unchanged (Verhulst and Schneidman, 1981; Lyketsos, Sakka and Mailis, 1983; Lilleleht and Lieblum, 1993). As with affective disorders, there are too few controlled investigations of nonmedicated patients. Studies of schizophrenic patients taking neuroleptics have shown an increased prevalence of low sexual desire and erectile and orgasmic difficulties compared with controls (Nestoros, Lehmann and Ban, 1981; Teusch et al., 1995; Kockott and Pfeiffer, 1996). Beyond the occurrence of sexual dysfunction, the sexuality of schizophrenic patients is influenced by the presence of negative symptoms such as flatness of affect, anhedonia and emotional isolation, by their bizarre behavior and interpersonal difficulties, and by the occurrence of hallucinatory and delusional experiences that not infrequently have a sexual content.

Conclusion

Sexuality, as the above selective review suggests, has been ignored despite the growth of information about the psychopathology of aging. And yet, clinical evidence indicates that even in chronic progressive disorders such as dementia, sexual issues are salient phenomena that need to be addressed for patient care to be adequate. Data, primarily from younger age groups, show the deleterious effects that depression and substance abuse may have on male sexuality. As the high prevalence of mood disorders in the aged is recognized, and pharmacological interventions are increasingly employed, the evaluation of psychiatrically impaired older men should include sexual function as a necessary component of a comprehensive management plan.

Case studies

Case study 10.1

Mr. M, a 67-year-old salesman, sought help for erectile problems which had begun 18 months before in the context of considerable upheaval resulting in marital separation. Sexually, the couple had had no problems during the 29 years they had been together. His sexual desire, after the marital break, was diminished but he continued to experience full erections when he 'tested himself' by masturbating and when awakening in the morning. The events that prompted him to seek help were his new partner's impatience for his consistent loss of erections as he attempted to penetrate, and his feeling that the future of his relationship depended on his ability to perform sexually. During the two sessions of evaluation Mr. M became tearful as he discussed the impending divorce and the fact that his daughter refused to see him. He felt sad, lonely, unable to concentrate, and his appetite was poor. His preoccupation with the break-up of his marriage interfered with his work capacity, leading to a one-third drop in income. Mr. M had experienced a transitory period of moderate depression ten years before, that had resolved spontaneously. A complete medical examination was negative.

With some reluctance the patient accepted pharmacotherapy for his depression. After four weeks of treatment with a selective serotonin-reuptake inhibitor (SSRI), he noticed a partial lifting of his depression, enhanced sexual desire, and a newly found ability to achieve vaginal insertion. To his great dismay, however, Mr. M found he was unable to ejaculate despite prolonged thrusting. Fortunately, the ejaculatory inhibition was resolved by decreasing the dose of antidepressant medication without recurrence of psychiatric symptoms.

Comment

This vignette illustrates an erectile dysfunction associated with clinical depression. Diagnostically, however, Mr. M's problem does not meet DSM-IV criteria for male erectile disorder because the erectile dysfunction is better accounted for by the presence of a major depressive disorder. The alleviation of the sexual symptoms with antidepressant medication confirmed the diagnosis; at the same time, the onset of ejaculatory impairment showed a substance-induced (SSRI) sexual dysfunction. There were clear psychological determinants at the basis of the sexual problem but, regretfully, the patient chose not to address them at that time.

Case study 10.2

Ms. N sought advice about changes in her husband's behavior that were generating increasing marital tension and consternation to their grown-up children. She appeared both embarrassed and perplexed as she described the problem; her husband had refused to join her for evaluation. They were both in their late 60s and had been married for over 40 years. Their marriage had been mutually satisfying and, after a life of professional hard work and many accomplishments, they were economically comfortable and enjoying retirement. She defined both herself and her husband as conservative and old-fashioned and described a life-long pattern of sexual interactions which had been infrequent but problem free. During the preceding two years, however, her husband had become demanding sexually, requesting sex several times daily, but becoming distracted and uninterested once she accepted his overtures. He was mostly able to gain erections but did not seek sexual release or his wife's satisfaction. His approach to sex had become uncharacteristically coarse and insensitive which 'turned her off'. The triggering event for her requesting help was his beginning to make sexual propositions to their maid and to one of her friends.

Ms. N was eventually able to have her husband join her for a second evaluation session. He appeared well dressed and behaved in a superficially appropriate manner. A mental status evaluation showed significant cognitive deficits including marked memory impairment. There was no evidence of delusions or depressed mood. Consultation with the couple's children revealed that Mr. N was becoming increasingly unable to handle the family finances, and carry usual activities of daily living. A medical evaluation was noncontributory.

Comment

The cognitive deficits and behavioral deterioration of Mr. N, including his sexual manifestations, met diagnostic criteria for dementia of the Alzheimer's type. Changes in the nature of the sexual interaction, at the early stages of the disease, can seriously strain marital relationships but they are infrequently discussed with health-care professionals. This demented patient's wife resented her husband's inappropriate sexual demands but also felt guilty about not meeting his expectations. Unexpectedly, she was more prone to complain about changes in her husband's sexual behavior than about his overall impairment in social adjustment. Components of a successful intervention included addressing Ms. N guilt about limit setting, sleeping in separate rooms, reframing the husband's behavior as a quest for affection and support, fostering physically affectionate but nongenital interactions and participation in a care-takers' support group.

Case study 10.3

Mr. and Ms. O, aged 61 and 55 respectively, were referred by a marital agency for treatment of their sexual difficulties. The couple denied having had sexual problems before he gradually began abusing alcohol at the age of 50. By 53 he was drinking more than one pint of gin daily; although he felt his drinking did not interfere significantly with his work as a salesman, it did impair his relationship with his wife and children to the point of threatened separation. Her distaste at having intercourse with her husband when drunk led her to a total refusal of engaging in sexual activity. This was an important 'turning point' in their marriage, resulting in his seeking treatment for his addiction. With the help of Alcoholics Anonymous (AA), he became sober and had remained completely abstinent for the past three years. Much to his regret, as the couple resumed sexual activities he was unable to penetrate. He had sexual desire but his erections during attempts at intercourse, masturbation and early morning awakenings were partial at best (rated at 4 on a 1–10 scale; 10 maximum tumescence). The couple reported having a loving, caring relationship and being at a good point in their lives, free from economic responsibilities and worries about children. He would like to reactivate sex with his wife but is discouraged by her lack of sexual interest and his own fear of failure. Ms. O is puzzled by her own loss of desire and speculates that it could be due to residual negative feelings stemming from the period of heavy alcohol abuse, which also coincided with the onset of the menopause. She expressed her willingness to engage in sexual counseling for her husband's sake; as for herself she could live without sex indefinitely.

A comprehensive medical evaluation was negative with the exception of leg paresthesias and decreased peripheral sensations; a urological examination was within normal limits. Blood chemistries, including hepatic liver function indices, were normal. Mr. O was studied in the sleep laboratory over three nights with the last one devoted to sequential blood sampling for hormonal assessments. Sleep architecture was normal and there was a considerable amount of tumescent activity, with an average of three erectile episodes per night, but none of them were full as noted by systematic awakenings. The endocrine results demonstrated that circulating levels of total testosterone, bioavailable testosterone and LH were all within the normal range. The erectile response to pharmaco-cavernosal testing was also normal.

Comment

The presence of persistent erectile problems encompassing all sexual activity, abnormal NPT recordings, with no penile rigidity during three nights of testing and peripheral neurological symptoms all indicate an organic erectile dysfunction. The evidence points to chronic alcoholism as the etiological determinant, possibly mediated by neuropathic changes of the penile nervous supply. There is no evidence that hormonal, metabolic and vascular factors play a contributory role in this case. An interesting feature we have previously noted in some couples is the onset of sexual problems following sobriety. The reason for this contra-intuitive observation remains unclear. Ms. O's loss of sexual desire may play a contributory role but it is unlikely to fully explain the extent of his impairment in erectile capacity.

References

American Psychiatric Association. *Diagnostic and Statistical Manual of Mental Disorders*, 4th edn (1994). Washington DC: American Psychiatric Association.

Anthony, J. C. and Aboraya, A. (1992). The epidemiology of selected mental disorders in later life. In *Handbook of Mental Health and Aging*, 2nd edn, ed. J. E. Birren, R. B. Sloane and G. D. Cohen, pp. 27–73. San Diego, CA: Academic Press.

Atkinson, R. M., Ganzini, L. and Bernstein, M. J. (1992). Alcohol and substance use disorders in the elderly. In *Handbook of Mental Health and Aging*, 2nd edn, ed. J. E. Birren, R. B. Sloane and G. D. Cohen, pp. 515–55. San Diego, CA: Academic Press.

Bannister, P. and Losowsky, M. S. (1987). Ethanol and hypogonadism. *Alcohol and Alcoholism* 22, 213–17.

Bedi, A. R. and Halikas, J. A. (1985). Alcoholism and affective disorders. *Alcoholism* 9, 133–44.

Blazer, D. (1995). Epidemiology of psychiatric disorders in late life. In *The American Psychiatric Association Textbook of Geriatric Psychiatry*, pp. 155–71. Washington DC: American Psychiatric Press.

Bozzola, F. G., Gorelick, P. B. and Freels, S. (1992). Personality changes in Alzheimer's Disease. *Archives of Neurology* 49, 297–300

Burns, A., Jacoby, R. and Levy, R. (1990). Psychiatric phenomena in Alzheimer's disease IV. Disorders of behavior. *British Journal of Psychiatry* 157, 86–94.

Collopy, B. (1988). Autonomy in long term care: some crucial distinctions. *Gerontologist* 28, 10–18.

Derogatis, L. R. and Melisaratos, N. (1979). The DSFI; a multidimensional measure of sexual functioning. *Journal of Sex and Marital Therapy* 5, 244–81.

Derogatis, L. R. and Melisaratos, N. (1983). The Brief Symptom Inventory: an introductory report. *Psychological Medicine* 13, 595–605.

Derogatis, L. R., Meyer, J. K. and King, K. M. (1981). Psychopathology in individuals with sexual dysfunction. *American Journal of Psychiatry* 138, 757–63.

Duffy, L. M. (1995). Sexual behavior and marital intimacy in Alzheimer's couples: a family theory perspective. *Sexuality and Disability* 13, 239–54.

Eysenck, H. J. (1971). Personality and sexual adjustment. *British Journal of Psychiatry* 118, 593–608.

Fagan, P. J., Wise, T. N., Schmidt, C. W. Jr. and Dupkin, C. N. (1987). Inhibited sexual excitement in the aging male. *Journal of Geriatric Psychiatry* 20, 153–63

Fagan, P. J., Schmidt, C. W. Jr., Wise, T. and Derogatis, L. R. (1988a). Sexual dysfunction and dual psychiatric diagnosis. *Comparative Psychiatry* 29, 278–84.

Fagan, P. J., Schmidt, C. W. Jr., Wise, T. and Derogatis, L. R. (1988b). Alcoholism in patients with sexual disorders. *Journal of Sex and Marital Therapy* 14, 245–52.

Feldman, H. A., Goldstein, I., Hatzichristov, D. G., Krane, R. J. and McKinlay, J. B. (1994). Impotence and its medical and psychological correlates: results of the Massachusetts Male Aging Study. *Journal of Urology* 151, 54–61.

Gambert, S. R. (1997). Alcohol abuse: medical effects of heavy drinking in late life. *Geriatrics* 52, 30–7.

Ganzini, L. and Atkinson, R. M. (1996). Substance abuse. In *Comprehensive Review of Geriatric Psychiatry* II, 2nd edn, ed. J. Sadavoy, L. W. Lazarus, L. F. Jarvik and G. T. Grossberg, pp. 659–92, Washington DC: American Psychiatric Press.

Gurland, B. (1996). Epidemiology of psychiatric disorders. In *Comprehensive Review of Geriatric Psychiatry* II, 2nd edn, ed. J. Sadavoy, L. W. Lazarus, L. F. Jarvik and G. T. Grossberg, pp. 3–41, Washington DC: American Psychiatric Press.

Haddad, P. M. and Benbow, S. M. (1993). Sexual problems associated with dementia; Part 1: Problems and their consequences. *International Journal of Geriatric Psychiatry* 8, 547–51.

Howell, J. R., Reynolds, C. F., Thase, M. E., Frank, E., Jennings, J. R., Houck, P. R., Berman, S., Jacobs, E. and Kupfer, D. J. (1987). Assessment of sexual function, interest and activity in depressed men. *Journal of Affective Disorders* 13, 61–6.

Jensen, S. B. (1979). Sexual function and dysfunction in alcoholics. *British Journal of Sexual Medicine* 10, 29–31.

Kockott, G. and Pfeiffer, W. (1996). Sexual disorders in nonacute psychiatric outpatients. *Comprehensive Psychiatry* 37, 56–61.

Konovsky, M. and Wilsnack, S. C. (1982). Social drinking and self esteem in married couples. *Journal of Studies on Alcohol* 43, 319–33.

Lichtenberg, P. A. and Strzepek, D. M. (1990). Assessment of institutionalized demented patient's competencies to participate in intimate relationships. *Gerontologist* 30, 117–20.

Lilleleht, E. and Leiblum, S. R. (1993). Schizophrenia and sexuality: a critical review of the literature. *Annual Review of Sex Research* 4, 247–76.

Lyketsos, G. C., Sakka, P. and Mailis, A. (1983). The sexual adjustment of chronic schizophrenics: a preliminary study. *British Journal of Psychiatry* 143, 376–82.

Mathew, R. J. and Weinman, M. L. (1982). Sexual dysfunctions in depression. *Archives of Sexual Behavior* 11, 323–8.

Maurice, W. L. and Guze, S. B. (1970). Sexual dysfunction and associated psychiatric disorders. *Comparative Psychiatry* 11, 539–43.

McKinlay, J. B. and Feldman, H. A. (1994). Age-related variation in sexual activity and interest in normal men: results from the Massachusetts Male Aging Study. In *Sexuality Across the Life Course*, ed. A. S. Rossi, pp. 261–85, Chicago, IL: University of Chicago Press.

Nestoros, J. N., Lehmann, H. E. and Ban, T. A. (1981).Sexual behavior of the schizophrenic male: the impact of illness and medication. *Archives of Sexual Behavior* 10, 421–42.

Nofzinger, E. A., Thase, M. E., Reynolds, C. F. III, Frank, E., Jennings, J. R., Garamoni, G. L., Fasiczka, A. L. and Kupfer, D. J. (1993). Sexual function in depressed men. *Archives of General Psychiatry* 50, 24–30.

O'Farrell, T. J., Choquette, K. A., Cutter, H. and Brichler, G. R. (1997). Sexual satisfaction and dysfunction in marriages of male alcoholics: comparison with non alcoholics, marital conflicted and non conflicted couples. *Journal of Studies on Alcohol* 58, 91–9.

Schiavi, R. C. (1990). Chronic alcoholism and male sexual dysfunction. *Journal of Sex and Marital Therapy* 16, 23–33.

Schiavi, R. C., Karstaedt, A., Schreiner-Engel, P. and Mandeli, J. (1992). Psychometric characteristics of individuals with sexual dysfunction and their partners. *Journal of Sex and Marital Therapy* 18, 219–30.

Schiavi, R. C., Stimmel, B. B., Mandeli, J. and White, D. (1995). Chronic alcoholism and male sexual function. *American Journal of Psychiatry* 152, 1045–51.

Schreiner-Engel, P. and Schiavi, R. C. (1986). Lifetime psychopathology in individuals with low sexual desire. *Journal of Nervous and Mental Disease* 174, 646–51.

Segraves, R. T. (1992). Overview of sexual dysfunction complicating the treatment of depression. *Journal of Clinical Psychiatry* (Monograph series 10) 2, 4–10.

Snyder, S. and Karacan, I. (1981). Effects of chronic alcoholism on nocturnal penile tumescence. *Psychosomatic Medicine* 43, 423–9.

Teusch, L., Scherbaum, N., Bohme, H., Bender, S., Eschmann-Mehl, G. and Gastpar, M. (1995). Different patterns of sexual dysfunctions associated with psychiatric disorders and psychopharmacological treatment *Pharmacopsychiatry* 28, 84–92.

Thase, M. E., Reynolds, C. F., Jennings, J. R., Frank, E., Howell, J. R., Houch, P. P., Berman, S. and Kupfer, D. J. (1988). Nocturnal penile tumescence is diminished in depressed men. *Biological Psychiatry* 24, 33–46.

Van Thiel, D. H., Gavaler, J. S., Eagan, P. K., Chiao, Y. B., Cobb, C. F. and Lester, R. (1980). Alcohol and sexual function. *Pharmacology, Biochemistry and Behavior* 13 [Suppl 1] 125–9.

Van Thiel, D. H., Gavaler, J. S. and Sanghvi, A. (1982). Recovery of sexual function in abstinent alcoholic men. *Gastroenterology* 84, 677–82.

Verhulst, J. and Schneidman, B. (1981). Schizophrenia and sexual functioning. *Hospital and Community Psychiatry* 32, 259–62.

Whalley, L. J. (1978). Sexual adjustment of male alcoholics. *Acta Psychiatrica Scandinavica* 58, 281–8.

Wise, T. N., Rabins, P. V. and Gahnsley, J. (1984). The older patient with a sexual dysfunction. *Journal of Sex and Marital Therapy* 10, 117–21.

Wright, L. K. (1991). The impact of Alzheimer's Disease on the marital relationship. *Gerontologist* **31**, 24–237.

Zeiss, A. M., Davies, H. D., Wood, M., Tinklenberg, J. R. (1990). The incidence and correlates of erectile problems in patients with Alzheimer's disease. *Archives of Sexual Behavior* **19**, 325–31.

Zeiss, A. M., Davies, H. D. and Tinklenberg, J. R. (1996). An observational study of sexual behavior in demented male patients. *Journal of Gerontology* M325–M329.

11   Effects of drugs and medications

Older persons consume a disproportionately high quantity of prescription and nonprescription drugs. Thirty-one per cent of all medications are prescribed to patients older than 65 while they comprise less than 12% of the total US population (Lamy, 1980). The high prevalence of chronic illness and elevated use of health-care services among the aged, and socioeconomic factors such as mass media promotion of medication use, to the exclusion of nondrug alternatives, contribute to the increased drug use. Heart disease, hypertension, and arthritis are common chronic conditions that, among others, afflict four out of five aged persons and occur about five times more frequently than in younger age groups (Soldo and Agree, 1988). Physician visits markedly increase with patient age, as do the frequency and total number of medications prescribed per visit (Stewart, 1988).

The ranking of specific drug categories administered to patients over 65 years of age has remained consistent over the years. Table 11.1 lists the most common drug classes identified in two studies of prescription drugs or combined prescription and nonprescription medication use in older persons (Task Force on Prescription of Drugs USDHEW, 1968; May et al., 1982). Most of the top-ranked drug categories are commonly associated with adverse reactions including sexual dysfunction.

Adverse drug effects have been reported two to three times more frequently among the aged than in the general population (Wade and Bowling, 1986). The risk of toxic drug reactions to specific drugs in the elderly requires that altered pharmacokinetics and age-related changes in organ response are considered. (Andrews, 1992). However, the notion that adverse drug reactions are a direct and unavoidable consequence of aging is supported by inconsistent data, mostly derived from inpatient studies (Nolan and O'Malley, 1988). Polypharmacy, multiple pathology, higher medication dosage, and chronic treatment and drug interactions contribute significantly to the higher rate of noxious drug effects in the elderly (Nolan and O'Malley, 1988; Cadieux, 1989). Important gender differences should also be considered; medication use and the rate of adverse effects to drug therapy are consistently higher in female than in male elderly populations.

Table 11.1. Comparative rankings of drug use

Rank	Prescription use*	Prescription and nonprescription medication use**
1	Cardiovascular drugs	Vitamins
2	Tranquilizers	Analgesics/antirheumatics
3	Diuretics	Cardiovascular drugs
4	Sedatives/hypnotics	Antihypertensives
5	Antibiotics	Sedatives/hypnotics
6	Analgesics	Cathartics
7	Hormones	Diuretics
8	Antiarthritics	Antacids
9	Diabetic medications	Thyroid medications
10	Antispasmodics	Anticoagulants

Notes:

* Task force on prescription drugs US Dep HEW, 1968; ** May, et al. (1982)

Adverse drug-induced sexual effects

A substantial number of publications, mostly focused on men, reflect a growing awareness of the deleterious consequences of drugs on sexual function [see Crenshaw and Goldberg (1996) for an extensive review of this literature]. They mainly consist of case reports or uncontrolled clinical series with little attention given to interacting causative variables such as aging, the underlying medical condition, psychological status, and relationship factors. Usually no information about the person's sexual activity and function before medication is gathered, making it difficult to determine the extent to which the sexual problem is attributable to aging, the medical condition or to the medication used for its treatment. There are few drug studies that provide conclusive evidence based on reproducible dose-related effects that stop when the medication is discontinued.

Ideally, accurate interpretation of the role of a drug in the etiology of sexual dysfunction should rest on knowledge of three things. First, the pharmacology of the drug, particularly how its distribution, metabolism, excretion, and target tissue sensitivity change with age. Second, the mechanisms that mediate sexual function and dysfunction, and third the interactive physiological and psychological effects of the medical illness on the sexual responses of the aged. While much has been achieved, our knowledge is limited by inadequate information on the specificity of drug action. Drugs may influence sexual responses by nonspecific effects on general well-being, energy level, and mood. They also have complex physiological consequences which, by acting on multiple neurotransmitters and hormonal processes, make it difficult to delineate the precise mechanism of action on sexual function. The problem of lack of specificity is frequently compounded by vague or inadequate characterization of the components of the sexual response that are impaired by the drug, i.e., sexual desire, subjective arousal, penile erection, seminal emission, ejaculation and/or orgasm.

Medication effects have been diagnosed in medical or geriatric clinics as the likely or contributing cause of erectile dysfunction in a significant but varying proportion of patients (Davis et al., 1985). For example, Slag et al. (1983), in a previously mentioned survey (Chapter 9), screened 1180 men from a medical outpatient clinic for the presence of erectile dysfunction. Out of 401 men with this diagnosis, 47% accepted further evaluation and, among those, medications were identified as responsible in 25% of the dysfunctional patients. These men reported preexisting normal sexual function and a temporal relationship between medication onset and the development of the sexual difficulties. Antihypertensives, diuretics, and vasodilators were the medications more frequently implicated. While confirming the high prevalence of chronic disorders associated with erectile failure, other investigators (Mulligan and Katz, 1989) identified causative adverse drug reactions in as few as 3.9% of the dysfunctional patients. The method of gathering information on adverse drug effects is an important source of variability. Studies that have used structured interviews or sexual questionnaires show higher prevalence rates of sexual dysfunction than those that rely on the spontaneous complaints of patients. There is limited information on the etiological role of drugs in the sexual problems of older men who attend sexual dysfunction clinics. A range of medications, mainly cardiovascular and antihypertensive agents, were frequently noted in our clinic to be associated with the sexual problems of male patients aged 60 years and older (see Chapter 8). However, as with surveys of medical clinics, the lack of systematic longitudinal assessment made it impossible to draw definite conclusions about the cause of the dysfunction.

What follows is a review of the most common medications prescribed to aged individuals, implicated as having adverse effects on male sexual function (Table 11.2).

Antihypertensive medications

The prevalence of mild to severe hypertension has been estimated to be as high as 64% in persons aged 65 to 74 years (The Working Group on Hypertension in the Elderly, 1986). Hypertension is a major contributor to the increased morbidity and mortality of the aged. It is associated with a higher risk of coronary disease, stroke, congestive and renal failure, and peripheral vascular pathology. Several large clinical trials have shown that antihypertensive medication has significant therapeutic

Table 11.2. Prescription drugs commonly associated with sexual dysfunction in older men

Class	Drugs
Antihypertensives	
Diuretics	Bendrofluazide, hydrochlorothiazide, spironolactone
Central adrenergic	Methyldopa, clonidine, reserpine
Peripheral adrenergic	Guanethidine
Beta-blockers	Propranolol, timolol, pindolol, metoprolol
Cardiovascular drugs	
Cardiac	Digitalis
Antiarrhythmic	Disopyramide, amiodarone
Hypolipidemic	Clofibrate, gemfibrozil
Psychotropic drugs	
Phenothiazines	Chlorpromazine, thioridazine, fluphenazine, trifluoperazine
Thioxanthenes	Thiothixene
Butyrophenones	Haloperidol
Tricyclic antidepressants	Imipramine, amitryptiline, clomipramine, doxepin
MAO inhibitors	Phenelzine, tranylcypromine
Serotonergic inhibitors (SSRIs)	Fluoxetine, sertraline, paroxetine
Mood stabilizers	Lithium, carbamazepine, valproate
Other antidepressants	Trazodone
Anxiolytics	Alprazolam, diazepam, lorazepam
Cytotoxic agents	
Alkylating agents	Chlorambucil, cyclophosphamide
Other cytotoxic agents	Procarbazine, vinblastine
Histamine-2 antagonists	Cimetidine
Carbonic anhydrase inhibitors	Acetazolamide, methazolamide , dichlorophenamide
Hormonal agents	GnRH agonists, antiandrogens, estrogens

Note:
MAO, Monoamine oxidase; GnRH, gonadotrophin releasing hormone.

effects on the cardiovascular sequelae of hypertension (Management Committee of the National Heart Foundation of Australia, 1981; Hypertension Detection and Follow up Program Cooperative Group, 1982; Medical Research Council Working Party, 1985). While the beneficial consequences of reducing high blood pressure are without question, adverse effects of antihypertensive drugs are relatively frequent and can interfere with treatment compliance. In a large, five-year study of antihypertensive drug effects involving over 5000 patients (Curb et al., 1985), 9.3% had discontinued treatment because of definite or probable side-effects; possible adverse reactions leading to treatment interruption were noted in an additional 23% of patients. Frequently reported side-effects included lethargy and drowsiness, gastrointestinal symptoms, dizziness and depression. Sexual problems, primarily impotence and decreased sexual drive, led to treatment discontinuation in 8.3% of male patients. Guanethidine, chlorthalidone, a thiazide-like diuretic, methyldopa, and reserpine were the drugs more commonly associated with sexual problems (Curb et al., 1985). Contrary to expectation, the five-year incidence of total side-effects did not increase with age.

Physicians, concerned with the cardiovascular state of their patients, may over-look the medication's less obvious effects on contentment. In a survey by Jachuck et al. (1982), the effect of hypotensive drugs (diuretics, methyldopa, and beta-blockers) on quality of life was assessed from reports of hypertensive patients, their treating physicians and sexual partners or close relatives. All the physicians found their patients to be improved based on adequate blood pressure control and no complaints of adverse effects. In contrast, on direct questioning, less than half of the patients felt better and 75% of close relatives indicated moderate or severe adverse changes after treatment. Deterioration after treatment was usually attrib-uted to declines in energy, general activity, and sexual interest. The high drop-out rates noted in major drug trials drew attention to the impact of antihypertensive therapy on quality of life and stimulated the development of less adverse therapeu-tic agents. Several investigators (Croog et al., 1986; Williams, 1988; Wassertheil-Smoller et al., 1991), although not all (Beto and Bansal, 1992), observed that antihypertensive medications significantly impaired the physical state, emotional well-being, and sexual and social functioning of patients. For example, Croog and collaborators (1986) found, in a randomized double-blind clinical trial, that three major agents, methyldopa, propranolol, and captopril (an angiotensin-converting enzyme inhibitor), had differential effects on validated quality of life measures. After six months, methyldopa and propranolol treatment, while effective at reduc-ing high blood pressure, resulted in lower scores in measures of emotional well-being, and more frequent sexual dysfunction and physical symptoms than the captopril group. Patients taking captopril were less likely to discontinue treatment because of adverse effects.

Quality of life is an important consideration in the selection of a treatment strat-egy from the array of effective antihypertensive agents currently available (Gandhi and Kong, 1996). Regretfully, little controlled data are available on the impact of antihypertensive treatment on sexual function, which is an important component of the quality of life of older patients. While there is evidence that the rate of sexual dysfunction in nontreated hypertensive patients is higher than in normotensive men (Bulpitt, Dollery and Carne, 1976; Bauer et al., 1981), the results are not grouped according to age, which complicates the interpretation of the side-effects of antihypertensive agents on the sexuality of the aged.

Diuretics

Thiazide diuretics continue to be widely prescribed alone or in combination with other agents in the management of hypertension in the elderly (Kligman and Higbee, 1989). Evidence from major controlled drug trials show that thiazide diuretics have deleterious effects on sexual functioning. The Medical Research Council treatment trial found, for example, that bendrofluazide is associated with a 23% rate of erectile complaints compared to 10% among the control group. In most patients the sexual problem resolved after discontinuation of the thiazide (Medical Research Council Working Party on Mild to Moderate Hypertension, 1981). A randomized, double-blind, study (Chang et al., 1991) was carried out to assess the effect of a thiazide diuretic (hydrochlorothiazide) on quality of life in hypertensive men aged 35–70 years. Significantly greater sexual problems, including decreased libido, difficulties getting and maintaining erections and ejaculating, were reported by the thiazide group than the placebo-treated hypertensive patients. Multivariate analysis showed that the findings were not accounted for by the confounding effects of age, potassium level or blood pressure changes. Prospective data (Williams et al., 1987) show that taking hydrochlorothiazide with other classes of antihypertensives (propranolol, methyldopa) increases the rate of sexual dysfunction and has a negative impact on the quality of life. The mechanism of action of thiazide diuretics on sexual function remains speculative. It has been proposed that thiazides may directly impair vascular smooth muscle erectile mechanisms (Muller et al., 1991).

Spironolactone, a potassium-sparing, aldosterone-antagonistic diuretic, is associated with a loss of sexual drive, erectile dysfunction and gynecomastia. The overall incidence of erectile problems, mostly based on case reports, has ranged widely from 4% to 30% (Spark and Melby, 1968; Brown et al., 1972); the changes appear to be dose related and reversible following treatment discontinuation. The side-effects on sexuality may be hormonally mediated because of its antiandrogenic action, elevated prolactin secretion or possible androgen receptor competition.

Sympatholytic agents

Adrenergic inhibitors, alone or in combination with diuretics, have been traditionally used in the treatment of hypertension in the aged (Kligman and Higbee, 1989). Methyldopa and clonidine are two commonly used centrally active sympatholytic drugs that have been frequently associated with erectile impairment and, to a lesser degree, diminished sexual drive (Buffum, 1992; Segraves and Segraves, 1992). Differences in medication dose, duration of treatment, patients' age and physical status, and the interacting effect of diuretics may contribute to the wide range of reports of erectile failure. Higher rates of erectile impotence were noted when sexual information was specifically requested.

Peripheral-acting adrenergic antagonists such as guanethidine have also been reported to cause loss of libido and erectile difficulties, but ejaculatory problems are the most frequent complaints, possibly because of their action on sympathetically mediated emission and ejaculatory mechanisms (Stevenson and Umstead, 1984; Deamer and Thompson, 1991). Prazosin decreases peripheral arterial resistance by blocking postsynaptic alpha-1 adrenergic receptors. The prevailing, although not entirely consistent, opinion is that this drug has relatively few adverse sexual effects (Buffum, 1992). Lipson (1985), in a single-blind study, found no differences in sexual side-effects between prazosin and placebo; the prevalence of erectile difficulties was lower for the prazosin-treated than for the methyldopa-treated group. However, in the Veterans Administration Cooperative Study Group on Hypertensive Agents (1982), sexual difficulties were reported more frequently with prazosin than hydralazine, a directly acting relaxant of vascular smooth muscle. The incidence of ejaculatory problems is rare but there have been several reports of priapism related to prazosin treatment (Stevenson and Umstead, 1984). The use of reserpine in older patients, an antihypertensive agent with both central and peripheral antiadrenergic effects, has markedly declined in recent years. It has been frequently associated with decreased sexual drive and erectile difficulties and, to a lesser extent, with ejaculatory failure (Papadopoulos, 1989). Clinical depression and increased prolactin secretion may contribute to the adverse effects of this drug on sexuality.

Beta-adrenergic blockers

Propranolol, a nonselective lipophilic beta-blocker drug, is that most commonly used to treat hypertension. There are numerous clinical reports of erectile impotence and diminished libido with propranolol treatment, particularly at higher doses (Rosen, 1991; Segraves and Segraves, 1992). The Medical Research Council Hypertension Study (1985) found that the drop-out rate of patients because of erectile complaints was significantly greater in the propranolol-treated than in the placebo control group. Kostis and collaborators (1990) conducted a prospective, placebo-controlled study comparing the effects of propranolol and clonidine in younger and older hypertensive males. Both drugs were found to impair nocturnal penile tumescence measures and to decrease subjective arousal. Propranolol decreased the amplitude of sleep erections but only in older patients. Although the data are limited, it appears that less lipophilic beta-blockers, such as atenolol or nadolol, with less access to the central nervous system, are associated with fewer side-effects on sexuality (Buffum, 1992). The pathway by which beta-blockers induce sexual side-effects is not known. They have been associated with a reduced circulating testosterone level (Rosen, Kostis and Jekelis, 1988), but their significance as a mediating mechanism remains to be determined.

Angiotensin-converting enzyme (ACE) inhibitors

Drugs such as captopril or enalapril, alone or in combination with a diuretic, have been suggested as a first line treatment to manage hypertension in the elderly because they have few side-effects and preserve quality of life (Kligman and Higbee, 1989). They act by inhibiting production of aldosterone, resulting in lowered peripheral vascular resistance and decreased blood pressure. There are relatively few reports of adverse sexual side-effects induced by this class of drug. In the previously mentioned randomized double-blind, quality-of-life study conducted by Croog et al. (1986) on 626 hypertensive men aged 21–65 years, the captopril group had fewer sexual side-effects, significantly less than the propranolol group.

Calcium channel blockers

Verapamil and nifedipine are among a relatively new class of drugs that reduce blood pressure by acting directly on arterial smooth muscle tone, and are considered effective as antihypertensive agents in the aged. There are few reports of adverse sexual reactions with these drugs. Morrissette and collaborators (1993) contributed the only prospective, placebo-controlled study on the effects of nifedipine and atenolol on the sexual function of older men. With the exception of a decrease in erectile firmness with nifedipine, neither drug had significant negative effects on a large array of sexual measures.

In summary, adverse sexual reactions have been noted in association with almost all antihypertensive drugs but only a small number of prospective, controlled studies have examined their effects on sexual function (Rosen and Weiner, 1997). Cumulative evidence, mostly clinically based, suggests that agents such as methyldopa, reserpine, guanethidine, propranolol or clonidine, alone or in conjunction with diazide diuretics, are the most likely to have adverse sexual effects. Other antihypertensives, such as ACE inhibitors or calcium antagonists, appear to be more benign sexually, but greater experience with these agents is required, particularly in the treatment of elderly hypertensive men.

Other cardiovascular drugs

Digoxin

This cardiovascular drug, frequently used in the aged, has been associated with significant decreases in libido and erectile problems when compared to a drug-free control group with comparable cardiac functional capacity (Neri et al., 1980). Decreased circulating testosterone and elevated estrogen levels may contribute to the decrease in sexual drive and to gynecomastia in some patients following long-term treatment (Neri et al., 1987).

Antiarrhythmic agents

Disopyramide induces erectile problems with full recovery of sexual function following treatment discontinuation (McHaffie, Guz and Johnston, 1977; Ahmad, 1980). There are few reports of an association between other antiarrhythmic drugs, such as amiodarone and mexiletine, and erectile impotence and further examination is required (Anastasiou-Nana et al., 1986).

Hypolipidemic agents

Clofibrate and gemfibrozil, drugs used to decrease serum cholesterol and triglyceride levels in patients unresponsive to dietary restriction, may cause decreased libido and erectile difficulties. In a placebo-controlled study of 1065 men on clofibrate, 14.1% reported decreased sexual drive or erectile problems, a rate that was significantly higher than the 10% incidence in the placebo group. (Coronary Drug Project Research Group, 1975). The adverse effects of clofibrate on sexual function may involve abnormalities of steroidogenesis and hepatic metabolism of sex steroids.

Psychoactive medications

Rational psychopharmacological treatment of aging patients needs to consider their increased prevalence of physical disease, the potential for noxious interactions with prescribed and over-the-counter medications, and age-related alterations in drug disposition. Changes in the rate of absorption, alterations in plasma protein binding, diminished hepatic metabolism and impaired renal clearance, for example, can have profound effects on the pharmacological action of psychotropic medications in the aged. Equally important are changes in central nervous system receptor-site sensitivity to psychiatric drugs, which may occur naturally in the course of aging or as a result of illness. Regardless of the mediating processes, older people, as a group, are increasingly sensitive to the therapeutic *and* the toxic effects of psychoactive drugs. Oversedation, extrapyramidal symptoms, anticholinergic toxicity, cardiovascular disturbances and cognitive impairment often occur at significantly lower psychotropic doses and blood levels than in younger adults. Sexual symptoms have been frequently noted as side-effects of psychotropic treatment, but the role of aging in the rate of adverse sexual reactions to psychiatric drugs has not been systematically explored.

Antipsychotic drugs (neuroleptics)

Neuroleptic drugs are frequently used when treating psychotic elderly patients and when managing behavioral disturbances associated with dementia and organic mental syndromes. Although there are few controlled studies, numerous case reports and clinical series document sexual side-effects with almost every class of antipsychotic medication, including the new atypical antipsychotics such as clozapine and risperidone (Buffum, 1992; Segraves and Segraves, 1992; Schiavi and Segraves, 1995). The sexual side-effects include diminished sexual desire, erectile problems, and orgasmic and ejaculatory impairments. In a systematic prevalence study of neuroleptic side-effects involving 1259 men, reduced sexual desire, erectile difficulties and ejaculatory dysfunction were reported by 36.6%, 21.5%, and 18.7% of patients respectively (Lingjaerde et al., 1987). The rate of reported sexual side-effects was highest among patients between 50 and 70 years of age, and was more frequent among those receiving high-dose neuroleptics such as chlorpromazine and thioridazine than high-potency, low-dose neuroleptics such as fluphenazine. Thioridazine is particularly deleterious to sexual function, having been associated with delayed or inhibited orgasm, lack of ejaculation at orgasm and painful ejaculation (Rosen, 1991; Buffum, 1992). Olanzapine, a new second-generation antipsychotic agent, appears to be an exception, in that few adverse sexual effects were reported by a large series of schizophrenic patients (Beasly, Tollefson and Tran, 1997). Several mechanisms are possibly implicated in the adverse effects of antipsychotic drugs on sexuality (Segraves, 1989; Brock and Lue, 1993). They include their central antidopaminergic receptor action, increased prolactin secretion resulting from dopamine D2 receptor blockade, decreased cholinergic activity and inhibited alpha-adrenergic function. Interference with alpha-adrenergic mechanisms may be responsible for the occurrence of priapism also noted in response to chlorpromazine and thioridazine.

Antidepressants and mood-stabilizing drugs

Depression, a common psychiatric disorder in older people, is frequently accompanied by anxiety, agitation, insomnia, bodily complaints, and impaired cognitive function. The effectiveness of antidepressant treatment in the elderly has been documented by controlled studies, but it is usually associated with adverse reactions such as orthostatic hypotension, sedation, anticholinergic toxicity, and impaired memory function (Young and Meyers, 1996). The occurrence of sexual symptoms, a well-known side-effect in the treatment of younger depressed patients, has not been studied systematically in the aged.

Sexual dysfunction has been reported with virtually all classes of antidepressants but, as with antipsychotic agents, there are few controlled studies. The interpretation of the evidence is confounded by conflicting information on the effects that affective disorders themselves have on sexual function. Nofzinger et al. (1993) and Thase et al. (1994) have shown that, compared to a control group, the most consistent problem of nonmedicated depressed patients is diminished sexual satisfaction, and not necessarily, as is commonly assumed, decreased sexual interest or activity. Successful treatment of depression with cognitive–behavioral interventions (not involving drug effects) enhanced sexual satisfaction but inconsistently changed sexual activity; in addition, erectile function, as measured by nocturnal penile tumescence, was not restored to normal levels. The lack of adequate baseline sexual information during the premedicated depressed state compromises the interpretation of drug effects on sexual activity.

Impaired sexual drive, erectile impotence, orgasmic and ejaculatory difficulties have all been noted in relation to tricyclic antidepressants, monoamine oxidase inhibitors (MAOIs) and the selective serotonin reuptake inhibitors (SSRIs) (Segraves, 1992). The reported incidence of adverse sexual effects of antidepressants has ranged from less than 10% to rates as high as 96%. There is no consistent evidence that, within each class of antidepressants, individual drugs differ in their type or rate of sexual side-effects. Possible exceptions are bupropion, a nontricyclic antidepressant, which appears to have few sexual side-effects (Gardner and Johnston, 1985; Rowland et al., 1997), trazodone which has been implicated in causing priapism (Buffum, 1992) and nefazodone (Feiger et al., 1996). Some, but not all, clinical studies have observed predominant deleterious effects of serotonergic antidepressants on orgasmic and ejaculatory function (Balon, Yeragani and Pohl, 1993; Gitlin, 1995; Lane, 1997). Although the data are limited (Schiavi and Segraves, 1995), lithium carbonate and carbamazepine, both used as mood stabilizers, are associated with decreased libido and erectile failure (see Case Study 11.1). Valproic acid, also used in the treatment of manic disorders in geriatric patients, appears to cause relatively few adverse sexual reactions. The mechanisms mediating the antidepressant effects on sexuality involve, presumably, their adrenergic, serotonergic and anticholinergic properties. Several case reports suggest that yohimbine, a presynaptic alpha-2 blocker, cyproheptadine, a serotonergic antagonist, and bethanechol, a cholinergic agent, may be effective at restoring sexual function in patients treated with antidepressants (Segraves, 1992; Gitlin, 1994).

Antianxiety agents

The primary anxiolytic agents are the benzodiazepines. This class of drug is also frequently used for their sedative and hypnotic actions. Despite the potential for toxic side-effects, such as sedation, ataxia and cognitive impairment, and for the risk of abuse and dependence, they are administered extensively to the aged

(Salzman and Nevis-Olesen, 1992). Their most common adverse sexual effect is a dampening of sexual drive, and to a lesser extent, particularly at higher doses, erectile and ejaculatory problems. The combination of lithium and benzodiazepines appears to be particularly deleterious to sexual function (Ghadirian, Annable and Belanger, 1992). Buspirone, a nonbenzodiazepine with 5-HT-1a (5-HT is 5-hydroxytryptamine, otherwise known as serotonin) receptor action, has been used to treat anxiety in the aged. The lack of reported negative sexual effects with this agent may reflect its recent introduction.

Other prescription drugs

Several additional agents with potentially adverse effects on sexuality are commonly used in the medical care of aging individuals.

Histamine-2 antagonists

Cimetidine is associated with decreased sexual drive, erectile difficulties and gynecomastia (Jensen, Collen and Pandol, 1983). These effects appear to be dose dependent and tend to disappear when treatment stops. Ranitidine, another antiulcer drug, is less likely to induce adverse sexual effects (Abramowicz, 1987). Cimetidine's action on sexual function may be because of its considerable antiandrogenic effects and the induction of elevated prolactin secretion in men.

Cancer chemotherapy agents

A wide range of cytotoxic agents, including alkylating drugs such as chlorambucil or cyclophosphamide, are associated with decreased libido, impotence, gynecomastia and infertility (Chapman, 1982; Balducci et al., 1988). Some of these effects may be the result of their toxic action on gonadal function. However, it is difficult to disentangle the direct effect of chemotherapeutic drugs from the nonspecific psychological consequences of the underlying disease and the general malaise associated with its treatment.

Carbonic anhydrase inhibitors

Acetazolamide, methazolamide and dichlorophenamide, drugs used to treat glaucoma, have been associated with decreased sexual drive and erectile problems (Epstein, Allen and Lunde, 1987). The sexual side-effects may be nonspecific, related to the dysphoria frequently induced by these medications.

Drugs with hormonal effects

The role of androgens in sustaining male sexual behavior was discussed in Chapter 3. It is possible, although not yet clearly demonstrated, that drugs such as digoxin, cimetidine and clofibrate affect sexual function by interfering with androgen metabolism, circulating steroids or prolactin secretion. Antiandrogens used in the treatment of carcinoma of the prostate can markedly impair sexual drive and erectile capacity. Flutamide, a nonsteroidal antiandrogen that blocks testosterone's action on target cell receptors, has adverse effects when used in combination with a luteinizing hormone releasing hormone (LHRH) agonist to treat metastatic prostate cancer (Pavone-Macaluso et al., 1990). LHRH analogs such as leuprolide acetate and buserelin can severely limit sexual function (Roila, 1989). Several drugs have been used to treat benign prostatic hyperplasia; while some have detrimental sexual actions (Meiraz et al., 1977), others of recent use, such as finasteride, appear to have more limited sexual side-effects (Wilton et al., 1996).

Drugs of abuse

Alcohol and nicotine are two drugs of abuse that are commonly used by the aged. The toxic effects of alcohol on sexual function was discussed in Chapter 10. Tobacco smoking has been linked with an increased prevalence of erectile disorders (see Case Study 11.2). Nakagawa, Watanabe and Nakao (1990) found, in a population study of Japanese males, that smokers had erectile problems twice as often as their age-matched nonsmoking controls. Regular tobacco users, smoking high-nicotine cigarettes had significantly lower penile tumescence increases during controlled exposure to erotic films (Gilbert, Hagen and D'Agostino, 1986). In another study, smoking two cigarettes inhibited the erectile responses induced by an intracavernous injection of papaverine (Glina et al., 1988). Nicotine, in addition to long-term effects on the development of atherosclerotic vascular disease, may acutely impair erectile responses, probably through its action on penile cavernous smooth muscles.

Conclusion

Epidemiological data on adverse drug reactions are limited by the low number of placebo-controlled studies that consider aging as a factor in the incidence of side-effects. Numerous case reports and clinical series show that several classes of drugs such as antihypertensives and psychotropic agents, which are commonly prescribed to the elderly, can impair sexual function, but information on the rate of sexual side-effects within drug classes varies widely. Discrepant findings probably reflect differences in demographic and clinical characteristics, medication dose, and the extent of treatment and drug interactions. Prescription drugs should be considered, along with chronic illness, as an important risk factor for sexual dysfunction in the aged. The effect of drugs on sexual function is determined not only by their pharmacological action on mediating physiological mechanisms and their interaction with the underlying disorder, but also by their nonspecific effects on well-being, energy level, and mood. In addition, patients' psychological characteristics, such as sexual attitudes and expectations, and the setting of drug administration may also influence individual responses to drug administration. Given the multiplicity of factors that mediate drug effects, the managing of adverse sexual responses remains largely empirical. Clinicians responsible for the treatment of older patients need to be guided by an accurate medical and drug history, knowledge of the pharmacology of the drugs chosen, and awareness of potential adverse effects. They should include sexual function in the medical history and recognize that sexual side-effects compromise compliance with adequate drug therapy as much in the aged as in younger patients.

Case studies

Case study 11.1

Mr. P, a 66-year-old divorced executive, was seen in consultation for his loss of sexual desire He suffered from a bipolar depressive disorder and had been under psychiatric care since the age of 30, treated with lithium. His past history was characterized by recurrent episodes of depression, usually because of noncompliance with medication, with the associated lack of sexual interest that remitted as he recovered from his mood disturbance. One year previously, lithium treatment had been discontinued because of renal complications and carbamazepine treatment was initiated. Although Mr. P remained free from depressive symptoms his sexual interest disappeared soon after the medication change. He continued to have intercourse, however, when his sexual partner, with whom he had been living over the past three years, initiated sexual experiences. He was pleased by his ability to satisfy her, but found it taxing to perform in the absence of sexual desire. Mr. P denied awareness of personal or relationship difficulties that could account for his loss of desire. He was puzzled by the problem and wondered whether it was because he was growing old. A complete medical evaluation, including hormonal testing, was not contributory.

Comment

This case illustrates the atypical clinical presentations that occasionally characterize the sexual complaints of older men with life-long psychopathology. It demonstrates the occurrence of loss of sexual drive as a symptom of depression, as well as the consequence of a medication used for its treatment. Although Mr. P's psychiatric assessment indicated full recovery from his last depressive episode, it remained possible that he continued to suffer from a subclinical depressive state. However, the short period between the start of carbamazepine treatment and the loss of sexual desire, in the absence of identifiable interpersonal problems, suggests that this drug was responsible for the sexual symptom. Unfortunately, the patient did not return to a follow-up clinic, so the differential diagnosis of either an adverse effect of medication or a lack of sexual desire as a residual depressive symptom was not clarified. The patient's capacity to engage in intercourse in the absence of sexual interest is an infrequent but not an exceptional observation. Although the cause of his loss of sexual drive remained uncertain, Mr. P was reassured that age per se could not account for it.

Case study 11.2

Mr. Q, a 66-year-old semiretired, obese executive was referred by his internist for his sexual problem. He denied any difficulty getting or maintaining full erections prior to two years previously when he developed a herniated lumbar disk that required full bed rest for a month. Four years earlier the patient had been diagnosed with hypertension and treated with a diuretic to which, at the time of the back episode, a beta-blocker was added. During the last two years Mr. Q noted a progressive decrease in the rigidity of his erections during coital and masturbatory attempts, resulting in a total inability to achieve vaginal insertion. His sexual desire and ejaculatory capacity were not impaired. The couple described a warm and committed marital relationship and denied that his wife's recent mastectomy could have contributed to his sexual difficulties. Of significance is a 20-year history of nicotine abuse (two packs per day), an addiction that he had been unable to relinquish. With the exception of his hypertensive condition, a medical evaluation that included neurological testing provided negative results.

Mr. Q had assumed that the erectile difficulties were caused by the hypertensive medication, but the sexual problem had persisted during a three-week discontinuation of hypertensive treatment. Changing to another class of antihypertensives did not ameliorate the sexual difficulties. The patient was strongly advised to seek the help of a nutritionist to lose weight and to address his nicotine addiction since it could contribute to his sexual problem. Mr. Q was successful in normalizing his weight and, with the help of group therapy, was able to decrease his smoking to four cigarettes per day. Blood pressure fell within normal limits and antihypertensive medication no longer became necessary. The restoration of his sexual function significantly reinforced his radical life-style change.

Comment

It is not possible to ascertain which was the active ingredient for therapeutic change: the loss of weight, the discontinuation of antihypertensive medication or the decreased nicotine intake. It is likely that all of these factors contributed to the successful sexual outcome. The possibility of a neurological impairment following the herniated lumbar disk did not prove to be a significant etiological determinant in Mr. Q's erectile disorder.

References

Abramowicz, M. (1987). Drugs that cause sexual dysfunction [Medical letter]. on *Drugs and Therapeutics* 29, 65–70.

Ahmad, S. (1980). Disopyramide and impotence. *Southern Medical Journal* 73, 958.

Anastasiou–Nana, M. I., Anderson, J. L., Nanas, J. N., Luz, J. R., Smith, R. A. and Anderson, K. P.

(1986). High incidence of clinical and subclinical toxicity associated with amiodarone treatment of refractory tachyarrhythmias. *Canadian Journal of Cardiology* 2, 138–45.

Andrews, P. H. (1992). Drugs and the elderly. In *Human Aging and Chronic Disease*, ed. C. S. Kart, pp. 267–85. London: Jones & Barlett Publishing.

Balducci, L., Phillips, D. M., Gearhart, J. G., Little, D. D., Bowie, C. and McGehce, R. P. (1988). Sexual complications of cancer treatment. *American Family Physician* 37, 159–72.

Balon, R., Yeragani, U. K. and Pohl, R. (1993). Sexual dysfunction during antidepressant treatment. *Journal of Clinical Psychiatry* 54, 209–12.

Bauer, G. E., Hunyor, S. N., Baker, J. and Marshall, P. (1981). Clinical side effects during antihypertensive therapy: a placebo controlled double blind study (special report). *Postgraduate Medical Communications* 1, 49–54.

Beasly, C. M. Jr., Tollefson, G. D. and Tran, P. V. (1997). Safety of olanzapine. *Journal of Clinical Psychiatry* 58 [Supplement 10], 13–17.

Beto, E. A. and Bansal, U. K. (1992). Quality of life in treatment of hypertension. A meta-analysis of clinical trials. *American Journal of Hypertension* 5, 125–33.

Brock, G. B. and Lue, T. F. (1993). Drug-induced male sexual dysfunction. *Drug Safety* 8, 414–26.

Brown, J., Davies, D. L., Ferris, J. G., Fraser, R., Haywood, E., Lever, A. F. and Robertson, J. I. S. (1972). Comparison of surgery and prolonged spironolactone therapy in patients with hypertension, aldosterone excess and low plasma renin, *British Medical Journal* ii, 729–34.

Buffum, J. (1992). Prescription drugs and sexual function. *Psychiatric Medicine* 10, 181–98.

Bulpitt, C. J., Dollery, C. T. and Carne, S. (1976). Changes in symptoms of hypertensive patients after referral to hospital clinic. *British Heart Journal* 38, 121–8.

Cadieux, L. (1989). Drug interactions in the elderly. How multiple drug use increases risk exponentially. *Postgraduate Medicine* 86, 186–7.

Chang, S. W., Fine, R., Siegel, D., Chesney, M., Black, D. and Hulley, S. B. (1991). The impact of diuretic therapy on reported sexual function. *Archives of Internal Medicine* 151, 2402–8.

Chapman, R. M. (1982). Effect of cytotoxic therapy on sexuality and gonadal function. *Seminars in Oncology* 9, 84–94.

Coronary Drug Project Research Group. (1975). Clofibrate and niacin in coronary heart disease. *Journal of the American Medical Association* 231, 360–81.

Crenshaw, T. L. and Goldberg, J. P. (1996). *Sexual Pharmacology*. New York: W.W. Morton.

Croog, S. H., Levine, S., Testa, M. A., Brown, B., Bulpitt, C. J., Jenkins, C. D., Klerman, G. L. and Williams, G. H. (1986). The effects of antihypertensive therapy on the quality of life. *New England Journal of Medicine* 314, 1657–64.

Curb, J. D., Borhani, N. O., Blaszkowski, T. P., Zimbaldi, N., Fotiu, S. and Williams, W. (1985). Long–term surveillance for adverse effects of antihypertensive drugs. *Journal of the American Medical Association* 253, 3263–8.

Davis, S. S., Viosca, S. P., Guralnik, M., Windsor, C. and Buttiglieri, M. W. (1985). Evaluation of impotence in older men. *Western Journal of Medicine* 142, 499–505.

Deamer, R. L. and Thompson, J. F. (1991). The role of medications on geriatric sexual function. *Clinics in Geriatric Medicine* 7, 95–111.

Epstein, R. J., Allen, R. C. and Lunde, M. W. (1987). Organic impotence associated with carbonic anhydrase inhibitor therapy for glaucoma. *Annals of Ophthalmology* **19**, 48–50.

Feiger, A., Kiev, A., Shrivastava, R. K., Wisselink, P. G. and Wilcox, C. S. (1996). Nefazodone versus sertaline in outpatients with major depression: focus on efficacy, tolerability, and effects on sexual function and satisfaction. *Journal of Clinical Psychiatry* **57** [Suppl 2], 53–62.

Gandhi, S. K. and Kong, S. X. (1996). Quality of life measures in the evaluation of antihypertensive drug therapy: reliability, validity and quality of life domains. *Clinical Therapy* **18**, 1276–95.

Gardner, E. A. and Johnston, J. A. (1985). Bupropion: an antidepressant without sexual pathophysiological action. *Journal of Clinical Pharmacology* **5**, 24–9.

Ghadirian, H. M., Annable, L. and Belanger, M. C. (1992). Lithium, benzodiazepines and sexual function in bipolar patients. *American Journal of Psychiatry* **149**, 801–5.

Gilbert, D. G., Hagen, R. L. and D'Agostino, J. A. (1986). The effects of cigarette smoking on human sexual potency. *Addiction Behavior* **11**, 431–4.

Gitlin, M. J. (1994). Psychotropic medications and their effects on sexual function: diagnosis, biology and treatment approaches. *Journal of Clinical Psychiatry* **55**, 406–13.

Gitlin, M. J. (1995). Effects of depression and antidepressants on sexual functioning. *Bulletin of the Menninger Clinic* **59**, 232–48.

Glina, S., Reichelt, A. C., Leao, P. P. and DosReis, J. M. (1988). Impact of cigarette smoking on papaverine-induced erection. *Journal of Urology* **138**, 438–9.

Hypertension Detection and Follow up Program Cooperative Group. (1982). Five-year findings of the hypertension detection and follow up program. III. A reduction in stroke incidence among persons with high blood pressure. *Journal of the American Medical Association* **247**, 633–8.

Jachuck, S. J., Brierley, H., Jachuck, S. and Willcox, P. M. (1982). The effect of hypotensive drugs on the quality of life. *Journal of the Royal College of General Practitioners* **32**, 103–5.

Jensen, R. T., Collen, M. J. and Pandol, S. J. (1983). Cimetidine-induced impotence and breast changes in patients with gastric hypersecretory states. *New England Journal of Medicine* **308**, 883–7.

Kligman, S. and Higbee, M. D. (1989). Drug therapy for hypertension in the elderly. *Journal of Family Practice* **28**, 81–7.

Kostis, J. B., Rosen, R. C., Holzer, B. C., Randolph, C., Taska, L. S. and Miller, M. H. (1990). CNS side effects of centrally-active hypertensive agents: a prospective, placebo-controlled study of sleep, mood state and cognitive and sexual function in hypertensive males. *Psychopharmacology* **102**, 163–70.

Lamy, P. P. (1980). *Prescribing for the Elderly*. Littleton, MA: PSG Publishing Co.

Lane, R. M. (1997). A critical review of selective serotonin reuptake inhibitor-related sexual dysfunction: incidence, possible etiology and implications for management. *Journal of Psychopharmacology (Oxford)* **11**, 72–82.

Lingjaerde, O., Ahlfors, V., Bech, P., Dencker, S. and Elgen, K. (1987). The UKU side effect rating scale. *Acta Psychiatric Scandinavia* **76**, [Suppl 334] 11–77.

Lipson, L. G. (1985). Treatment of hypertension in diabetic men: problems with sexual dysfunction. *American Journal of Cardiology* **53**, 46A–50A.

Management Committee of the National Heart foundation of Australia. (1981). Treatment of mild hypertension in the elderly. *Medical Journal of Australia* 2, 398–402.

May, F. F., Steward, R. B., Hale, W. E. and Marks, R. G. (1982). Prescribed and nonprescribed drug use in an ambulatory elderly population. *Southern Medical Journal* 75, 522–8.

McHaffie, D. J., Guz, A. and Johnston, A. (1977). Impotence in patients on disopyranide. *Lancet* i, 859.

Medical Research Council Working Party. (1985). MRC trial of treatment of mild hypertension: principal results. *British Medical Journal* 291, 97–104.

Medical Research Council Working Party on Mild to Moderate Hypertension. (1981). Adverse reaction to bendrofluazide and propranolol for the treatment of mild hypertension. *Lancet* 2, 539–43.

Meiraz, D., Margolin, Y., Lev-Ran, A. and Lazebnik, J. (1977). Treatment of benign prostatic hyperplasia with hydroxyprogesterone-caproate. *Urology* 9, 144–8.

Morrissette, D. L., Skinner, M. H., Hoffman, B. B., Levine, K. E. and Davidson, J. M. (1993). Effects of antihypertensive drugs atenolol and nifedipine on sexual function in older men: a placebo-controlled, crossover study. *Archives of Sex Behavior* 22, 99–109.

Muller, S. C., El-Damanhoury, H., Ruth, J. and Lue, T. F. (1991). Hypertension and impotence. *European Urology* 19, 29–34.

Mulligan, T. and Katz, P. G. (1989). Why aged men become impotent. *Archives of Internal Medicine* 149, 1365–6.

Nakagawa, S., Watanabe, H. O. and Nakao, M. (1990). Sexual behavior in Japanese males relating to area of occupation, smoking, drinking and eating habits. *Andrologia* 22, 21–8.

Neri, A., Aygen, M., Zukerman, Z. and Baharh, L. (1980). Subjective assessment of sexual dysfunction of patients on long-term administration of digoxin. *Archives of Sexual Behavior* 9, 343–7.

Neri, A., Zukerman, Z., Aygen, M., Lidor, Y. and Kaufman, D. (1987). The effects of long-term administration of digoxin on plasma androgens and sexual dysfunction. *Journal of Sex and Marital Therapy* 18, 58–63.

Nofzinger, E. A., Thase, M. E., Reynolds, C. F., Frank, E., Jennings, J. R., Garamoni, G. L., Fasiczka, A. L. and Kupfer, D. J. (1993). Sexual function in depressed men: assessment by self report, behavioral and nocturnal penile tumescence measures before and after treatment with cognitive behavioral therapy. *Archives of General Psychiatry* 50, 24–30.

Nolan, L. and O'Malley, K. (1988). Prescribing for the elderly. Part I: Sensitivity of the elderly to adverse drug reactions. *Journal of the American Geriatrics Society* 36, 142–9.

Papadopoulos, C. (1989). Cardiovascular drugs and sexuality. In *Sexual Aspects of Cardiovascular Disease. Sexual Medicine* vol. 10, ed. C. Papadopoulos, pp 69–90. New York: Praeger Publishing.

Pavone-Macaluso, M., Serretta, V., Daricello, G. and Pavone, C. (1990). Is there a role for pure antiandrogens in the treatment of advanced prostatic cancer. *Progress in Clinical and Biological Research* 350, 149–58.

Roila, F. (1989). Buserelin in the treatment of prostatic cancer. *Biomedical Pharmacotherapy* 43, 279–85.

Rosen, R. C. (1991). Alcohol and drug effects on sexual response: human experimental and clinical studies. *Annual Review of Sex Research* 2, 119–80.

Rosen, R. C. and Weiner, D. N. (1997). Cardiovascular disease and sleep related erections. *Journal of Psychosomatic Research* 42, 517–30.

Rosen, R. C., Kostis, J. B. and Jekelis, A. W. (1988). Beta-blocker effects on sexual function in normal males. *Archives of Sexual Behavior* 17, 241–55.

Rowland, D. L., Myers, L., Culver, A. and Davidson, J. M. (1997). Bupropion and sexual function: a placebo controlled prospective study on diabetic men with erectile dysfunction. *Journal of Clinical Psychopharmacology* 17, 350–7.

Salzman, C. and Nevis-Olesen, J. (1992). Psychopharmacologic treatment. In *Handbook of Mental Health and Aging*, 2nd edn, pp. 721–58. New York: Academic Press.

Schiavi, R. C. and Segraves, R. T. (1995). The biology of sexual function. *Psychiatric Clinics of North America* 18, 7–23.

Segraves, R. T. (1989). Effects of psychotropic drugs on human erection and ejaculation. *Archives of General Psychiatry* 46, 275–84.

Segraves, R. T. (1992). Overview of sexual dysfunction complicating the treatment of depression. *Journal of Clinical Psychiatry Monograph* 10, 4–10.

Segraves, R. T. and Segraves, K. (1992). Aging and drug effects on male sexuality. In *Erectile Disorders, Assessment and Treatment*, ed. R. C. Rosen and S. R. Leiblum, pp. 96–138. New York: The Guilford Press.

Slag, M. F., Morley, J. E., Elson, M. K., Trence, D. L., Nelson, C. J., Nelson, A. E., Kinlaw, W. B., Beyer, S., Nuttall, F. Q. and Shafer, R. B. (1983). Impotence in medical clinic outpatients. *Journal of the American Medical Association* 249, 1736–40.

Soldo, B. J. and Agree, E. M. (1988). *Population Bulletin America's Elderly*, vol. 43, no. 3. Washington, DC: Population Reference Bureau, Inc.

Spark, R. F. and Melby, J. C. (1968). Aldosteronism in hypertension. *Annals of Internal Medicine* 69, 685–91.

Stevenson, J. G. and Umstead, G. S. (1984). Sexual dysfunction due to antihypertensive agents. *Drug Intelligence and Clinical Pharmacy* 18, 113–21.

Stewart, R. B. (1988). Drug use in the elderly. In *Therapeutics in the Elderly*, ed. J. C. Delafuente and R. B. Stewart, pp. 50–63. Baltimore, MD: Williams and Wilkins.

Task Force on Prescription of Drugs. (1968). *US Department of Health, Education and Welfare: The Drug Users*, Washington, DC: US Government Printing Office.

Thase, M. E., Nofzinger, E., Reynolds, C. F. III, Fasiczka, A. L., Jennings, J. R. and Frank, E. (1994). Effect of antidepressant treatment on sexual function in depressed men. *Psychopharmacology Bulletin* 30, 83.

The Working Group on Hypertension in the Elderly. (1986). Statement on hypertension in the elderly. *Journal of the American Medical Association* 256, 70–4.

Veterans Administration Cooperative Study Group on Antihypertensive Agents. (1982). Comparison of propranolol and hydrochlorthiazide for the initial treatments of hypertension. *Journal of the American Medical Association* 248, 2004–11.

Wade, B. and Bowling, A. (1986). Appropriate use of drugs by elderly people. *Journal of Advanced Nursing* 11, 47–55.

Wassertheil-Smoller, S., Blaufox, M. D., Oberman, A., Davis, B. R., Swencionis, C., O'Connell, M., Hawkins, C. M., Langford, H. G. for the TAIM Research Group. (1991). Effect of anti-hypertensives on sexual function and quality of life: the TAIM study. *Annals of Internal Medicine* 114, 613–20.

Williams, G. H. (1988). Beyond blood pressure control. Effect of antihypertensive therapy on quality of life. *American Journal of Hypertension* 1, 363S–365S.

Williams, G. H., Croog, S. H., Levine, S., Testa, M. A. and Sudilousky, A. (1987). Impact of anti-hypertensive therapy on quality of life: effect of hydrochlorothiazide. *Journal of Hypertension* 5 [Suppl 1], 529–35.

Wilton, L., Pearce, G., Edet, E., Freemantle, S., Stephens, M. D. and Mann, R. D. (1996). The safety of finasteride used in benign prostatic hypertrophy: a non-interventional observational cohort study in 14772 patients. *British Journal of Urology* 78, 379–84.

Young, R. C. and Meyers, B. S. (1996). Psychopharmacology. In *Comprehensive Review of Geriatric Psychiary*, 2nd edn, ed. J. Sadavoy, L. W. Lazarus, L. F. Jarvik and G. T. Grossberg, pp. 755–99. Washington, DC: American Association of Geriatric Psychiatry.

12   Role of psychosocial factors; coping and adaptation

The sexuality of aging is best understood by considering physiological evidence, personal history and beliefs, individual circumstances, and sociocultural expectations, throughout the individual's life. Aging is viewed traditionally in the Western world as a decline and loss: decline of functional capacities and loss of close attachments, health, and social status. This pessimistic, but culturally ingrained, view is consistent with several studies which found that the most common major life events reported by the aged are medical problems and illness or death of the spouse (Ruth and Coleman, 1996). Decline models of aging have been balanced most recently by models that emphasize processes of adaptation, as reflected by the perceived quality of life of people in their older years. This adaptation, positive or negative, is shaped by personal commitments, cognitive appraisal and coping responses, in keeping with the significance of events in the context of the person's life.

We have discussed, in preceding chapters, the impact that a wide range of medical illnesses and drugs have on male sexual function. We will now elaborate on the relationship between aging and disease as well as the processes of adaptation and their relevance to individual well-being, contentment, and health-care behaviors. There is a vast amount of literature in these areas, most of it recently published. However, its relevance to human sexuality has been neglected and there is virtually no research on psychosocial geriatrics and health–behavior relationships pertinent to male sexuality. The discussion that follows is oriented by a model pictured in Figure 12.1. It focuses on several processes: the association between aging and chronic illness, the relevance of appraisal and coping mechanisms to sexual changes in aging and to the consequences of disease, and finally on the adaptive and health-care consequences of these interactions.

Aging and chronic illness

The increase in life expectation due, in part, to the successful treatment of acute medical illnesses, based upon the one-germ, one-disease, one-treatment model, has been paralleled by an elevated prevalence of chronic disease. Chronic disorders, such as cardiovascular disease, cancer and diabetes, contribute to eight of the ten most common causes of death in the elderly population. These diseases as well as

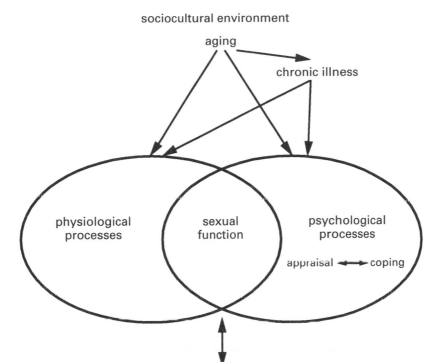

sociocultural environment

Figure 12.1   A framework of psychosexual adaptation to aging and chronic illness. Reproduced in modified form from Anderson and Wolf (1986) *Journal of Consulting and Clinical Psychology* **54**, 168–75, with permission from American Psychological Association, Washington DC.

other chronic conditions such as arthritis, bone disease, visual and hearing impairments markedly limit the quality of life in later years. The close interrelation between aging, chronic illness and disability has fostered a negative view of aging and the perception of aging as a medical problem.

It is important for clinical and research reasons to draw a distinction between disease and aging. Busse (1969) defined primary aging as irreversible changes inherent to the aging process and distinguished it from secondary aging, caused by illness-induced changes that are correlated with age but usually reversible. According to Kohn (1985), changes that occur during normal aging are universal, progressive and inevitable and occur even under optimal genetic and environmental circumstances. There is considerable evidence of age-related physiological declines in variables considered to represent 'normal aging', such as bone density, cardiovascular and pulmonary function, in individuals carefully selected to exclude pathological conditions. To this list we may add age-related decreases in male sexual arousal assessed physiologically during wakefulness and sleep in nondiseased individuals as discussed in Chapter 3.

There is marked physiological variability that often increases as age progresses, not only between individuals but also among organ systems within the same individual. Rowe and Devons (1996) discuss the importance of differentiating, within the 'normal', nonpathological group, two subsets. One subgroup of individuals is described as aging 'successfully', and is characterized by minimal age-related physiological losses and optimal functional adjustment. The other is a larger subgroup, termed the 'usual aging group', with significant impairments that place them at risk of disease and disability. The interaction between aging and disease may be viewed as a continuum from age-related physiological alterations without clinical relevance, to changes that have direct clinical consequence. An example of a physiological change without obvious clinical relevance is the decrease in testosterone secretion with increasing age, which, unless it reaches threshold levels, is inconsequential for male sexual behavior. An example from the opposite end of the spectrum is arteriosclerosis, a thickening of the arterial walls which may be considered 'normal' because it is unavoidable and occurs universally with advancing age, but that has direct clinical impact as manifested by increased systolic blood pressure and possibly by decreased erectile capacity.

Distinguishing between aging and disease has theoretical and clinical relevance. Conceptually, dichotomous views of health and illness derived from medical tradition are given ground to a paradigm shift that avoids placing elderly people in arbitrary diagnostic categories. Instead their status is assessed by the progress of any pathophysiological change and their adaptive response to it. Clinically, the nature and effectiveness of adaptive responses are critically important for successful individual adjustment to chronic illness, as evidenced by the preservation of functional capacities and inner contentment. In addition, evidence that habits and life-style factors such as smoking, heavy drinking and diet contribute to decrements in sexual function, previously considered as an intrinsic aspect of aging, opens a new perspective within the scope of behavioral medicine on the modifiable contributors to the sexual problems of the aging male (McKinlay and Feldman, 1994).

Appraisal and coping

Individuals, as they age, variously experience changes in their appearance, physical capacity, physiological function, health, interpersonal relationships, and social status. Sexuality is closely interwoven with each of these aspects, since it is influenced by, and in turn shapes, the subjects' reactions to them. Lazarus and Folkman (1994) worked out a conceptual framework, based on cognitive theory, that is valuable for understanding the highly individualized process of aging. Two interrelated processes are considered: appraisal and coping.

Cognitive appraisal

This is defined as how a person construes the significance of an event for his or her well-being. How the individual appraises a situation influences the impact of the event, the emotional, physiological and behavioral reactions, and the way of coping with it. A particular situation is considered threatening or stressful when it is viewed as taxing or exceeding the person's adaptive resources. External factors that shape appraisal include the strength and imminence of an event, and ambiguity. Obvious sexual examples of situational influences are the degree and rate of change in erectile function and the anticipated partner's reaction to it. However, it is not merely the presence of external stressors but also their subjective meaning or significance viewed in the context of the individual's life that affects adaptation. Personal factors include motivational characteristics, beliefs about self and the world, and intellectual resources and skills. The nature and strength of motivations and commitments determine vulnerability, and influence expectations and the appraisal of a threat. The degree of threat posed by an age-related decline in sexual performance depends on the value placed on sex by the individual, the extent of their sexual interest and its significance for personal relationships. Declines in sexual performance may be ignored or considered irrelevant when they happen at the same time as sexual interest diminishes or when sexual expression becomes less of a priority in a relationship. Beliefs, as defined by Lazarus and Folkman (1994), are personally formed or culturally determined notions about reality that help to organize the appraisal of situations and shape their interpretation. A common and deeply ingrained belief places sexual behavior at the center of individuals' identity, sense of value and worth. Age-related and disease- or drug-induced changes in sexual function may be appraised as stressful or threatening to the extent that they challenge self-identity and self-esteem. Beliefs about personal control also influence stress appraisal depending on the individual's conviction that they have the resources for effective coping and that the environment will be responsive to it. A change in sexual function may be particularly threatening since its meaning is frequently ambiguous and the individual's own perception of control uncertain. Cognitive appraisal is also influenced by the prevailing cultural belief that a decline in sexual function is the result of growing old, ignoring the deleterious effect of illness or, conversely, by attributing to illness what is actually a natural physiological decrease in sexual function.

Case vignette: Mr. R, a 66-year-old, divorced, successful business man derived considerable pride from his appearance, his excellent physical shape, and his list of sexual conquests. Sexuality was an important component of his self-esteem, as was his need to maintain control over life situations. Although he was having intercourse regularly with different partners, he was distressed by a small but gradual decrease in erectile capacity. He was action oriented and not prone to introspection. He reacted by self-medicating with multivitamins, engaging in a strenuous course of physical exercise and finally by concluding that 'there is something physically wrong with me'. Mr. R was not persuaded by the repeatedly negative medical and urological findings and decided to have a penile prosthetic implant. He was reassured by the predictability of his postsurgical erectile capacity but disappointed by the less-than-enthusiastic reception by his partners.

Coping

Coping is defined as, 'constantly changing cognitive and behavioral efforts to manage specific external and/or internal demands that are appraised as taxing or exceeding the resources of the person' (Lazarus and Folkman, 1994). Coping strategies may be divided into two groups according to their function: one aims at changing the environment or manipulating the conditions that generate the threat (problem solving), and the other involves individual processes directed at minimizing emotional distress generated by the threat (emotion-regulating coping). Problem-focused coping is directed at the environment, altering external pressures, or at the self. Examples of problem-oriented coping are the gathering of sexual information, discussing sexual concerns with the spouse, engaging in experiences that enhance sexual arousal, developing coital strategies that compensate for the decline in sexual function, finding alternative modes of gratification, and seeking consultation and treatment.

Among the emotion-focused forms of coping directed at lessening emotional distress are strategies such as avoidance, minimization, denial, selective attention and cognitive reappraisal, where the meaning of a situation is changed without altering objective reality. Examples of emotion-regulating coping include cognitive restructuring (accepting a decrease in sexual functioning as a natural aspect of aging), minimizing the value of sexuality, focusing on personal attributes or activities that makes a person advantaged compared to others, sexual avoidance, projection of the source of the sexual difficulty onto the partner, and denial of sexual changes. Denial of sexual changes may be related to denial of aging as individuals strive to maintain younger self-images compared to the stereotyped characteristics of old persons (Bultena and Powers, 1978).

Problem- and emotion-focused coping functions often occur concurrently. In a study of coping in a middle-aged community sample (Folkman and Lazarus, 1980), problem-solving and emotion-focused coping were both used in response to stressful events of daily living over the course of one year. Problem- and emotion-focused coping were influenced differently by situational factors such as the context and persons involved in the coping event, and how it was appraised. Situations that were assessed as requiring more information or that could be modified favored problem-focused coping, whereas those that the person thought had to be accepted favored emotion-focused coping. Emotion-focused coping was used more frequently in response to physical illness and disability, to minimize anxiety and fear and to enhance interpersonal relationships. The following example illustrates the sequential use of emotion and problem-focused coping.

Case vignette: Sexuality was an important component of marital adjustment and satisfaction for this older couple. The onset of diabetes, accompanied by a marked decrease in erectile capacity, was extremely disturbing to Mr. S who reacted by withdrawing emotionally and abusing alcohol during the increasingly frequent evenings spent 'with the boys'. Attempts by his wife to discuss the sexual problem were met with anger and denial. Ms. S finally confronted her husband with an 'ultimatum': either he would refrain from alcohol use and take better care managing his diabetes or she would move to her sister's home. His acceptance to join a diabetic couples' support group was considerably helpful, and they learnt about the disease, seeking effective medical treatment, fostering marital communication about the sexual problem, and eventually developing alternate modes of sexual gratification. His coping responses shifted from emotional withdrawal and denial to an active, problem-solving confrontation of his sexual disability.

Aging and coping

Evidence of change in coping strategies over a lifetime is inconsistent. Earlier investigations suggest that age-related differences in coping are a function of the different types of stressors associated with aging rather than age per se (Folkman and Lazarus, 1980; McCrae, 1982). Recent evidence (Folkman et al., 1987), comparing younger and older people, showed that younger subjects use proportionally more interpersonal, problem-based forms of coping (problem solving, confrontation, seeking social support) and that older subjects use proportionally more passive, intrapersonal, emotion-oriented ways of coping (distancing, acceptance of responsibility and positive reappraisal). These findings held up regardless of differences in the nature of the encounters experienced by both age groups. It would appear that the coping strategies of the younger and older groups are developmentally appropriate to their stage of life, with the older people appraising life events as less changeable compared with their younger counterparts. Brandtstadter and Renner (1990) distinguished two alternative modes of coping that are possibly relevant to aging and sexuality: assimilative coping and accommodative coping. Discrepancies between actual and desired preferences in personal development over a life-time can be eliminated by actively modifying one's circumstances to personal preferences (assimilative coping) or by adjusting personal preferences and expectations to situational constraints (accommodative coping). Accommodative coping includes adjusting one's aspirations, using cognitive reappraisal to change the meaning of an event, and modifying self-criticism. The authors provided cross-sectional evidence, from a sample of 890 subjects aged 34–63 years, of a gradual shift with increasing age from assimilative to accommodative strategies of coping. The increasing dominance of accommodative modes of coping with age may account for the maintenance of well-being and sexual satisfaction despite the increased occurrence of aversive events during the later stages of life.

There is some evidence that reminiscence, defined as reviewing personal memories of a distant past, has adaptational value (Butler, 1974). Wong and Watt (1991) developed a taxonomy of reminiscence which they applied to the study of successful aging, defined as higher than average mental and personal health and adjustment. Successful agers engaged in significantly more integrative reminiscence (accepting one's past as worthwhile, reconciling the discrepancy between ideal and reality) and instrumental reminiscence (recollecting past attempts at overcoming difficulties) and in less obsessive reminiscence (ruminations on problematic past experiences) than their unsuccessful counterparts. Although causality is not demonstrated, this study is consistent with the adaptive benefit of positive reappraisal in aging.

Case vignette: Mr. and Ms. T described a stable and successful marriage. After a passionate few years during the early stages of their life together, they had settled into a comfortable relationship characterized by satisfying companionship but only sporadic sexual interactions. Following his retirement at age 68, Mr. T, a lawyer who had had multiple affairs during the course of his successful career, found himself shifting to a more contemplative life-style that included pursuing his vocation as a short-story writer. He began incorporating memories of his past extramarital experiences into his stories and, much to Ms. T's surprise, became increasingly active sexually, having found his sexual interest in her reawakened. He indicated, in private, that his hectic sexual life was a thing of the past and expressed some regret at having ignored the pleasure of a more sedate marital sexual life.

Coping with chronic disease

Moos (1977), in a study of coping with physical illness, identified the following problem focused and emotion focused strategies: (1) seeking relevant information, (2) setting concrete, limited goals, (3) rehearsing alternate outcomes to the problem, (4) seeking emotional support and reassurance from others, (5) denying or minimizing the seriousness of the problem and (6) searching for a generalized purpose or meaning of the event. Felton, Revenson and Hinrichsen (1984), in a factor-analyzing study of coping responses of middle-aged and older adults with chronic illnesses, identified six dimensions: (1) information seeking, (2) cognitive restructuring, (3) emotional expression, (4) wish-fulfilling fantasy, (5) self-blame and (6) minimizing threat. Some, but not all, of these strategies contribute to positive adaptation and are components of comprehensive treatment approaches to the sexual problems of the aged (see Chapter 14). It has been stated that older people use a wide repertoire of coping strategies, and that it is not age but the specific demands of the illness, and personal beliefs and characteristics that determine their response (Felton and Revenson, 1984). Other investigators, however, have noted age-related differences in coping with chronic illness, but the nature of the differences varied across studies. Older people have been described as engaging in more health-promoting practices and are more likely to comply with therapeutic regimens (Prohaska et al., 1985). Conversely, they have been described as being more passive than younger adults and less likely to seek help or information, or use other such active strategies to cope with chronic disorders (Felton and Revenson, 1987). Felton and Revenson (1987) have shown that affective responses to chronic illness decrease with age. Also, it has been suggested (Neugarten and Datan, 1973) that their anticipating health-related stresses and declining health expectations may make the aged less emotionally reactive than younger individuals to the insults of illness.

The cross-sectional design of most of these studies needs to be considered when interpreting the data. For example, the reported age-related decrease in information-seeking may be a cohort effect, insofar as people born at the beginning of the twentieth century may have been socialized into greater self-reliance and may be less prone to seek health assistance. The specific type of chronic disease has frequently been ignored as contributing to differences in cognitive appraisal. The nature of the chronic illnesses and their treatment are likely to be variously associated with appraisals of the threat to gender and sexual identity, body image, personal control over body functions and sexual intimacy, and to be an important determinant of coping responses (Anderson and Wolf, 1986). Decreased erectile function, for example, may impair self-worth, resulting in sexual avoidance when caused by diabetes, or may lead to poor medication compliance when interpreted as being caused by treatment of hypertension.

Adaptational outcomes

Discrepant definitions of successful adaptation are reflected in the many different outcome measures that have been used. Recently, emphasis has been placed on multicriteria approaches that incorporate subjective as well as objective indicators of a successful outcome (Baltes and Baltes, 1990). The most frequently studied aspects of coping adaptiveness in older people are satisfaction with life, social relationships, and health. Palmore and Kivett (1977) conducted a longitudinal study of changes in satisfaction with life among a sample of 378 community residents,

46–70 years old. Life satisfaction was assessed in relation to self-rated health, social activities, 'productive hours' measured by the number of hours spent working, and sexual enjoyment. There were no significant changes in average life satisfaction for the total group within the four-year period of the study, although substantial changes were noted in about one-quarter of the subjects. Significant predictors of life satisfaction were self-rated health, sexual enjoyment and number of hours spent in social activity. However, other authors (Larson, 1978; Diener, 1984) have noted low and inconsistent relationships between life satisfaction and objective indicators, such as social status, wealth and health. Costa and McCrae (1980) suggested that individuals tend to habituate to distressing conditions of life and to develop personal norms that shape their subjective experiences to a greater extent than objective reality. The frequently noted persistence of life or sexual satisfaction despite age or illness-induced functional declines may be viewed, within the cognitive framework, as a form of emotion-focused coping.

There is evidence that social relationships play a significant, mediating impact on adaptation to stress. Weiss (1983), for example, examined the effect of intimacy, operationally defined and measured, on adaptation to major life stressors in a sample of community volunteers aged 21–72 years old. Older people who were not very intimate with their spouses were less apt to adapt to increasing stress. The mediating effect of intimacy on adaptation to stress was not observed in younger people and was less effective among friends than among older married couples. The results suggest that intimacy between older couples may have a mediating or buffering influence on adaptation to stress.

It is difficult to assess the adaptability of coping outcomes to illness, because of differences in the nature of the disease, the time frame of the study, personal characteristics and how coping is measured. Among the factors identified by Cohen and Lazarus (1983) as relevant variables for an adaptive outcome are active versus passive coping strategies, personal control and expression versus inhibition of emotion. Their adaptive effectiveness depend to a large extent on when the assessment is made (illness stage), under what circumstances (hospitalized or outpatient) and on the controllability of physical progress and medical routines. It is important to note that successful adaptation in some measures may be achieved at the expense of other adaptive outcomes.

Case vignette: Mr. and Ms. U had a committed relationship and had accommodated to a lack of sexual experiences caused by his organic erectile dysfunction and her postmenopausal loss of sexual interest. However, following involuntary retirement, Mr. U, prompted by a TV program on erectile impotence, decided, without discussion with his wife, to be evaluated for a penile prosthetic implant. The surgical restoration of coital capacity markedly enhanced his self-esteem but led to a significant destabilization of marital adjustment.

Health-care behaviors

The notion of health-care behavior encompasses the manner in which people perceive bodily changes, interpret their symptoms, adopt remedial measures, and utilize the health-care system (Mechanic, 1983). The sociocultural environment shapes individual beliefs about the nature of the aging process and determines how older people view their physical problems and the actions they contemplate. Epidemiological surveys have found that the nature and severity of physical symptoms, the degree of distress, gender, inclination to use medical facilities and faith in doctors are significant factors in health-care behaviors (Siegler and Costa, 1990). These surveys are, however, of limited value in explaining individual differences in the help-seeking process. The way bodily changes are perceived and how individuals evaluate their symptoms, attribute them to physical or psychological causes, and make health decisions are important for understanding behavior during illness. There is considerable evidence that psychological distress enhances the probability of seeking medical care. Labeling a vague bodily complaint as a symptom of illness and searching for health-care may be, for some, a culturally acceptable way of coping with stressful events and seeking external support. Many symptoms and illnesses are highly prevalent in the population and do not prompt people to seek treatment; this decision is frequently triggered by events surrounding the perception of symptoms (Mechanic, 1983). This is exemplified by the, not too uncommon, observation of older men with a nonpathological, age-related, long-standing decline in sexual function whose search for help with the self-diagnosis of 'impotence' is precipitated by a marital crisis, retirement or work-related difficulties.

Among the factors that influence individual appraisal and patients' responses are the ambiguity and perceived seriousness of the symptoms, the knowledge and cultural assumptions of the person, and the existence of needs or beliefs that interfere with the acceptance of an illness' definition. For example, men may ignore urological symptoms or delay seeking treatment for fear that prostatic cancer will be diagnosed or that their surgical treatment will result in erectile impotence. There are limited data on how these factors influence the health practices of the aged. Elderly adults, in a health survey (Prohaska et al., 1985), considered themselves more vulnerable to disease than younger respondents and reported higher frequencies of health-promoting practices and avoidance of emotional stress. It has been proposed that older persons are averse to taking risks, and that they engage in active coping to minimize the intensity of the emotional reactions and negative affects associated with illness (Leventhal, Leventhal and Schaefer, 1992). However, bodily changes or symptoms that are ambiguous or that occur slowly may be attributed to age rather than to illness. There is evidence that older persons are more likely to self-diagnose vague symptoms of slow onset as signs of aging, an attribution that may lead to a delay in seeking treatment (Prohaska et al., 1987). They may attribute a gradual decline in erectile function to aging, for example, ignoring a change that is symptomatic of a serious problem, such as diabetes.

The extent to which an individual attributes a change in sexual function to physical illness, psychological distress or aging determines the care they may seek. The assessment of the patient's condition by health-care professionals is the outcome of a selective flow influenced not only by signs and symptoms but also by the attitudes of the patient and the orientation of the clinic. Frequently ignored in the literature of health behavior is the concept of self-care. Self-care has been defined as the range of health and illness behavior engaged by individuals on behalf of their own health (Dean, 1992). It reflects findings from adult populations that a large proportion of symptoms are not brought to the attention of the medical care system but are treated by individuals and their lay networks (Dean, 1984; Haug, Wykle and Namazi, 1989). Self-care behaviors may include self-medication, sex manuals, home remedies, dietary practices, alcohol abuse, participation in health-care programs or avoidance behaviors, such as discontinuation of prescribed medications. Self-care is an important aspect of health-related behavior concerning chronic illness and aging sexuality that has yet to be investigated.

Conclusion

Individuals do not suddenly become old. Growing old is a process shaped by adaptational responses to biological changes and internal and external conditions as the individuals strive to maintain continuity in their life and to adjust their priorities to the altered meaning of events and experiences as they grow old. The individuals' success at preserving self-worth, self-esteem and satisfaction with life depends, in some measure, on how they appraise sexual changes, sexual commitments and beliefs, and on the nature of their coping responses. Successful coping in the aged may not only depend on modifying external circumstances but also on adjusting personal preferences and expectations to situational constraints, and on developing compensatory strategies to maximize adaptation. The frequently reported persistence of well-being and sexual satisfaction despite marked functional declines demonstrates the importance of exploring the cognitive and emotional significance of sexuality for the aged rather than interpreting sexual changes according to performance-oriented agendas. Cognitive theory provides a heuristic framework for understanding adaptation throughout life, including the impact of illness on behavior. How individuals appraise bodily changes, evaluate and label their symptoms determine in great measure the interaction with the health-care professions and the perspective that will orient their medical evaluation and treatment.

References

Anderson, B. J. and Wolf, F. M. (1986). Chronic physical illness and sexual behavior: psychological issues. *Journal of Consulting and Clinical Psychology* 54, 168–75.

Baltes, P. B, and Baltes, M. M. (1990). Psychological perspectives on successful aging: the model of selective optimization with compensation. In *Successful Aging: Perspectives for the Behavioral Sciences*, ed. P. B. Baltes and M. M. Baltes, pp. 1–34. Cambridge, UK: Cambridge University Press.

Brandtstadter, J. and Renner, G. (1990). Tenacious goal pursuit and flexible goal adjustment: explication and age-related analysis of assimilative and accommodative strategies of coping. *Psychology of Aging* 5, 58–67.

Bultena, G. L. and Powers, E. A. (1978). Denial of aging: age identifications and reference group orientations. *Journal of Gerontology* 33, 748–54.

Busse, E. W. (1969). Theories of aging. In *Behavior and Adaptation in Later Life*, ed. E. W. Busse and E. Pfeiffer, pp. 11–32. Boston, MA: Little Brown.

Butler, R. N. (1974). Successful aging and the role of the life review. *Journal of the American Geriatrics Society* 22, 529–35.

Cohen, F. and Lazarus, R. S. (1983). Coping and adaptation in health and illness. In *Handbook of Health, Health Care and the Health Professions*, ed. D. Mechanic, pp. 608–35. New York: The Free Press.

Costa, P. T. Jr. and McCrae, R. R. (1980). Influence of extraversion and neuroticism on subjective well-being: happy and unhappy people. *Journal of Personality and Social Psychology* 38, 668–74.

Dean, K. (1984). Influence of health beliefs on lifestyles: what do we know? *European Monographs in Health Education Research* 6, 127–51.

Dean, K. (1992). Health-related behavior: concepts and methods. In *Aging, Health and Behavior*, ed. M. G. Ory, R. P. Abeles and P. D. Lipman, pp. 27–56. Newbury Park: Sage Publication.

Diener, E. (1984). Subjective well-being. *Psychological Bulletin* 95, 542–75.

Felton, B. J. and Revenson, T. A. (1984). Coping with chronic illness: a study of illness controllability and the influence of coping strategies on psychological adjusment. *Journal of Consulting and Clinical Psychology* 52, 343–53.

Felton, B. J. and Revenson, T. A. (1987). Age differences in coping with chronic illness. *Psychology and Aging* 2, 164–70.

Felton, B. J., Revenson, T. A. and Hinrichsen, G. A. (1984). Stress and coping in the explanation of psychological adjustment among chronically ill adults. *Social Science Medicine* 18, 889–98.

Folkman, S. and Lazarus, R. S. (1980). An analysis of coping in a middle-aged community sample. *Journal of Health and Social Behavior* 21, 219–39.

Folkman, S., Lazarus, R. S., Pimley, S. and Novack, J. (1987). Age differences in stress and coping processes. *Psychology of Aging* 2, 171–84.

Haug, M. R., Wykle, M. L. and Namazi, K. H. (1989). Self-care among older adults. *Social Science and Medicine* 29, 171–84.

Kohn, R. R. (1985). Aging and age-related diseases: normal processes. In *Relations between Normal Aging and Disease*, ed. H. A. Johnson, pp. 1–43. New York: Raven Press.

Larson, R. (1978). Thirty years of research on the subjective well being of older Americans. *Journal of Gerontology* 33, 109–25.

Lazarus, R. S. and Folkman, S. (1994). *Stress, Appraisal and Coping.* New York: Springer Publishing Company.

Leventhal, H., Leventhal, E. A. and Schaefer, P. M. (1992). Vigilant coping and health behavior. In *Aging, Health and Behavior,* ed. M. G. Ory, R. P. Abeles and P. D. Lipman, pp. 109–39. Newbury Park: Sage Publishing.

McCrae, R. R. (1982). Age differences in the use of coping mechanisms. *Journal of Gerontology* 37, 454–60.

McKinlay, J. B. and Feldman, H. A. (1994). Age-related variation in sexual activity and interest in normal men: results from the Massachusetts Male Aging Study. In *Sexuality Across the Life Course,* ed. A. S. Rossi, pp. 261–85. Chicago, IL: University of Chicago Press.

Mechanic, D. (1983). The experience and expression of distress: the study of illness behavior and medical utilization. In *Handbook of Health, Healthcare and the Health professions,* ed. D. Mechanic, pp. 591–60. New York: The Free Press.

Moos, R. (1977). *Coping with Physical Illness.* New York: Plenum Press.

Neugarten, B. L. and Datan, N. (1973). Sociological perspectives on the life cycle. In *Life-span Developmental Psychology: Personality and Socialization,* ed. P. B. Baltes and K. W. Schaie, pp. 53–69. New York: Academic Press.

Palmore, E. and Kivett, V. (1977). Change in life satisfaction: a longitudinal study of persons aged 46–70. *Journal of Gerontology* 32, 311–16.

Prohaska, T. R., Leventhal, E. A., Leventhal, H. and Keller, M. L. (1985). Health practices and illness cognition in young, middle aged and elderly adults. *Journal of Gerontology* 40, 569–78.

Prohaska, T. R., Keller, M. L., Leventhal, E. A. and Leventhal, H. (1987). Impact of symptoms and aging attributions on emotions and coping. *Health Psychology* 6, 495–514.

Rowe, J. W. and Devons, C. A. J. (1996). Physiological and clinical considerations of the geriatric patient. In *The APA Textbook of Geriatric Psychiatry,* ed. E. W. Busse and D. G. Blazer, pp. 25–47. Washington DC: American Psychiatric Press.

Ruth, J.-E. and Coleman, P. (1996). Personality and aging: coping and management of the self in later life. In *Handbook of the Psychology of Aging,* 4th edn, ed. J. E. Birren and K. W. Schaie, pp. 308–22. San Diego: Academic Press.

Siegler, I. C. and Costa, P. T. (1990). Health behavior relationships. In *Handbook of the Psychology of Aging,* ed. E. Birren and K. W. Schaie, pp. 144–66. San Diego: Academic Press.

Weiss, L. J. (1983). Intimacy and adaptation. In *Sexuality in the Later Years: Roles and behavior,* ed. R. B. Weg, pp. 147–66. New York: Academic Press.

Wong, P. T. P. and Watt, L. M. (1991). What types of reminiscence are associated with successful aging? *Psychology and Aging* 6, 272–9.

13   Assessment of sexual problems

Population surveys have consistently shown in cross-sectional analysis a decrease in sexual function, primarily erectile capacity, associated with aging in men. Individual responses, as discussed in the previous chapter, are variably shaped by attitudes and expectations that contribute personal significance to the sexual change. Although the aged with sexual complaints approach the health-care system in increasing numbers, the majority of older men do not seek sexual help, even though they may experience significant decrements in sexual function (Feldman et al., 1994). Slag et al. (1983) screened over 1000 patients in a medical outpatient clinic for the presence of erectile dysfunction and found that half of the patients with erectile difficulties declined to be examined for this problem. The investigators speculated that older age and the greater number of medical problems noted in this subgroup of patients may have contributed to their lack of interest in pursuing evaluation of their sexual difficulties.

There is limited information on the reasons that lead men to seek clinical assistance for their sexual concerns. Perez, Mulligan and Wan (1993) conducted a large survey of a random sample of male veterans aged 30–99 to assess variables that may contribute to their interest in a sexual evaluation. A hierarchical regression analysis that included measures of sexual function, emotional state, physical state and demographic characteristics showed that the perception of erectile and orgastic difficulties only partially predicted the desire to be referred for medical assessment. Diminished sexual interest and demographic traits (older age, never married, and nonwhite) had significant negative effects on men's motivation to seek a sexual evaluation. The observation that, in this regression model, 40% of predictive significance for interest in a sexual evaluation remained unexplained demonstrates the complexity of the factors involved when deciding whether to seek sexual help.

Clinical experience shows that a wide range of psychological and relationship factors, in addition to a decline in sexual capacity, may trigger the decision to contact the health-care system with a sexual complaint. Common contributors to sexual dissatisfaction in older men are emotional depression, marital difficulties and life experiences, such as physical problems or retirement, that challenge the individual's self-worth and self-esteem. The evaluation of a sexual complaint, primarily erectile problems, is frequently flawed by the tendency to diagnose patients into mutually exclusive psychogenic or organic categories. Attempts have been made to avoid this dichotomous approach by categorizing dysfunctional patients on a bipolar scale from primarily organic to primarily psychogenic. Inherent in this conceptualization is the risk of ignoring alternative contributors to the dysfunction once a physiological or psychological cause has been identified. For example, for an older men a moderate impairment in the vascular supply to the penis may render him vulnerable to erectile problems in response to psychological difficulties. The decision to engage in an invasive intervention may result in the neglect of psychological approaches to try and restore his sexual function. Conceptually, the literature on the evaluation of male sexual problems is influenced by a categorical (either–or) and mechanistic (single cause–single effect) approach to health and illness. In recent years a dramatic turnabout has been taking place, with traditional boundaries between disciplines being bridged and new interdisciplinary fields, such as behavioral medicine, emerging. This shift reflects the realization that problems of health and illness are complex, best addressed by adopting a multifactorial, interactive conceptual and research model that includes biological, psychological and social determinants (Schwartz, 1982). This systemic approach, characteristic of behavioral medicine, has yet to be fully applied to the area of sexual dysfunction.

Older patients with sexual complaints are likely to approach their primary care physician first. Their sexual concerns may remain unexpressed unless the clinician, in a sensitive and nonjudgmental manner, offers an opportunity for sexual discussion in the context of the overall medical evaluation. Although sexual problems commonly occur in patients with chronic illness, they are infrequently identified and addressed in daily clinical practice (Schover and Jensen, 1988). Clinicians' conflicting attitudes about exploring the sexuality of older individuals, lack of expertise and practical limitations of time all contribute to the avoidance of sexual issues. The primary care-giver is well placed to address sexual concerns, identify the existence of sexual problems, and provide limited sexual counseling (Kligman, 1991; Schover, 1992). In practice, patients with sexual disorders, primarily of erectile nature, are frequently referred to specialized centers where, depending on their type, they may follow different evaluation pathways. Ideally, a comprehensive evaluation of the sexual disorders of older patients is best implemented in multidisciplinary clinics where there is integrated access to medical, urological and psychological expertise (Tiefer and Melman, 1989; Buvat et al., 1990). While there is no universally agreed diagnostic protocol, a problem-oriented sexual, medical and psychosocial history is an essential component of the evaluation of male patients with sexual problems.

The assessment interview

The main objectives of the clinical interview are to inquire about the sexual complaint, identify the existence and course of the sexual problem, explore the causes and contributing factors to the disorder and begin to elaborate possible strategies of intervention.

The nature and course of the sexual problem

The sexual dissatisfaction that triggers the call for help of older couples may not necessarily be due to a sexual dysfunction, but may reflect faulty sexual expectations or individual or relationship problems unrelated to natural age-related decreases in sexual function. The clinical assessment focuses first on a detailed description of the sexual difficulties, the couple's thoughts about possible causes and the reason for seeking help at the time. Erectile concerns are common presenting complaints in older men. Valuable diagnostic information is provided by inquiring about the onset and duration of the erectile problem, the degree and persistence of erectile failure, its relation to possible psychological difficulties, life events, or health issues, and the presence of other sexual disorders. A sudden onset of erectile failure during intercourse at a time of psychosocial stress, a dysfunction that is partner related, or the existence of adequate spontaneous, masturbatory or early morning erections all indicate a psychological contribution while not excluding organic involvement. Because of the tendency to report erections as all or none, we routinely ask patients to rate erectile rigidity on a 1–10 scale with 5 being adequate for penile insertion with manual assistance. Psychological participation is suggested by discrepancies in erectile capacity in coital versus noncoital situations, particularly when adequate morning erections are noted (Segraves, Segraves and Schoenbeg, 1987). A report of a gradual, progressive decline in erectile capacity encompassing all forms of sexual expression has less diagnostic significance because of the difficulty of distinguishing natural age-related decreases in sexual function from organic pathology. It is important, when assessing older men, to evaluate sexual desire and to determine if a loss of sexual interest contributes to or is a consequence of erectile difficulties. A primary loss of sexual drive leading to secondary erectile failure may reflect normal aging phenomena or be caused by endocrine pathology, depression or interpersonal difficulties. Ejaculatory impairments, loss of penile sensitivity or painful intercourse is occasionally reported by older patients and may be indicative of neurological abnormalities. Premature ejaculation, infrequently noted in aging men, may be the result of the increased penile stimulation required to obtain an adequate erection. Frequently ignored in the evaluation of older couples is the assessment of sexual satisfaction. It is not uncommon, in general medical practice, to note the persistence of satisfying sexuality in the context of significant declines of erectile function. For some couples, nonproblematic sexual impairments are the consequence of sexual ignorance, negative biases or resignation, but for others it is an adaptive adjustment that needs to be respected. Patients' perceptions about sexual change, their expectations and motivation are of considerable relevance to treatment planning.

Behavioral, cognitive, and psychosocial assessment

It is valuable to obtain detailed behavioral information about the sexual interaction. Aging men may engage sexually in a restricted or routine manner that, while sufficient in younger years, no longer provides the necessary sexual stimulation to sustain adequate erections. The role of cognition in sexual function and satisfaction was discussed in Chapter 12. How individuals appraise age-related sexual change and the effectiveness of the coping strategies are significant areas of inquiry with predictive relevance for therapeutic planning. Equally important is the evaluation of emotional states such as anger, anxiety, guilt and depression, because of their destructive consequences for sexual interest, arousal, and pleasure. The natural decline in sexual drive and erectile capacity render men, as they age, more vulnerable, sexually, to psychosocial stresses such as those commonly observed at that stage of life: marital discord, retirement, bereavement, professional disappointments or health-related concerns.

The medical history

Any illness that causes weakness, discomfort or psychological distress is likely to have nonspecific effects on sexuality. As discussed in Chapter 9, particular attention should be paid to cardiovascular, neurological, hormonal, metabolic, and postsurgical risk factors because of their possible impact on the mechanisms that mediate sexual function. A medication and drug history should be obtained which includes the assessment of life-style influences such as alcohol and tobacco consumption.

Partner assessment

Inclusion of the patient's partner, when available, in the evaluation is of considerable value in defining the problem and developing appropriate interventions (Tiefer and Melman, 1983). Interviewing the sexual partner serves to corroborate the patient's sexual complaint, and provides independent evidence about the role of the relationship and the partner's own sexual function in the couple's sexual adjustment. It also permits exploration of the partner's motivation or capacity to engage in treatment. There is a poor therapeutic prognosis if the sexual partners hold discrepant views about the nature of the sexual problem. Often, the partner's own lack of sexual interest and sexual disengagement contribute significantly to the patient's sexual dysfunction. It is valuable to allow a separate interview with the patient's partner to permit discussion of confidential information that he or she may be reluctant to mention otherwise.

Psychiatric and psychometric assessment

The evaluation of older individuals should assess mood and cognitive disorders. Administering a standardized, self-administered, sexual and health history questionnaire before the first interview can help the initial evaluation by sensitizing patients to the nature of the topics to be explored, obtaining subjective information about sexual pleasure and satisfaction, and steering the clinician to problematic areas of inquiry (Gregory, 1993). Several psychological instruments of demonstrated validity and reliability may contribute quantifiable information on dimensions relevant to sexual function and marital interaction (Schiavi et al., 1979; Ackerman and Carey, 1995). We have included in the evaluation package, depending on clinical requirements, the Brief Sexual Function Questionnaire (Reynolds et al., 1988), the Derogatis Sexual Functioning Inventory (Derogatis and Melisaratos, 1975), the Locke–Wallace Marriage Inventory (Locke and Wallace, 1959), the Dyadic Adjustment Scale (Spanier, 1976), the Beck Depression Inventory (Beck et al., 1961) and the 'Mini-mental State' for the assessment of cognitive function (Folstein, Folstein and McHugh, 1975). In addition to their clinical relevance, these instruments permit comparison of information across patient's groups or assessment of individuals at different times. A recently available, multidimensional, self-administered scale for the assessment of erectile dysfunction, validated cross-culturally, assesses five domains (erectile function, orgasmic function, sexual desire, intercourse satisfaction and overall satisfaction; Rosen et al. 1997). However, most sexual questionnaires are standardized on young or middle-aged population samples, and scores from older patient groups should be interpreted with caution. The use of psychological measures to discriminate between psychogenic and organic erectile disorders has provided contradictory findings and have limited diagnostic significance (Conte, 1986).

Physical examination

A physical examination of all aged men with sexual difficulties should be carried out. It looks for the existence of peripheral vascular disease, including femoral pulses and bruits, assesses secondary sexual characteristics such as the pattern of hair distribution, genital development and presence of gynecomastia, and tests for knee and ankle reflexes, testicular and penile sensitivity and when, peripheral neuropathy is suspected, perineal sensation. The genitalia are examined for evidence of penile curvature or plaques indicative of Peyronie's disease and abnormalities in testicular size and consistency. A rectal examination, a worthwhile preventative measure to detect unsuspected prostatic abnormalities, may be used to assess anal sphincter tone. The bulbocavernosus reflex may be elicited as evidence of pudendal nerve function but false-negative results are common. A blood-screen complements the physical examination with a complete blood count, a serum chemical profile, including a fasting blood sugar and a lipid panel, a morning serum testosterone and urinalysis.

Specialized diagnostic approaches

Depending on the results of the clinical interview, medical history and physical examination, several additional diagnostic procedures may be considered. They include specialized testing of hormonal, vascular and neurological mediating mechanisms and noninvasive approaches such as nocturnal penile tumescence and visual stimulation methods for the objective assessment of erectile capacity (Schiavi, 1992).

Hormonal assessment

Hormonal screening of all aging men with sexual dysfunction should be carried out. Androgen deficiency is the most common endocrine abnormality found in 1.7–15.6% of men with erectile dysfunction in urological studies (Govier, McClure and Kramer-Levien, 1996; Buvat and Lemaire, 1997). Wide variations in the reported prevalence of hypogonadism are probably due to differences in sample characteristics such as age, referral patterns, and diagnostic criteria. As described in Chapter 3, aging is associated with a decline in circulating testosterone, but hormonal concentrations usually remain above the level required to sustain normal sexual function. Hormonal testing is important when there is clinical evidence of hypogonadism or loss of sexual drive. Blood testosterone, because of its diurnal variation and pulsatile release, is best measured in the morning, and the result confirmed by repeated samplings when the levels are below the 3ng/ml level. Determination of bioavailable testosterone enhances the clinical significance of the hormonal test by assessing the physiologically active free and loosely bound hormonal fractions. Several conditions such as hyperthyroidism and hepatic cirrhosis may increase plasma proteins, resulting in androgen deficiency despite normal total testosterone concentrations. No further hormonal testing may be necessary when total and bioavailabe testosterone levels are normal in the absence of clinical evidence of endocrinopathy. When testosterone levels are low, luteinizing hormone (LH) measurements are necessary to differentiate hypergonadotrophic from hypogonadotrophic hypogonadism. LH is elevated when there is a primary testicular failure and it is either normal or decreased when the hypogonadal condition is caused by a pituitary or hypothalamic disorder. Aging men with partial testicular failure and borderline hypogonadism may have a compensatory increase in LH with testosterone levels within normal limits.

There is controversy regarding the need to screen all sexually dysfunctional men for serum prolactin levels. The prevalence of hyperprolactinemia in men with erectile disorders is relatively low ranging from 1.8% (Govier, McClure and Kramer-Levien, 1996) to 6.2% (Nickel et al., 1984). Because of cost-effective considerations, prolactin determinations may be reserved for patients with low circulating testosterone, gynecomastia and/or diminished sexual drive (Govier, McClure and Kramer-Levien, 1996; Buvat and Lemaire, 1997). When increased diagnostic precision is required, prolactin determinations may be included in the initial hormonal screening because some hyperprolactinemic patients do have normal or borderline testosterone levels.

Vascular assessment

Vasculogenic factors associated with erectile dysfunction in older men commonly involve impairment of the arterial supply to the penis, the functional integrity of the corpora cavernosa or veno-occlusive mechanisms. A large arterial supply reserve capacity to the penis exists and hemodynamic mechanisms must be severely impaired before they become the primary etiological cause of the erectile dysfunction (Oates et al., 1995). Several tests are available to assess the arterial and venous physiological components of penile rigidity.

Intracorporal pharmacological testing

An important diagnostic and therapeutic contribution was made by the discovery that intracavernosal injection of papaverine, a vasoactive agent, can induce rigid erections in healthy men. The development of full and sustained penile responses in patients with erectile problems was viewed as indicative of normal erectile hemodynamics, suggesting that the dysfunction was due to psychological or neurological factors (Virag et al., 1984). Vascular problems were suspected when the erections were delayed, partial or absent. Recent evidence has shown that the diagnostic significance of this test is less clear-cut than initially believed. A positive erectile response to intracorporal pharmacological testing indicates adequate veno-occlusive function but does not necessarily demonstrate normal arterial hemodynamics (Buvat et al., 1991; Cormio et al., 1996). Pescatory et al. (1994), for example, identified arterial disease in 19% of patients who had been carefully screened as having positive intracavernous tests. Conversely, deficient erectile responses to pharmacological testing, possibly mediated by increased adrenergic constrictor tone, may be caused by psychological reasons (Buvat et al., 1986; Aversa et al., 1996). Kim and Oh (1992) found significantly elevated noradrenaline levels in patients with psychological erectile dysfunction, especially those who did not respond to papaverine. Van der Borght, Vanderschueren and Demyttenaere (1995) studied the effects of stress and coping style on the diagnostic responses of men with erectile dysfunction to intracavernous injection of prostaglandin E1. They found that coping mechanisms such as avoidance, but not anxiety per se, were associated with significant decreases in penile responses to intracavernosal injection. Manual, audiovisual and vibratory stimulation are used in conjunction with penile injections to minimize psychological inhibition and enhance smooth muscle relaxation, but their effects on diagnostic accuracy are not clear.

Diagnostic intracavernosal testing is presently carried out in highly variable ways across laboratories. Patients are usually injected with papaverine (alone or in combination with phentolamine, an alpha-adrenergic blocking agent) or with prostaglandin E1 into the lateral side of one corpus cavernosum. Penile changes are assessed at various intervals and the time of onset of the response, the angle of the erection, and the degrees of tumescence and rigidity are recorded. The Rigiscan methodology is useful for documenting erectile changes in response to intracavernosal agents (Ogrinc and Linet, 1995). Patients are instructed to monitor the duration of the erection and to inform the clinician if the erection lasts longer than four to six hours. Prostaglandin E1, among all vasoactive drugs, appears to be the most effective diagnostic agent, with the rate of prolonged erectile responses being as low as 0.1%. However, its use is occasionally accompanied by pain or discomfort (Goldstein, 1994). In general, older men require higher doses of vasoactive agents to obtain an erection. The combined effects of aging and antihypertensive medication predict poor intracavernosal responses to prostaglandin E1 in men with erectile failure (Purvis, Brekke and Christiansen, 1996). In conclusion, although the diagnostic validity of intracorporal testing has been questioned, the elicitation of adequate erections has clear therapeutic implications suggesting, when positive responses occur, an opportunity for intervention. When there is interest in clarifying the pathogenesis of erectile failure, particularly when surgical interventions are considered, additional invasive vascular procedures are required.

Color Duplex ultrasonography

Duplex ultrasonography permits the corpora cavernosa and cavernosal arteries to be visualized, and measurement of blood flow in the penile vessels during flaccidity and in response to erections induced by intracorporal administration of vasoactive substances. The duplex system includes an ultrasound transducer that measures changes in the inner diameter of the cavernosal arteries, and a pulsed Doppler transducer that can be focused on a predetermined artery to measure blood flow.

The addition of color imaging helps vessel identification and peak flow velocity measurement. A defective arterial dilatation and minimal changes in mean peak systolic flow velocity (<25 cm/s), measured five minutes following intracavernosal challenge, has been considered suggestive of arterial disease (Lue et al., 1985; Shabsigh et al., 1989). However, the diagnostic criteria of arteriogenic erectile dysfunction vary considerably across laboratories (Meuleman and Diemont, 1995). Duplex ultrasonography and pulsed Doppler analysis are sensitive procedures that require considerable time and experience for reliable use. Diagnostic interpretations are based on the combined evaluation of several parameters, and determining the accuracy of these judgments requires the development of a normative data base and explicit criteria.

Cavernosometry and cavernosography

An impaired response to intracavernosal pharmacological testing may be caused not only by inadequate arterial inflow, but also by venous insufficiency. The techniques of cavernosometry and cavernosography assess cavernosal venous outflow resistance; they are more invasive and are more appropriate for younger patients who are candidates for vascular surgery. Cavernosometry involves infusing saline into the corpora cavernosa and monitoring the perfusion rates required to obtain and maintain an artificial erection while the intracavernosal pressure is measured. An elevated infusion flow rate and low intracavernosal pressures indicate venous incompetence. Cavernosography involves the infusion of contrast media into the corpora cavernosa to visualize the site of venous leakage and identify possible abnormalities requiring surgical intervention (Meuleman and Diemont, 1995). Both procedures should always be carried out after pharmacologically induced complete relaxation of the cavernous smooth muscle. Inhibiting psychological stress may lead to an incomplete drug-induced cavernous relaxation and to an overestimation of the degree of structural veno-occlusive dysfunction (Montague and Lakin, 1992; Vickers, Benson and Dluhy, 1992). These techniques have not been standardized yet, and there is no agreement about the physiopathological significance of venous leakage as diagnosed by these methods, particularly in instances of moderately elevated maintenance flow rates (Lue, 1996).

In summary, intracorporal pharmacological testing may be considered as a screening procedure for patients with suspected vasculogenic erectile dysfunction, in the knowledge of the problems of interpretation mentioned above. An impaired response may be followed up with Duplex ultrasonography testing. Cavernosometry and cavernosography are more invasive and are best reserved for younger patients, when there is evidence of veno-occlusive dysfunction, and before surgery.

Neurological assessment

The medical history and neurological examination provide the most valuable approach for identifying neurogenic erectile dysfunction, a diagnosis that is usually reached by exclusion of other pathogenic factors. There are no direct techniques that assess the integrity of the autonomic components of erection. Some investigators have developed clinical tests of autonomic status based on assessing cardiovascular reflexes, but the results have limited diagnostic and prognostic specificity (Berger, Rothman and Rigaud, 1994). More research needs to be done to validate the proposition that assessing electrical activity by needle electrodes from the cavernous smooth muscles directly measures autonomic erectile mechanisms (Wagner, Gerstenberg and Levin, 1989). Most of the tests currently used to investigate neurogenic participation assess the afferent, pudendally mediated components of the erectile reflex.

Penile biothesiometry

This procedure measures the threshold of vibratory perception in the glans and penile shaft using an electromagnetic device. Since there is an age-related decrease in penile sensitivity, possibly caused by pacinian degeneration and collagen infiltration, abnormal results need to be interpreted by comparison with data from age-appropriate controls (Rowland and Slob, 1995; Padma–Nathan, 1995). Approximately 50% of patients with abnormal biothesiometric results were found to have abnormal somatosensory-evoked potentials (Padma–Nathan and Levine, 1987). Biothesiometry has been proposed as a useful, noninvasive screening test of penile sensory afferent pathways (Padma–Nathan, 1988), but more empirical information is needed to determine its diagnostic value.

Dorsal nerve conduction velocity

This electrophysiological technique measures conduction of the dorsal nerve of the penis, a terminal branch of the pudendal nerve that may be involved in penile sensory loss. Bradley, Lin and Johnson (1984) developed this procedure to permit direct evaluation of penile neuropathy in men with erectile disorders, but its practical use will require further standardization and validation.

Bulbocavernosus reflex latency

This test, one of the earliest employed to diagnose neurogenic impotence, consists of recording the latency of the electromyographic (EMG) response of the bulbocavernosus muscles to electrical stimulation of the dorsal nerve of the penis. Absent or prolonged reflex latency is interpreted as indicative of neuropathological changes within the reflex arc, which includes the afferent and efferent components of the pudendal nerve and sacral segments S2, S3 and S4 of the spinal cord.

Variations of this test include measuring the conduction latency from the dorsal nerve to the distal urethral sphincter, measuring the latency from the distal urethral sphincter to the anal sphincter, and determining the sensory thresholds of the dorsal nerve and the posterior urethra (Parys, Evans and Parsons, 1988). There is conflicting evidence about the diagnostic value of this test. Some investigators have described it as a sensitive and useful diagnostic procedure (Parys, Evans and Parsons, 1988), whereas others have found it of doubtful validity and limited predictive value in discriminating between neurogenic (diabetic) and nonorganic erectile dysfunction (Lavoisier et al., 1989) or between diabetics with and without erectile problems (Buvat et al., 1985).

Somatosensory-evoked potential

The procedure records the evoked potential waveforms of the cerebral cortex (electroencephalogram, EEG), elicited by electrical stimulation of the dorsal nerve of the penis. The total conduction time is thought to be a measure of peripheral as well as central pudendal afferent pathways. Padma–Nathan (1988) has reported that this test permits the further evaluation of patients with erectile dysfunction identified by abnormal biothesiometric responses. In some individuals, the erectile dysfunction may be caused by defective sensory input from the penis to cerebral structures that activate efferent lumbosacral erectile reflexes. These patients are described as having normal nocturnal penile tumescence patterns and difficulty in sustaining (but not in gaining) erections. More information is required to define this syndrome further, and to evaluate the significance of somatosensory-evoked potential testing for the diagnosis of erectile disorders.

In summary, the relevance and diagnostic value of neurophysiological tests of erectile dysfunction are presently uncertain because they do not evaluate the autonomic control of genital vasocongestion. They may be considered, however, when the erectile disorder is associated with clinical evidence of neurological impairment, in the knowledge of limitations posed by lack of age-related normative information.

The nocturnal penile tumescence (NPT) method

The NPT method provides a valuable diagnostic approach to assess erectile capacity objectively. The working assumption is that in psychogenic impotence, erections during rapid eye movement (REM) sleep are normal, in marked contrast to the patient's daytime performance, whereas in organic impotence, nocturnal erections are impaired, corresponding closely to the patient's deficient waking erectile function. The procedure for NPT testing, as evolved in our sleep laboratory (Schiavi, 1994), is usually carried out over two or preferably three recording nights. EEG activity, eye movements, muscle tone and erectile tumescence are recorded continuously. Penile rigidity is assessed during systematic awakenings by visual ratings, photographic documentation or a device that applies a known pressure to the erected penis and measures the force required to make it buckle. Sleep records are scored according to standardized criteria, and the amount and distribution of sleep stages are determined. Frequency, duration and degree of penile circumferential increases are quantified based on calibrated penile strain-gauge recordings. Despite the wide utilization of the NPT method few studies have evaluated its diagnostic accuracy. The diagnostic efficiency of the method, assessed in our laboratory by the ability of the test to identify diabetic men both with and without organic pathology, minimizing false-positive and false-negative results, ranged from 77.8% to 88.9%, depending on the decision rules chosen for discrimination (Schiavi et al., 1985). These findings may not apply to other causes of organic dysfunction or to older patients.

Lack of consideration of methodological and conceptual issues from evolving NPT research may compromise the accuracy of diagnostic interpretations. Since some of these issues are discussed in detail elsewhere (Schiavi, 1988; Meisler and Carey, 1990; Moore, Fishman and Hirshkowitz, 1997), they are only briefly mentioned here. Age should always be considered in the diagnostic interpretation of apparently atypical observations of older subjects. We have previously mentioned, in a study of healthy aging volunteers, significant decreases in NPT in men who reported satisfactory intercourse (Schiavi et al., 1990). The paucity of NPT norms in men older than 65 years of age raises a note of caution about the significance of NPT findings in this age group, since the results may not indicate pathological conditions but rather reflect the normal physiological decreases associated with aging. The importance of assessing sleep architecture for the interpretation of NPT cannot be underestimated. Any illness, pharmacological agent or psychological problem associated with abnormal sleep and REM activity is likely to disrupt NPT and lead to false diagnostic conclusions. In addition, sleep disorders (sleep apnea and periodic leg movements), frequently noted in aging individuals, may be associated with abnormal NPT or result in NPT's monitoring artifacts that may be overlooked in the absence of respiratory and EMG measures (Schiavi et al., 1991). NPT is more responsive to psychological phenomena than was once thought. Clinical depression, anxiety and loss of sexual desire may be associated with NPT abnormalities in physically healthy individuals. Anxiety should be considered when there is evidence of sleep fragmentation, frequent arousals, or diminished REM sleep associated with depressed NPT activity. Although individual responses are highly variable, some subjects have inhibited erections during the first study night or when they are aware that they will be woken for rigidity verification.

The discrepancy between penile tumescence and rigidity during NPT episodes requires systematic awakenings to observe penile firmness and the use of a device that measures the pressure required for the penis to buckle. The technical difficulties of carrying out observations at the optimum time of maximum rigidity, as well as the problem of sleep disruption have fostered the development of devices for the continued monitoring of rigidity. The Rigiscan (Dacomed Corp. Minneapolis, MN, USA) is a portable computerized instrument that has gained increasing acceptance for the electronic measurement of both tumescence and rigidity (Bradley et al., 1985). It is based on periodic and automatic checks of radial loading using loop transducers placed around the penis. This method is an important methodological development, but its results should be interpreted with caution because of insufficient validity and reliability studies and a lack of concurrent polygraphic sleep information (Licht et al., 1995). Diagnostic categorizations are usually based on face validity criteria, i.e., the presence or absence of sleep erections of adequate rigidity and duration for vaginal penetration and satisfactory completion of intercourse (Wasserman et al., 1980), but its practical use varies considerably across laboratories. We have required, for the diagnosis of patients with organic erectile dysfunction, a mean frequency of less than one full erection per night, lasting a minimum of five minutes. These criteria may be sufficient to permit distinctions between nonoverlapping conditions, but are less than adequate when psychogenic and organic factors coexist, or when there are gradual changes in NPT associated with illness or aging.

In summary, the NPT method with rigidity monitoring remains a valuable diagnostic test but the interpretation of results needs to consider the normality of sleep architecture, age-related normative information and the interaction with emotional states such as clinical depression or excessive anxiety. The observation of normal REM erections has diagnostic significance, since it suggests that mediating physiological mechanisms are intact. Abnormal REM erections, on the other hand, may not only be indicative of organic pathology but may also reflect psychological inhibition.

The audio-visual sexual stimulation method

This test assesses penile polygraphic or Rigiscan recordings of erectile responses to controlled audio-visual presentation of erotic stimuli. Erotically induced erections may reflect more closely the physiological mechanisms that mediate sexual arousal during wakefulness. It records penile *and* subjective responses, and has the further advantage of being simpler and less costly than NPT recordings. While evidence of full erections suggests psychogenicity, partial or no responses have limited diagnostic significance. An important factor is the difficulty that a substantial proportion of physically normal, mainly older, men have in becoming aroused under laboratory conditions (Earls, Morales and Marshall, 1988; Wincze et al., 1988). Zuckerman et al. (1985), and Wincze et al. (1988) also observed, in patients with psychogenic erectile difficulties, a discrepancy between low erectile responses in the laboratory and normal NPT activity. Some investigators have attempted to enhance erectile responses to erotic videotaped presentations by self-stimulation, vibrotactile stimulation or intracavernosal injection of small doses of vasoactive agents with unpredictable results in older patients (Incrocci, Hop and Slob, 1996) Obviously, the subjects' attitudes toward visual erotica and masturbation are important factors in the applicability of this method, a consideration particularly relevant to older individuals.

Conclusion

There is no uniformly agreed protocol for evaluating male sexual problems, as evidenced by the diverse algorithms suggested to guide the sequence of testing procedures (Bancroft and Wu, 1985; Shabsigh et al., 1989; Buvat et al., 1990; Rosen and Leiblum, 1992; Lewis and King, 1994). A carefully obtained psychosexual interview, preferably involving the partner, a medical evaluation and routine laboratory tests most often suffice to identify clinically significant psychological determinants, relevant medical conditions, risk factors, and drug effects. A tentative formulation of contributing causes to the sexual problem is discussed with the patient/couple and, depending on their expectations and motivation, further diagnostic testing and treatment options are considered. The choice of ancillary diagnostic procedures is determined by:

1   An informed opinion of likely causal determinants and potential for reversing the sexual problem.
2   Data on the validity, reliability, and predictive value of individual tests.
3   Practical considerations, such as the degree of methodological complexity, patient's acceptance, and cost.

Patients with clear evidence of psychological determinants, depression, or relationship difficulties may be offered further psychological evaluation and therapy. Endocrine assessment, including total and bioavailable testosterone measurement, is indicated when there is evidence of hypogonadism and loss of sexual drive. If low bioavailable testosterone levels are obtained repeatedly, prolactin and LH measurements may follow to further identify the nature of the endocrinopathy. Intracavernosal testing of vascular function should be considered when the pattern of erectile dysfunction suggests an organic origin, particularly for patients with a history of cardiovascular difficulties. A positive erectile response to intracavernosal testing, although not ruling out arteriogenic factors, indicates adequate venoocclusive mechanisms and suggests the option of penile injection therapy. A negative erectile response, however, is not diagnostic of vasculogenic dysfunction, since it can be caused by inhibitory psychological states. Further vascular testing involving duplex ultrasonography and invasive procedures, such as cavernosometry, cavernosography and angiography, are usually reserved for younger patients before considering vascular reconstruction, and are best carried out in specialized centers. NPT/rigidity monitoring in the sleep laboratory has a valuable diagnostic role in assessing the erectile capacity of patients whose primary cause is thought to be psychological, of patients who have sleep disorders, or before invasive interventions. Interpretation of abnormal NPT findings should be made in the context of age-related normative information and consideration of the occurrence of emotional states such as clinical depression or excessive anxiety and sleep disorders. The diagnostic value of neurological testing is uncertain because these methods do not evaluate the autonomic control of genital vasocongestion and, with the exception of biothesiometry, have limited practical applicability at the present time.

Laboratory methods for assessing sexual dysfunction have advanced our knowledge of mediating physiological processes involved in erectile disorders. Their diagnostic significance will be increased by much-needed information on test validity, accuracy, and age-related norms. The tendency to neglect the contribution of psychological factors when interpreting test results and planning therapy for older individuals should be minimized by enhanced awareness of the complex nature of sexual dysfunction. The importance of a multidisciplinary approach to patients' sexual difficulties is illustrated by the cases that follow.

Case studies

Case study 13.1

Mr. V, a 67-year-old married engineer, dated the sudden onset of erectile impotence to five years ago when he returned from his father's funeral in Israel. Although prohibited by religious rules from intercourse for one month, he acceded to his wife's desire for sex and experienced considerable anger and guilt afterwards. Since that time, he has been unable to have intercourse, and his wife discouraged further attempts because, 'she didn't want to get frustrated'. His sexual desire is not impaired and he occasionally ejaculates by rubbing against her body. He follows strict religious principles, does not masturbate, smoke or drink alcohol, and denies extramarital experiences. Mr. and Ms. V's sexual life had been problematic since the beginning of their marriage, because of premature ejaculation and her lack of sexual interest, unwillingness to engage in foreplay and orgasmic difficulties. Before the onset of his current problem, Mr. V had noticed a gradual decrease in erectile firmness, which he attributed to aging and to lack of sexual stimulation by his wife, which had not prevented vaginal penetration.

Mr. V had been diagnosed with hypertension three years before, treated with hydrochlorothiazide and had had cardiac bypass surgery for angina one year before this evaluation. The physical examination was noncontributory. Hormonal assessments, glucose tolerance test and penile blood pressure measures were normal. The results of two NPT recording nights, visual sexual stimulation, and intracavernosal pharmacological testing demonstrated only partial erections, suggesting an organic impairment of erectile capacity. Modification of the antihypertensive treatment did not improve Mr. V's erectile function. Because of considerable marital upheaval, it was decided to accept this couple for combined marital–sex therapy on a trial basis. Partial resolution of destructive marital interactions, mutual recriminations and guilt as well as removal of some of Ms. V's sexual inhibitions that had prevented effective sexual stimulation resulted in improved erectile capacity which, although not full, permitted sexual intercourse and enhanced sexual satisfaction.

Comment

This case study illustrates the interaction of causal determinants in Mr. V's sexual problem. The medical history and physiological testing suggest an organic, probably vascular, participation in his erectile impairment. It is likely that this functional limitation rendered Mr. V vulnerable to a traumatic experience, following the death of his father, that gained significance in the context of life-long marital problems, many centered around sexual issues. Ms. V's own sexual difficulties had a clear pathogenic influence on her husband's sexual dysfunction. Attempting to categorize the problem as mostly organic or mostly psychogenic risks distorting our view of the constellation of factors that contributed to this older couple's call for help.

Case study 13.2

Mr. W is a 63-year-old divorced pharmacist who recently married his 40-year-old sexual partner, after they had been living together for four years. Coital difficulties began soon after marriage when they decided to have a child and both felt under pressure, feeling that her fertile years would soon be over. He had been remarkably free from sexual difficulties, with the exception of a four-month period of ejaculatory incompetence ten years before, around the period of his divorce. Mr. W had noticed a progressive decrease in erectile rigidity prior to his remarriage but it had not prevented his having intercourse on regular basis. At the time of the evaluation his sexual desire and ejaculatory capacity were not impaired and both Mr. and Ms. W, described a caring and sexually rich relationship.

Mr. W's medical evaluation was significant for diabetes mellitus and moderate obesity. The diabetes mellitus had been diagnosed six years before, did not have nonsexual complications, and was treated with insulin. NPT testing showed considerable erectile activity but no full tumescence, while intracavernosal testing resulted in normal erectile responses. The couple decided to enter a course of intracavernosal pharmacotherapy with the primary aim of conceiving. Soon after Ms. W became pregnant they discontinued prostaglandin injections, and to their considerable pleasure they regained, over a period of six months, and without further treatment, the capacity to have intercourse.

Comment

This is another case in which physiological and psychological determinants interact in the development of erectile dysfunction. It is likely that diabetes alone or in association with age-related changes in erectile capacity were contributing factors, to which was added the performance demands associated with the couple's desire to have a child. The observation that erectile function is restored following discontinuation of intracavernosal treatment is not unusual and suggests the participation of inhibitory psychological influences.

References

Ackerman, M. C. and Carey, M. P. (1995). Psychology's role in the assessment of erectile dysfunction: historical precedents, current knowledge, and methods. *Journal of Consulting and Clinicical Psychology* **63**, 862–76.

Aversa, A., Rocchietti, M. M., Caprio, M., Giannini, D., Isidori, A. and Fabbri, A. (1996). Anxiety induced failure in erectile response to intracorporeal prostaglandin E1 in non-organic male impotence: a new diagnostic approach. *International Journal of Andrology* **19**, 307–13.

Bancroft, J. and Wu, F. C. (1985). Erectile impotence. *British Medical Journal* **290**, 1566–8.

Beck, A. T., Ward, C. H., Mendelsohn, M., Mock, J. and Erbaugh, J. (1961). An inventory for measuring depression. *Archives of General Psychiatry* **4**, 561–71.

Berger, R. E., Rothman, I. and Rigaud, G. (1994). Nonvascular causes of impotence. In *Impotence: Diagnosis and Management of Erectile Dysfunction*, ed. A. H. Bennett, pp. 10626. Philadelphia: WB Saunders Co.

Bradley, W. E., Lin, J. T. Y. and Johnson, B. (1984). Measurement of the conduction velocity of the dorsal nerve of the penis. *Journal of Urology* **131**, 1127–9.

Bradley, W. E., Timm, G. W., Gallagher, J. M. and Johnson, B. K. (1985). New method for continuous measurement of nocturnal penile tumescence and rigidity. *Urology* **26**, 4–8.

Buvat, J. and Lemaire, A. (1997). Endocrine screening of 1022 men with erectile dysfunctin: clinical significance and cost-effective strategy. *Journal of Urology* **158**, 1764–7.

Buvat, J., Lemaire, A., Buvat–Herbaut, M., Guieu, J. D., Bailleul, J. P. and Fossati, P. (1985). Comparative investigations in 26 impotent and 26 non impotent diabetic patients. *Journal of Urology* **133**, 34–8.

Buvat, J., Buvat–Herbaut, M., Dehaene, J. L. and Lemaire, A. (1986). Is intracavernous injection of papaverine a reliable screening test for vascular impotence? *Journal of Urology* **135**, 476–8.

Buvat, J., Buvat–Herbaut, M., Lemaire, A., Marcolin, G. and Quittelier, M. (1990). Recent developments in the clinical assessment and diagnosis of erectile dysfunction. *Annual Review of Sex Research* **1**, 265–308.

Buvat, J., Buvat–Herbaut, M., Lemaire, A., Marcolin, G. and Dehaene, J. L. (1991). Diagnostic value of intracavernosus injections of 20 µg of prostaglandin E1 in impotence. *International Journal of Impotence Research* **3**, 113–17.

Conte, H. R. (1986). Multivariate assessment of sexual dysfunction. *Journal of Consulting and Clinical Psychology* **54**, 149–57.

Cormio, L., Nisen, H., Selvaggi, F. P. and Ruutu, M. (1996). A positive pharmacological erection test does not rule out arteriogenic erectile dysfunction. *Journal of Urology* **156**, 1628–30.

Derogatis, L. R. and Melisaratos, N. (1975). The DSFI: a multidimensional measure of sexual functioning. *Journal of Sex and Marital Therapy* **5**, 244–81.

Earls, C. M., Morales, A. and Marshall, W. L. (1988). Penile sufficiency: an operational definition. *Journal of Urology* 139, 536–8.

Feldman, H. A., Goldstein, I., Hatzichristou, D. G., Krane, R. J. and McKinlay, J. B. (1994). Impotence and its medical and psychological correlates: results from the Massachusetts Male Aging Study. *Journal of Urology* 151, 54–61.

Folstein, M. F., Folstein, S. F. and McHugh, P. R. (1975). 'Mini-Mental State': a practical method for grading the cognitive state of patients for the clinician. *Journal of Psychiatric Research* 12, 189–98.

Goldstein, I. (1994). Impotence [editorial]. *Journal of Urology* 152, 1119–20.

Govier, F. E., McClure, R. D. and Kramer–Levien, D. (1996). Endocrine screening for sexual dysfunction using free testosterone determinations. *Journal of Urology,* 156, 405–8.

Gregory, A. (1993). Questionnaires and rating scales. In *Impotence. An Integrated Approach to Clinical Practice,* ed. A. Gregoire and J. P. Pryor, pp. 97–105. Edinburgh: Churchill Livingstone.

Incrocci, L., Hop, W. C. J. and Slob, A. K. (1996). Visual erotic and vibrotactile stimulation and intracavernous injection in screening men with erectile dysfunction: a 3 year experience with 406 cases. *International Journal of Impotence Research* 8, 227–32.

Kim, S. C. and Oh, M. M. (1992). Norepinephrine involvement in response to intracorporeal injection of papaverine in psychogenic impotence. *Journal of Urology* 147, 1530–2.

Kligman, E. W. (1991). Office evaluation of sexual function and complaints. *Geriatric Sexuality* 7, 15–39.

Lavoisier, P., Proulx, J., Courtois, F. and deCarufel, F. (1989). Bulbocavernosus test: its validity as a diagnostic test of neurogenic impotence. *Journal of Urology* 141, 311–14.

Lewis, R. W. and King, B. F. (1994). The diagnostic algorithm. In *Impotence: Diagnosis and Management of Erectile Dysfunction,* ed. A. H. Bennet, pp. 42–51. Philadelphia: WB Saunders Co.

Licht, M. R., Lewis, R. W., Wollan, P. C. and Harris, C. D. (1995). Comparison of rigiscan and sleep laboratory nocturnal penile tumescence in the diagnosis of organic impotence. *Journal of Urology* 154, 1740–3.

Locke, H. and Wallace, K. (1959). Short marital adjustment tests: their reliability and validity. *Marriage and Family Living* 21, 251–5.

Lue, T. F. (1996). Veno-occlusive dysfunction of corpora cavernosa: comparison of diagnostic methods. *Journal of Urology* 155, 786–7.

Lue, T. F., Hricak, H., Marich, K. W. and Tanagho, E. A. (1985). Evaluation of vaculogenic impotence with high resolution ultrasonography and pulse Doppler spectrum analysis. *Radiology* 155, 777–81.

Meisler, A. and Carey, M. P. (1990). A critical reevaluation of nocturnal penile tumescence monitoring in the diagnosis of erectile dysfunction. *Journal of Nervous and Mental Disease* 178, 78–89.

Meuleman, E. J. and Diemont, W. L. (1995). Investigation of erectile dysfunction. *Urologic Clinics of North America* 22, 803–39.

Montague, D. K. and Lakin, M. M. (1992). False diagnoses of venous leak impotence. *Journal of Urology* 148, 148–52.

Moore, C. A., Fishman, I. J. and Hirshkowitz, M. (1997). Evaluation of erectile dysfunction and sleep related erections. *Journal of Psychosomatic Research* 42, 531–9.

Nickel, J. C., Morales, A., Condra, M., Fenemore, J. and Surridge, D. H. C. (1984). Endocrine dysfunction in impotence: incidence, significance and cost effective screening. *Journal of Urology* 13, 40–6.

Oates, C. P., Pickard, R. S., Powell, P. H., Murthy, L. N. S. and Whittingham, T. A. W. (1995). The use of Duplex ultrasound in the assessment of arterial supply to the penis in vasculogenic impotence. *Journal of Urology* 153, 354–7.

Ogrinc, F. G. and Linet, O. I. (1995). Evaluation of real-time rigiscan monitoring in pharmacological erection. *Journal of Urology* 154, 1356–9.

Padma–Nathan, H. (1995). Erectile dysfunction [editorial]. *Journal of Urology* 153, 1494–5.

Padma–Nathan, H. (1988). Neurologic evaluation of erectile dysfunction. *Urologic Clinics of North America* 15, 77–80.

Padma–Nathan, H. and Levine, F. (1987). Vibrating testing of the penis. *Journal of Urology* 137, 201A.

Parys, B. T., Evans, C. M. and Parsons, K. F. (1988). Bulbocavernosus reflex latency in the investigation of diabetic impotence. *British Journal of Urology* 61, 59–62.

Perez, E. D., Mulligan, T. and Wan, T. (1993). Why men are interested in an evaluation for a sexual problem. *Journal of the American Geriatrics Society* 41, 233–7.

Pescatori, E. S., Hatzichristou, D. G., Nambury, S. and Goldstein, I. (1994). A positive intracavernous injection test implies normal veno-occlusive but not necesarily normal arterial function: a hemodynamic study. *Journal of Urology* 151, 1209–16.

Purvis, K., Brekke, I. and Christiansen, E. (1996). Determinants of satisfactory rigidity after intracavernosal injection with prostaglandin E1 in men with erectile failure. *International Journal of Impotence Research* 8, 9–16.

Reynolds, C. F. III, Frank, E., Thase, M. E., Houck, P. R., Jennings, J. R., Howell, J. R., Lilienfeld, S. O. and Kupfer, D. J. (1988). Assessment of sexual function in depressed, impotent, and healthy men: factor analysis of a Brief Sexual Function Questionnaire for men. *Psychiatric Research* 24, 231–50.

Rosen, R. C. and Leiblum, S. R. (1992). Erectile disorders: an overview of historical trends and clinical perspectives. In *Erectile Disorders; Assessment and Treatment*, pp. 3–26, ed. R. C. Rosen and S. R. Leiblum. New York: The Guilford Press.

Rosen, R. C., Riley, A., Wagner, G., Osterloh, I. H., Kirpatrick, J. and Mishra, A. (1997). The international index of erectile function (IIEF): a multidimensional scale for assessment of erectile dysfunction. *Urology* 49, 822–30.

Rowland, D. L. and Slob, A. K. (1995). Understanding and diagnosing sexual dysfunction: recent progress through psychophysiological and psychophysical methods. *Neuroscience and Behavioral Reviews* 19, 201–9.

Schiavi, R. C. (1988). Nocturnal penile tumescence in the evaluation of erectile disorders: a critical review. *Journal of Sex and Marital Therapy* 14, 83–96.

Schiavi, R. C. (1992). Laboratory methods for evaluating erectile dysfunction. In *Erectile Disorders; Assessment and Treatment*, ed. R. C. Rosen and S. R. Leiblum, pp. 141–70. New York: The Guilford Press.

Schiavi, R. C. (1994). The role of the sleep laboratory in the evaluation of male erectile dysfunction. *The Mount Sinai Journal of Medicine* **61**, 161–5.

Schiavi, R. C., Derogatis, L. R., Kuriansky, J., O'Connor, D. and Sharpe, L. (1979). The assessment of sexual function and marital interaction. *Journal of Sex and Marital Therapy* **5**, 169–224.

Schiavi, R. C., Fisher, C., Quadland, M. and Glover, A. (1985). Nocturnal penile tumescent evaluation of erectile function in insulin-dependent diabetic men. *Diabetologia* **28**, 90–4.

Schiavi, R. C., Schreiner-Engel, P., Mandeli, J., Schanzer, H. and Cohen, E. (1990). Healthy aging and male sexual function. *American Journal Psychiatry* **147**, 766–71.

Schiavi, R. C., Mandeli, J., Schreiner-Engel, P. and Chambers, A. (1991). Aging, sleep disorders and male sexual function. *Biological Psychiatry* **30**, 15–24.

Schover, L. R. (1992). Erectile failure and chronic illness. In *Erectile Disorders; Assessment and Treatment*, ed. R. C. Rosen and S. R. Leiblum, pp. 341–67. New York: The Guilford Press.

Schover, L. R. and Jensen, S. B. (1988). *Sexuality and Chronic Illness: A Comprehensive Approach.* New York: The Guilford Press.

Schwartz, G. E. (1982). Testing the biopsychosocial model: the ultimate challenge facing behavioral medicine? *Journal of Consulting and Clinical Psychology* **50**, 1040–53.

Segraves, K. A., Segraves, R. T. and Schoenberg, H. W. (1987). Use of sexual history to differentiate organic from psychogenic impotence. *Archives of Sexual Behavior* **16**, 125–37.

Shabsigh, R., Fishman, I. J., Quesada, E. T., Seale-Hawkins, C. K. and Dunn, J. K. (1989). Evaluation of vaculogenic erectile impotence using penile duplex ultrasonography. *Journal of Urology* **142**, 1469–74.

Slag, M. F., Morley, J. E., Elson, M. K., Trence, D. L., Nelson, C. J., Nelson, A. E., Kinlaw, W. B., Beyer, S., Nuttall, F. Q. and Shafer, R. B. (1983). Impotence in medical clinic outpatients. *Journal of the American Medical Association* **249**, 1736–40.

Spanier, G. B. (1976). Measuring dyadic adjustment: new scales for assessing the quality of marriage and similar dyads. *Journal of Marriage and the Family* **38**, 15–28.

Tiefer, L. and Melman, A. (1989). Comprehensive evaluation of erectile dysfunction and medical treatments. In *Principles and Practice of Sex Therapy. Update for the 1990s*, ed. S. Leiblum and R. C. Rosen, pp. 207–36. New York: The Guilford Press.

Tiefer, L. and Melman, A. (1983). Interview of wives: a necessary adjunct in the evaluation of impotence. *Sexuality and Disability* **6**, 167–73.

Van der Borght, W., Vanderschueren, D. and Demyttenaere, K. (1995). The effects of stress and coping upon the diagnostic intracavernous injection in men with erectile dysfunction. *Journal of Psychosomatic Research* **39**, 865–73.

Vickers, M. A. Jr., Benson, C. B., Dluhy, R. G. et al. (1992). The current cavernosometric criteria for corporovenous dysfunction are too strict. *Journal of Urology* **147**, 614–17.

Virag, R., Frydman, D., Legman, M. and Virag, H. (1984). Intracavernosus injection of papaverine as a diagnostic and therapeutic method in erectile failure. *Angiology* **35**, 79–83.

Wagner, G., Gerstenberg, T. and Levin, R. J. (1989). Electrical activity of the corpus cavernosum during flaccidity and erection of the human penis: a new diagnostic method? *Journal of Urology* **142**, 723–5.

Wasserman, M. D., Pollak, C. P., Spielman, A. J. and Weitzman, E. D. (1980). Theoretical and technical problems in the measurement of nocturnal penile tumescence for the differential diagnosis of impotence. *Psychosomatic Medicine* 42, 575–85.

Wincze, J. P., Bansal, S., Malhotra, C., Balko, A., Susset, J. G. and Malamud, M. (1988). A comparison of nocturnal penile tumescence and penile response to erotic stimulation during waking states in comprehensively diagnosed groups of males experiencing erectile difficulties. *Archives of Sexual Behavior* 17, 333–48.

Zuckerman, M., Neeb, M., Ficher, M., Fishkin, R. E., Goldman, A., Fink, P., Cohen, S. N., Jacobs, J. A. and Weisberg, M. (1985). Nocturnal penile tumescence and penile responses in the waking state in diabetic and non-diabetic sexual dysfunctionals. *Archives of Sexual Behavior* 14, 109–29.

14 Management and treatment of sexual problems

The general considerations for treatment outlined in the National Institutes of Health, Impotence Consensus Statement (1992) remain valid to this day:

1 Psychotherapy and/or behavioral therapy may be useful for patients with erectile dysfunction without evident organic origin or as an adjunct to medical/urological interventions.

2 Treatment should be individualized to meet patient's desires and expectations, preferably including both partners in treatment plans.

3 Although there are several effective therapies, their long-term efficacy is relatively low and there is a high rate of voluntary discontinuation for all forms of erectile dysfunction treatment.

The sexual problems and concerns that lead aging men to approach health-care professionals are not limited, however, to erectile difficulties. As mentioned in previous chapters, life events such as medical illness or retirement, psychological problems such as depression and marital difficulties may induce sexual dissatisfaction which may, or may not, be accompanied by erectile difficulties. The generic model developed by Baltes and Baltes (1990) named selective optimization with compensation, described in Chapter 1, includes a set of propositions that help organize our views about the management and treatment of the sexual problems of aging individuals. The element of *selection* refers to concentration on those domains that are of high priority for the individual, which may or may not include, depending on the circumstances, sexual expression. It may also entail adjustment of goals and expectations to maximize sexual satisfaction and the sense of control. The element of *optimization* may involve enhancing the quality of sexual experiences by cognitive, emotional or interpersonal interventions or by modifying life-style factors in accordance to the priority given to sexuality. The third element, *compensation*, entails sexual behavior changes and technological approaches such as medication, intracavernosal injections or the use of vacuum constrictive devices that may contribute to sexual satisfaction. In the sections that follow we shall review psychological, behavioral, medical and surgical approaches for the management and treatment of male sexual problems, ending with a discussion of strategies of intervention and illustrative case histories.

Psychological and behavioral interventions

The sexual problems that bring older couples to the attention of health-care professionals are, in essence, not dissimilar to younger couples' difficulties. There are, however, some distinctions that influence evaluation and treatment strategies. Most frequently, older men with sexual concerns, usually erectile difficulties, approach a general practitioner or internist with the belief that, 'something is physically wrong' and the expectation that a medical intervention, hopefully a pill, 'will fix the problem'. Their acculturation discourages open discussion of emotions and exploration of relationship issues, which, when sexual, are particularly unwelcome for both the patient and his partner. Older couples are usually reluctant to implement a psychological referral, and referral to a medical specialist frequently leads to a cursory psychological evaluation, usually not involving the partner, followed, even in the presence of negative medical findings, by medical or surgical approaches.

It is important, as discussed in the previous chapter, to evaluate the nature of the sexual complaint. The evaluation should ensure that the older patient is not mislabeling a natural, gradual decrease in erectile rigidity as 'impotence', that there is no evidence of intellectual deficits that may complicate treatment, that the erectile impairment is not secondary to another problem, such as loss of sexual desire or mood disorder, and that it is not caused by interpersonal difficulties. Psychological interventions should be individualized and include the sexual partner to any extent possible. Educational, cognitive, behavioral and interpersonal components may be combined on the basis of the patient/couple's characteristics, the therapist's theoretical orientation and the treatment setting.

Educational component

Inadequate information and inaccurate beliefs and myths about sexuality are important targets for intervention. Frequently noted among men (and their partners) is ignorance about male and female anatomy and function, the normality of sexual expression at all ages, the existence of age-related decreases in erectile firmness, increases in the duration of the refractory period following ejaculation and greater need for direct penile stimulation as age progresses. Common dysfunctional beliefs are overvalued expectations about male sexual performance, intercourse and orgasm to the neglect of sexual communication between partners, sex play, pleasure and satisfaction. Older couples are usually receptive to an educational approach, which may include open discussion, audiovisual materials and appropriate books (for example, McCarthy's *Male Sexual Awareness*, 1984; Zilbergeld's *The New Male Sexuality*, 1992). Embedded in the provision of accurate sexual information is the aim to initiate an attitudinal change that may facilitate successful implementation of other therapeutic interventions.

Cognitive components

The close relationship between cognitive and behavioral therapeutic components makes distinction between them somewhat arbitrary. We discussed in Chapter 12 cognitive appraisal and coping strategies in relation to aging and sexuality. An age-related decrease in sexual function may be appraised as stressful when it threatens a culturally ingrained belief that places sexual performance at the center of men's identity, competence and self-worth. Coping responses may be adaptive, aimed at problem-solving such as acquiring information or new skills, or at minimizing emotional distress such reframing the significance of a sexual interaction as a pleasure and not a success. They may also be maladaptive, stemming from sexually destructive cognitions concerning sexual function and performance. Rosen, Leiblum and Spector (1994) listed the following common cognitive distortions:

All or nothing thinking: labeling the total interaction as a failure if one aspect is problematic.

Overgeneralization: viewing a single negative event as a never-ending pattern.

Disqualifying the positive: minimizing or rejecting the value of positive experiences.

Mind reading: projecting one's negative thoughts onto the partner.

Fortune-telling: anticipating that an event will have a negative outcome.

Emotional reasoning: assuming that the negative emotions experienced reflect reality.

Categorical imperatives: setting up behavioral standards dominated by 'shoulds' and 'musts'.

Catastrophizing: exaggerating out of proportion the distressing consequences of an event.

The therapeutic challenge is to help the patient recognize the hidden thoughts and cognitions that link a sexual event to unpleasant emotional reactions, to determine the unreasonable nature of the distortions and to reconsider negative qualities or events in a different light (reframing). Several authors have contributed valuable information on the implementation of this approach (Beck, 1988; Hawton, 1982).

Behavioral components

Identification of maladaptive cognitions is facilitated by engaging in behavioral experiences aimed at fostering mutually reinforcing cognitive and behavioral change. Considerable attention should be given to the timing and nature of behavioral exercises suggested to older couples. Premature behavioral suggestions to individuals with rather rigid sexual attitudes and beliefs may evoke resistance and compromise therapeutic effectiveness. Interventions should be individualized, taking into account the patients' willingness to experiment and expand patterns of sexual interaction. Commonly observed among older couples are routine and predictable sexual encounters that result in sexual boredom and loss of desire. While in younger days sexual arousal could be expected to occur in less than optimal conditions and with minimal sexual stimulation, this is, for many aging couples, no longer sufficient. An important behavioral objective is to help couples generate alternative sexual interactions, taking into account preferences, expectations and motivation, in order to enhance comfort and pleasure and minimize performance concerns (Hawton, 1982). Considerable creativity is required to adapt the behavioral assignments used in sex therapy to older couples. The partners are invited to engage in a progressive series of sensual and sexual tasks in the context of an initial proscription of intercourse. The sequence of behavioral steps for the treatment of erectile difficulties may include nongenital stimulation with emphasis on mutuality and communication, and gradual incorporation of genital pleasuring, during which erectile concerns are minimized. Eventually, if and when appropriate, vaginal insertion occurs, usually at the woman's initiative, with a continued focus on sexual enjoyment. The underlying aims of the behavioral experiences are to reduce performance anxiety, provide a means for enhanced learning, improve communication between partners, develop sexual skills, and modify destructive sexual cognitions. How the couple reacts to the behavioral assignments has valuable diagnostic and prognostic significance. Audiovisual materials directed at older couples and erotic literature may be helpful for generating discussion, expanding the range of sexual activities, and stimulating arousing sexual fantasies that may replace obsessive concerns about the state of the penis. Tact and sensitivity should be exercised, however, in keeping with the traditional and conservative background of many older couples.

Interpersonal components

Often, the sexual problem that brings men to clinical attention is caused by relationship issues that may, or may not, be recognized by the patient or the couple. Some of these issues, such as inadequate communication about sexual preferences or performance pressure because of the female's overemphasis on intercourse, may be easily resolved by the strategies previously discussed. On the other hand, conflicts concerning trust, power, control, and intimacy may be particularly salient for some aging couples, and pose difficult clinical decisions. Therapeutic strategies vary widely and include focusing first on the relationship problems, combining sex and couple's therapy or engaging the couple in individual psychotherapy sessions prior to sex therapy. Empirical evidence on the relative merits of these approaches is limited and contradictory, and the therapist is frequently guided by clinical experience rather than by a specific theoretical system (Leiblum and Rosen, 1992). Case study 14.1 illustrates a combined approach involving education, brief sexual counseling and a targeted intervention with the sexual partner.

Interventions for men without partners

Older men are frequently alone when they approach a clinician about a sexual problem. Many are recently separated, divorced or widowed, and others are initially unwilling to enlist the participation of their sexual partner, or their partner is not interested in treatment. The evaluation of men without partners should pay particular attention to the presence of mood disorders, low self-esteem, feelings of inadequacy, fears of failure and rejection, and misconceptions about aging. Treatment should be carefully individualized and may include educational and cognitive components, as discussed above, anxiety-reduction strategies and social skills training (Reynolds, 1991; McCarthy, 1992; Cole and Gregoire, 1993). While clinical evidence demonstrates the value of psychoeducational and cognitive approaches for inducing attitudinal changes and minimizing sexual anxiety, other techniques used with single men, such as guided imagery, masturbatory exercises, modeling and behavioral rehearsal, are of questionable applicability to aged patients.

Several authors have examined the effect, on older individuals and couples, of psychoeducational group interventions with the aim of improving knowledge and inducing positive attitudinal changes to sexuality (Rowland and Haynes, 1978; White and Catania, 1982; Goldman and Carroll, 1990; Wiley and Bortz, 1996). In general, time-limited, structured, instructional programs have resulted in significant improvements in sexual knowledge, attitudes and satisfaction, but have had limited effects on sexual performance.

Sexual counseling and chronic illness

Chronic illness makes a major contribution to the decline in male sexual function as age progresses. In addition to their specific effects on mediating physiological mechanisms, medical problems can impair sexuality through generalized psychological effects on well-being and self-perception. As discussed on Chapter 12, how individuals appraise threats to sexual identity, sexual intimacy, body image and control over bodily functions determines the nature of their adaptive responses. Older people avail themselves of a wide range of coping strategies, and it is not age but the specific challenges imposed by illness and personal characteristics that influence their adjustment to disease and response to treatment (Moos, 1977; Felton, Revenson and Hinrichsen, 1984).

Psychological treatment of sexual problems associated with medical disorders is based on implementing the following guiding principles, where appropriate (Schiavi, 1980):

1   Provision of information about normal sexual responses and the impact of the illness on sexual function.

2   Change of attitudes, from exclusive emphasis on intercourse to acceptance of behaviors that enhance mutual pleasure and erotic arousal.

3   Development of coping skills that contribute to sexual satisfaction.

4   Increased mutual communication about erotic preferences and needs.

5   Reduction of psychological factors that inhibit sexual responses.

6   Facilitation of acceptance and adjustment to the limitations imposed by the organic impairment.

Schover (1988; Schover and Jensen, 1992) has written extensively about sexual counseling for patients with chronic illness. Most of the aims outlined above may be successfully obtained with sexual counseling by a mental health clinician working, ideally, in collaboration with the practitioners responsible for the patient's medical care. It is best implemented by providing the relevant information to both partners, with the assistance of patient-educational materials, and by graduated, sensual 'homework' exercises. These exercises contribute to break the pattern of sexual avoidance, diminish sexual fears and anxiety, address technical problems generated by the physical handicap and facilitate the couple's adjustment to the impact of the illness. Specific advice is provided to help deal with the safety concerns about resuming sex of men with cardiovascular disease, fears of loss of control and embarrassment by patients with bowel or bladder ostomies, movement restrictions caused by arthritis or hemiparesis, and decreased penile skin sensitivity caused by multiple sclerosis. Sexual counseling may be supplemented with direct interventions such as intracavernosal injections or vacuum devices for motivated patients with organic erectile disorders. More intense, specialized, psychological or pharmacological treatment may be required to resolve destructive psychological or marital issues or mood disorders precipitated by the medical illness.

Summary

Successful implementation of psychological and behavioral modalities of intervention depends on a comprehensive biopsychosocial assessment and individualized approaches involving the sexual partner whenever possible. Although there is considerable clinical evidence for the value of psychological therapies for enhancing sexual function and satisfaction as part of an overall treatment plan, there is little objective evidence of their effectiveness in older individuals. Outcome studies of psychological treatment effectiveness have included older patients but their results are not grouped by age. Most studies have significant methodological limitations and show wide differences in outcome, ranging, for example, from no evidence of efficacy to successful response rates of up to 81% in the treatment of erectile dysfunction (Hawton, 1992; Cole, 1993). Progress has been made in identifying prognostic indicators of a good response to psychological treatment of erectile disorders. Contributing to good prognosis is evidence of inadequate sexual stimulation, overdependence on penile erections for female sexual satisfaction, lack of information on age-related changes in sexual functioning, and unrealistic demands for sexual performance (LoPiccolo, 1992). Positive prognostic factors identified in a prospective study by Hawton, Catalan and Fagg (1992) were: the overall quality of the couple's relationship, increased motivation for therapy, absence of psychiatric disorders in the female partner and more active engagement in homework assignments during the early stages of treatment.

Medical and surgical interventions

The first line of approach is to address medical conditions causally related to the sexual disorder and to evaluate and possibly change pharmacological regimens that contribute to sexual dysfunction. Strategies of intervention for male sexual disorders include, in addition, a range of therapeutic options such as hormone treatment, oral agents, intracavernosal pharmacotherapy, external vacuum devices, penile prosthetic implants, and vascular reconstructive surgery.

Endocrine treatment

There is consensus that, in the presence of normal sexual desire, testosterone is not therapeutically effective in eugonadal men with erectile dysfunction (Bancroft, 1988). As discussed in previous chapters, serum testosterone does decrease progressively in healthy aging men, but the clinical consequences of this decline remain uncertain, since relatively few older men reach hypogonadal criteria. Although it has been speculated that the threshold required to sustain the behavioral and physiological effects of testosterone may increase with age, there are no solid data supporting the therapeutic effects of androgen administration to aging men with sexual dysfunction (Schiavi et al., 1997). The National Institutes of Health Conference on Impotence (1992) reached the conclusion that androgen replacement therapy is only indicated for men with erectile disorders associated with hypogonadism and/or abnormally low testosterone levels. Androgen administration may cause deleterious effects on the prostate, cardiovascular system and contribute to fluid retention and sleep apnea. Long-term clinical studies are needed to assess the risk/benefit profile for hormonal supplementation in older men with borderline circulating testosterone levels (Tenover, 1995). Long-acting injectable preparations such as testosterone enanthate or testosterone cypionate are the most widely prescribed forms for replacement therapy. Oral preparations are more acceptable but have higher risks of hepatotoxicity and elevated serum lipid levels (Morales, 1995).

Oral drugs

Considerable interest is being attracted by the development and testing of drugs to treat sexual dysfunction (Garcia-Reboll, Mulhall and Goldstein, 1997). The availability of safe and effective oral agents could eventually have profound consequences for overall treatment strategies, in view of patients' expectation and demand for noninvasive modalities.

Yohimbine

This alpha 2-adrenoceptor antagonist is the oral agent that received the earliest attention for the treatment of erectile disorders. Its therapeutic value remains controversial despite the numerous studies that have been carried out to demonstrate its efficacy. (Rosen, 1991; Gregoire, 1993). Recently, Carey and Johnson (1996) carried out four meta-analyses on data from controlled as well as uncontrolled clinical trials using yohimbine alone or in combination with other drugs. The results of 25 studies reported from 1966 to 1993 suggested that yohimbine is therapeutically effective, but serious methodological limitations and overall patient heterogeneity severely restrict confidence in this conclusion and its appropriateness to older patient groups.

Trazodone

This serotonergic antidepressant with alpha-blocking activity may induce increased sexual drive unrelated to mood changes and, on rare occasions, priapism (Rosen, 1991). It has been used to treat erectile dysfunction but its clinical efficacy has yet to be experimentally demonstrated.

Apomorphine

Apomorphine is a short-acting dopamine receptor agonist which may induce erections in normal men and in patients with psychogenic erectile dysfunction. Its clinical use has been limited by adverse effects such as nausea, vomiting and hypotension. A sublingual form of apomorphine hydrochloride is undergoing a phase III clinical trial (Heaton et al., 1995).

Sildenafil

This drug – a selective inhibitor of guanosine 3',5'-cyclic monophosphate (cGMP) type-V phosphodiesterase, an enzyme present in human corpora cavernosa – holds considerable promise for the treatment of male erectile dysfunction. The results of a phase III, multi-institutional trial have shown that the drug facilitates the development of erections in response to sexual stimulation (Garcia-Reboll, Mulhall and Goldstein, 1997; Keith Light, 1997). Preliminary data indicate that the drug, taken by men with erectile dysfunction approximately one hour before intended sexual activity, results in harder and longer-lasting erections and that it is well accepted by patients; mentioned side-effects are headache, dyspepsia, flushing, and abnormal vision (Guirguis, 1998). Results from a double-blind, placebo-controlled study of sildenafil at 25 to 100 mg dose levels showed significant enhancement in erectile function in men aged 65 and older (Wagner, Mayton, Smith and the multicentre study group, 1998). The drug is contraindicated in patients who concurrently take organic nitrates. More information is required to substantiate the long-term efficacy, safety and clinical indications of this agent.

Antidepressant treatment of premature ejaculation

Premature ejaculation, independent of erectile difficulties, is not a usual complaint among older patients. The lack of convincing long-term therapeutic efficacy of traditional behavioral approaches, particularly in older individuals, and the observation that delayed ejaculation is a common side-effect of antidepressants led to exploration of the use of antidepressants for its treatment. Selective serotonin reuptake inhibitors (SSRIs), such as clomipramine, paroxetine, sertraline and fluoxetine, have emerged as relatively safe and effective treatment options in terms of increased ejaculatory latency and individual and partner satisfaction (Balon, 1996).

Topical and transurethral drug therapy

Testosterone

Recently, Arver and collaborators (1996) experimented with the effects of a transdermal testosterone delivery system on the sexual function of hypogonadal men. This system, which achieves more physiologically normal circadian hormonal variations than intramuscular administration, was effective at improving subjective and objective erectile measures when compared to the pretreatment hypogonadal state.

Prostaglandin E$_1$

Prostaglandin E$_1$ pellets are introduced into the distal urethra which, following absorption, induces relaxation of the cavernosal smooth muscle. The results of a double-blind, placebo-controlled medication study involving 1500 men with organic erectile dysfunction showed a 62% successful response rate, allowing intercourse on at least one occasion when used at home, compared to 10% in the placebo group. Adverse effects include local pain, burning sensations and hypotension but the discontinuation rate in this phase III drug trial was low (Padma-Nathan et al., 1997).

Intracavernosal injection therapy

Injection of vasoactive agents into the corpora cavernosa of the penis has become a commonly used treatment of erectile dysfunction (Montague, 1996). Patients or their partners are trained to carry out the penile injection procedure at home following titration in the doctor's office of the lowest dosage required to induce adequate rigidity. The drugs that have been most frequently used, either singly or in combination in urological practice, are papaverine, phentolamine, and prostaglandin E_1 (Gee et al., 1996). In 1995 prostaglandin E_1 received approval from the Food and Drug Administration for the treatment of erectile dysfunction. There is convincing evidence that intracavernous therapy is effective for organic, mixed or psychogenic erectile problems. Patients with a neurogenic dysfunction appear to have increased sensitivity, while men with vasculogenic dysfunction respond less well to vasoactive drugs. Significant side-effects are priapism, fibrotic nodules, bruising, pain, transient hypotension, and liver function abnormalities. Prostaglandin E_1 is becoming the first line of therapy because of its relatively low association with priapism (1%), penile fibrotic complications (2%), ecchymosis (8%), and liver function safety (Linet, Ogring, for the Alprostadil Study Group, 1996). Papaverine with phentolamine, or a combination of both drugs with prostaglandin E_1, is being reserved for patients who cannot tolerate the penile pain and burning sensations frequently induced with prostaglandin E_1 alone. No differences in the efficacy and safety of intracavernosal injections were noted between younger (mean age 47 years) and older patient (mean age 70 years) groups (Kerfoot and Carson, 1991). Although self-injection with vasoactive agents induces significant improvements in erectile rigidity, sexual satisfaction, and overall quality of life (Willke et al, 1997), it is associated with high discontinuation rates, ranging from 11 to 80%. In a study of intracavernosal injection therapy by Gupta et al. (1997), that included over 1000 patients, the overall attrition rate occurring mostly during the first two months of treatment was 37.6% (27.5% among prostaglandin E_1 users). The most frequent reasons for dropping out were complaints of ineffectiveness, penile scarring, penile pain, fear of injections, and inconvenience or lack of spontaneity. The observation that a significant number of patients discontinue intracavernosal injections for reasons independent of this treatment modality, and do not seek further therapy even when available, suggests the relevance of psychosocial factors to overall treatment outcome (Sexton, Benedict and Jarow, 1998). Further studies are required to identify, during the pretreatment stage and follow-up period, potential clinical and psychosocial predictors that may improve patient screening and comprehensive counseling. See Case study 14.2 for illustration of a comprehensive approach that includes psychopharmacology, sex therapy, and intracavernosal therapy.

External vacuum therapy

These devices generate negative pressure within a plastic cylinder that is placed around the flaccid penis, thereby drawing blood into the corpora cavernosa. Rubber constriction bands are then placed around the base of the penis limiting venous outflow and maintaining rigidity. Very little pretreatment testing is required and the overall clinical success rate is over 80%. Contraindications to the use of vacuum therapy are limited, mainly to unexplained intermittent priapism and bleeding disorders. The most common complaints are difficulties in the application of the device, lack of spontaneity, discomfort, and, in some patients, impaired ejaculation (Gregoire, 1993). Despite these problems, patients' acceptance of vacuum therapy is high, and the long-term drop-out rate, while significant, appears to be less than in intracavernosal pharmacotherapy. A prospective, randomized, crossover study comparing the effectiveness, side-effects, and patient satisfaction between external vacuum devices and intracavernosal injections showed a trend favoring injection therapy that was most significant in younger patients and in those with an erectile dysfunction of shorter duration (Soderdahl, Thrasher and Hansberry, 1997). Comparison of the sexual satisfaction of female partners of men treated with vacuum therapy or self-injections showed both groups to be equally satisfied with these approaches (Althof et al., 1992). Patients should receive individual training in the use of vacuum devices, preferably with their partners, and anticipate a learning period to achieve optimal results (Lewis and Witherington, 1997).

Penile prosthetic implants

Prosthetic implants currently available fall into three types: malleable, semirigid, and inflatable. Their use is primarily reserved for patients with severe organic erectile disorders who do not respond to less invasive approaches (Shabsigh, 1998). Age is not a significant factor when selecting the type of prosthesis. Inflatable prostheses have a more natural appearance but they require sufficient manual dexterity to be used successfully, are more expensive, and have higher mechanical failure rates. Semirigid prostheses are preferable for patients at greater medical risks of surgery because of their lower necessity of reoperation. Perioperative infections and erosions are complications that occur regardless of the prosthetic type. Adequate evaluation of candidates for prosthetic implants and sexual counseling are important if the objective is not only achieving penile rigidity but also enhancing sexual enjoyment (Melman and Tiefer, 1992). Ideally, the initial screening should involve both partners with attention placed on inaccurate expectations and on issues that contribute to postimplantation dissatisfaction. Among these factors are the coexistence of other dysfunctions (e.g., hypoactive sexual desire, premature ejaculation), poor sexual communication, overemphasis on penile size and rigidity for sexual pleasure, and decreased orgasmic intensity (Schover and von Eschenbach, 1985) (see Case study 14.3).

Surgical procedures

Surgery for erectile disorders includes the correction of penile curvature (Peyronie's disease), arterial revascularization and surgery for veno-occlusive dysfunction. Peyronie's disease is not uncommon in older men and its surgical correction is usually successful in selected patients following diagnostic intracavernosal testing and color Doppler ultrasonography. Arterial bypass surgery for vasculogenic erectile disorders is reserved for patients younger than 60 who are free from diabetes mellitus and cardiovascular disease, have no evidence of venous corporal incompetence and an abnormal pudendal angiogram (Melman and Tiefer, 1992). Suitable candidates are usually young patients with congenital or post-traumatic vascular insufficiency. Surgery for venous corporal incompetence is carried out to correct an abnormal leakage of blood from the penis; it requires a preoperative evaluation that includes pharmaco-cavernosometry and cavernosography to identify the presence and location of the lesion. Venous surgical repair has not achieved consistent satisfactory results (Pryor, 1993). The National Institutes of Health Consensus on Impotence (1992) recommended further efforts at improving diagnostic standardization prior to vascular surgery which may best be carried out in specialized medical centers.

Treatment guidelines

The growing array of evaluation and treatment alternatives may be confusing to health-care professionals when approached by aging men with sexual complaints, the most frequent being erectile dysfunction. The aim of treatment should be improvement of sexual satisfaction for the patient, alone or with his partner, and not be limited to restoring erectile capacity. The overall therapeutic strategy is based on an integrated approach with equal attention given to medical and psychological issues, and a step-wise evaluation involving the minimal amount of testing required for treatment implementation. Medically, it includes diagnosis and treatment of underlying chronic disorders as well as reversible medical conditions such as hypogonadism, medication effects, alcohol and tobacco abuse. Psychologically, it involves assessing the nature of the sexual problem, identifying possible emotional and relationship issues, the presence of a mood disorder, and exploring sexual expectations and motivation for treatment. A careful assessment of both aspects usually suffices to formulate preliminary notions about what is contributing to the problem and alternative courses of action. It is critically important, in order for the patient to reach an informed decision, to provide an unbiased view of the nature of the difficulty and discuss advantages and limitations of appropriate therapeutic options. Sexual counseling, behavioral or marital therapy should be offered first to patients/couples with evidence of significant psychological involvement in the sexual dysfunction. Oral drugs are the patients' usual preferred medical approach but the effectiveness and safety of currently approved oral agents remains to be firmly established. Intracavernosal pharmacotherapy, or vacuum devices may be recommended, alone or in conjunction with counseling, to patients with organic erectile disorders or to individuals who do not respond to, or are unmotivated by, psychological interventions. Penile prostheses should be reserved for selected patients after careful screening and counseling. Vascular surgery remains an exceptional procedure for sexually dysfunctional older men.

This strategy, in its general outline, is in keeping with the goal-directed approach first described by Lue (1990), but differs in its greater psychological emphasis. Lue proposed a minimum diagnostic evaluation based on the patient's therapeutic preferences with little attention given to psychological factors. Two outcome studies of this primarily medical approach showed that most patients preferred, but were disappointed by, oral medications, and that intracavernosal injections were the second most selected therapy. However, long-term follow-up revealed that the majority of patients dropped-out of intracavernosal injections or refused further treatment (Jarow et al., 1996; Hanash, 1997). New oral agents such as 5-phosphodiesterase inhibitors, if proven effective and safe during long-term treatment, may become a major breakthrough in the management of erectile dysfunction. It is and will remain important when assessing and following-up older patients and partners to be attentive to their sexual motivation and expectations, and to provide education and counseling with the aim of optimizing sexual satisfaction and reducing relapse rates.

Case studies

Case study 14.1

Mr. X, aged 76, was a retired stock broker living in Connecticut with his wife aged 68. They reported a good marriage without major emotional upheavals, excellent health and a rewarding involvement in community activities. They had continued to engage in problem-free intercourse that had gradually decreased from three times per week at the beginning of their marriage 35 years ago, to twice per month. Sex had become a comfortable and predictable activity devoid of surprises, a necessary but not important aspect of their lives. This attitude, however, changed, as he found himself to have progressive erectile problems at a time of stress caused by a drop in the value of his investments. His financial worries were compounded by his frustrated sexual attempts, driven by a need for reassurance rather than desire. Five months before contacting our program Mr. X had consulted with a urologist who advised intracavernosal prostaglandin injections, a recommendation that he did not follow.

The most significant finding during our evaluation, in addition to his considerable performance anxiety, was a mild depression that by itself did not warrant pharmacological intervention. With some reluctance Mr. X agreed to return with his wife for a second evaluation session. When interviewed alone she disclosed, with embarrassment, her aversion to touching his penis since the beginning of their marriage, requiring his rubbing against her body in order to gain an erection sufficient for penetration. Therapeutic intervention consisted of sexual counseling for the couple, addressing the need of direct penile stimulation, and individual psychotherapy for Ms. X, focusing on early traumatic experiences that were at the root of her sexual aversion. Three months later the couple had reestablished regular coital activity in the context of a more balanced and effective sexual interaction.

Comments

This vignette illustrates the interplay of common causal determinants of erectile failure in the aged: insufficient sexual stimulation, depression and performance anxiety. The onset of a subclinical depression was sufficient to decompensate the marginal sexual adjustment of an older man who was relying on suboptimal sexual interactions with his wife. It also demonstrates the importance of bringing the sexual partner into the evaluation process. Mr. X acknowledged during therapy his own discomfort at providing detailed sexual information as well as his desire to protect his wife from having to disclose her sexual inhibitions.

Case study 14.2

Mr. Y is a 66-year-old man who sought help for loss of sexual desire and progressive erectile difficulties which started two years before, at a time of severe personal and financial stress caused by the bankruptcy of his printing business. Lack of sexual interest, fear of failure and apprehension at disappointing his wife had resulted in sexual avoidance during the preceding six months. The patient was no longer aware of early morning erections and when he attempted to masturbate to 'test himself' he only noticed minimal tumescence at the moment of ejaculation. Mr. Y reported a problem-free sexual life prior to the current episode. He had married for the second time five years before a woman 20 years his junior. Both described a warm and caring relationship and, although they were no longer sexual with one another, they felt physically close and affectionate. Mr. Y described himself as a 'type A' personality and as a workaholic who likes 'struggle and bustle', and felt that he could not live without it. However, during the preceding year his work efficiency had decreased, he had problems concentrating and at times felt overwhelmed by self-recrimination and guilt associated with his business and sexual failures.

The medical history was notable in that he had had double bypass heart surgery 15 years before from which he fully recovered, mild untreated hypertension, alcohol abuse averaging three pints of hard liquor a week over the last two years, and a family history of diabetes. The patient was not taking any medication other than aspirin. The physical examination revealed an atrophic right testis which the patient stated he had had for as long as he could remember, and decreased tibial and dorsalis pedis pulses.

Physiological assessment

The patient was studied in the sleep laboratory over two consecutive nights. He had five erectile episodes in each of the study nights but none of them was a maximum erection (less than 80% of full tumescence). The visual sexual stimulation test resulted in erections graded as 60% of full tumescence. Evaluation of penile blood pressure showed a penile to brachial systolic index of 0.65 after exercise, considered below the lower limit of normal. He also had a positive glucose tolerance test consistent with the diagnosis of diabetes mellitus. The blood hormone measures were within normal limits (prolactin: 11.5 ng/ml; testosterone: 5.0 ng/ml).

Formulation and treatment approach

A constellation of psychological and organic determinants singly or in combination are probable etiological contributors to the loss of sexual desire and erectile problems. Most revealing among the psychological factors is the onset of sexual difficulties after his financial debacle, resulting in clinically significant depression with associated cognitive difficulties, self-recrimination, and guilt. The medical evaluation and physiological assessment suggested, in addition, an organic limitation of erectile capacity involving neurovascular mechanisms possibly associated with diabetes. An additional contributor is alcohol abuse triggered by the stress of his business failure, and reactive depression. The treatment strategy was implemented in three phases. Mr. Y accepted with some reluctance to focus first on his affective disorder compelled by the aggravation of his depressive mood. He responded well to tricyclic antidepressants with elevation of mood, enhanced sexual desire, increased ability to work and sobriety. However, after four months his erectile function was not restored and he continued to be dominated by fear of failure and apprehension that his wife might leave him. The antidepressant medication was gradually withdrawn without erectile improvement. The second treatment phase involved a short course of sex therapy aimed at minimizing performance anxiety, enhancing the effectiveness of sexual stimulation, and improving marital communication. Although their sexual experiences became freer and more enjoyable, and insertion and intravaginal ejaculation was occasionally possible, Mr. Y remained dissatisfied by the unpredictable nature of his erections. He decided against his wife's wishes, who was content with the nature of their sexual experiences, to begin intracavernosal treatment with prostaglandin E_1. Mr. Y's erectile capacity was fully restored and for a period of about four months they engaged in intercourse on a once-a-week basis. Eventually, he discontinued intracavernosal injections feeling that it was 'too much trouble' and became more accepting of his erratic erectile capacity and satisfied with the shared pleasure of noncoital sexual interactions.

Comment

This vignette illustrates the multiplicity of causal determinants of sexual dysfunction commonly seen in the aged, and the value of developing a therapeutic strategy based on the integrated conceptualization of the problem. The sequential approach, involving psycho-pharmacology, sex therapy, and intracavernosal treatment, helped to clarify the pathogenic significance of potential contributors while implementing a multidisciplinary treatment plan. The patient's positive response to antidepressants demonstrated that a mood disorder was at the basis of the loss of sexual drive but it did not explain his impaired erectile function. Sex therapy reactivated the couple's sexual life and enhanced the quality of their sexual interaction but his erections, although improved, remained subnormal, limited by organic pathology. While intracavernosal pharmacotherapy corrected the erectile disability it did not contribute to the long-term expectations of this couple, who eventually chose to remain sexually active and to enjoy their experiences despite the vagaries of his penis.

Case study 14.3

Mr. Z is a 64-year-old retired pharmacist who came to our Program for consultation because of the imminence of separation from his 40-year-old wife, four months after penile prosthetic implantation. The progressive development of erectile difficulties over an eight-year period had not prevented his having satisfying sexual experiences prior to his marriage one year before. During the three years they had lived together before marriage they engaged in frequent sex play followed by his manually stimulating her to orgasm, and her manually assisting penile vaginal penetration to ejaculation. The onset of his total inability to achieve intercourse had occurred soon after their marriage after Ms. Z expressed her desire to become pregnant. His medical history included severe hypertension treated with verapamil and diuretics. Nocturnal penile tumescence assessment over two nights revealed a normal erectile pattern with adequate (sufficient for penetration without manual assistance) but not rigid erections. Doppler assessment with intracavernosal testing was suggestive of vasculogenic impotence. Change of the patient's antihypertensive regimen did not improve his erectile function. Intracavernosal injection treatment was initiated with prostaglandin E_1 later modified, because of intense pain, by combining it with papaverine and phentolamine. The patient experienced considerable anxiety about self-injecting (or being injected by his wife) and found himself, following penile injections, unable to ejaculate intravaginally, despite prolonged thrusting. He decided, without consulting with his wife, to have a malleable prosthesis implanted which resulted in a firm and reliable erection, but also in considerable marital upheaval since his wife resented not having been involved in the decision and felt 'turned off' because the coital experiences were 'too mechanical'. It required extensive sexual counseling before the couple could integrate the prosthesis into satisfying sexual experiences and, eventually, achieve intravaginal ejaculation.

Comment

Possible contributors to this patient's sexual problems include the interacting effects of vasculogenic factors associated with hypertension, the uncertain role of medication as well as the psychological pressure induced by his younger wife's frustrated desire to become pregnant. Achieving a full erection and intercourse was not the solution to Mr. Z's difficulty. Mr. Z's attempts to please his wife, despite serious reservations to have a child at this late stage of life, were defeated by his anxiety about sexual performance and fear of penile injections.

Although it may be tempting to explain his ejaculatory incompetence as the consequence of his ambivalence about paternity, a behavioral analysis of their sexual interaction disclosed that Mr. Z engaged in intercourse soon after achieving an erection following penile injections when not fully aroused. Mr. Z's impulsive decision to seek a prosthetic implant, without adequate advice or his wife's involvement in the decision, was unwarranted and destructive for the marital equilibrium. The couple's sexual counseling involved behavioral interventions to restore pleasure in their sexual interactions as well as open discussion of his unexpressed negative feelings about fatherhood. The vignette emphasizes the importance of considering psychological and relationship issues in the evaluation of patients with evidence of organic involvement as well as the value of long-term follow-up to help patients adjust to invasive interventions, particularly when it involves an irreversible approach such as prosthetic implantation.

References

Althof, S. E., Turner, L. A., Levine, S. B., Bodner, D., Kursh, E. D. and Resnick, M. I. (1992). Through the eyes of women: the sexual and psychological responses of women to their partner's treatment with self–injection or external vacuum therapy. *Journal of Urology* 147, 1024–7.

Arver, S., Dobs, A. S., Meikle, A. W., Allen, R. P., Sanders, S. W. and Mazer, N. A. (1996). Improvement of sexual function in testosterone deficient men treated for 1 year with a permeation enhanced testosterone transdermal system. *Journal of Urology* 155, 1604–8.

Balon, R. (1996). Antidepressants in the treatment of premature ejaculation. *Journal of Sex and Marital Therapy* 22, 85–96.

Baltes, P. B. and Baltes, M. M. (1990). Psychological perspectives on successful aging: the model of selective optimization with compensation. In *Successful Aging*, ed. P. B. Baltes and M. M. Baltes, pp. 1–34. Cambridge: Cambridge University Press.

Bancroft, J. (1988). Reproductive hormones and male sexual function. In *Hanbook of Sexology*. ed. J. M. A. Sitson, pp. 297–315, Amsterdam: Elsevier.

Beck, A. T. (1988). *Love is Never Enough*, New York: Harper Perennial.

Carey, M. P. and Johnson, B. T. (1996). Effectiveness of yohimbine in the treatment of erectile disorder: Four meta-analytic integrations. *Archives of Sexual Behavior* 25, 341–60.

Cole, M. (1993). Psychological approaches to treatment. In *Impotence. An Integrated approach to Clinical Practice*, ed. A. Gregoire and J. P. Pryor, pp. 129–64. Edinburgh: Churchill Livingston.

Cole, M. and Gregoire, A. (1993). The impotent men without a partner. In *Impotence. An Integrated Approach to Clinical Practice*, pp. 215–27, Edinburgh: Churchill Livingstone.

Felton, B. J., Revenson, T. A. and Hinrichsen, G. A. (1984). Stress and coping in the explanation of psychological adjustment among chronically ill adults, *Social Science Medicine* 18, 889–98.

Garcia–Reboll, L., Mulhall, J. P. and Goldstein, I. (1997). Drugs for the treatment of impotence. *Drugs and Aging* 11, 140–51.

Gee, W. F., Holtgrewe, H. L., Alberstein, P. C., Litwin, M. S., Manyak, M. J., O'Leary, M. P., Painter, M. R., Blizzard, R. T., Fenninger, R. B. and Emmons, L. (1996). Practice trends of American urologists in the treatment of impotence, incontinence and infertility. *Journal of Urology* 156, 1778–80.

Goldman, A. and Carroll, J. (1990). Educational intervention as an adjunct to treatment of erectile dysfunction in older couples. *Journal Sex and Marital Therapy* 16, 127–41.

Gregoire, A. (1993). Pharmacological treatments for impotence. In *Impotence. An Integrated Approach to Clinical Practice*, ed. A. Gregoire and J. P. Pryor, pp. 165–184. Edinburgh: Churchill Livingston.

Guirguis, W. R. (1998). Oral treatment of erectile dysfunction. *Journal of Sex and Marital Therapy* 24, 69–73.

Gupta, R., Kirschen, J., Barrow, R. C. and Eid, J. F. (1997). Predictors of success and risk factors for attrition in the use of intracavernous injection. *Journal of Urology* 157, 1681–6.

Hanash, K. A. (1997). Comparative results of goal oriented therapy for erectile dysfunction. *Journal of Urology* 157, 2135–8.

Hawton, K. (1982). The behavioral treatment of sexual dysfunction. *British Journal of Psychiatry* 140, 94–101.

Hawton, K. (1992). Sex therapy research: has it withered on the vine? *Annual Review of Sex Research* 3, 49–72.

Hawton, K., Catalan, J. and Fagg, J. (1992). Sex therapy for erectile dysfunction. characteristics of couples, treatment outcome and prognostic factors. *Archives of Sexual Behavior* 21, 161–75.

Heaton, J. P., Morales, A., Adams, M. A., Johnston, B. and El–Rashidi, R. (1995). Recovery of erectile function by the oral administration of apomorphine. *Urology* 45, 200.

Jarow, J. P., Nana–Sinkam, P., Sabbagh, M. and Eskew, A. (1996). Outcome analysis of goal directed therapy for impotence. *Journal of Urology* 155, 1609–12.

Keith Light, J. (1997). Impotence [editorial]. *Journal of Urology* 157, 2139.

Kerfoot, W. W. and Carson, C. C. (1991). Pharmacologically induced erections among geriatric men. *Journal of Urology* 146, 1022–4.

Leiblum, S. R. and Rosen, R. C. (1992). Couples therapy for erectile disorders: operative procedures and psychological issues. In *Erectile Disorders: Assessment and Treatment*, pp. 226–54. New York: The Guilford Press.

Lewis, R. W. and Witherington, R. (1997). External vacuum therapy for erectile dysfunction: use and results. *World Journal of Urology* 15, 78–82.

Linet, O. I., Ogring, F. G., for the Alprostadil Group. (1996). Efficacy and safety of intracavernosal alprostadil in men with erectile dysfunction. *New England Journal of Medicine* 334, 873–7.

LoPiccolo, J. (1992). Postmodern sex therapy for erectile failure. In *Erectile Disorders: Assessment and Treatment*, ed. R. C. Rosen and S. R. Leiblum, pp. 171–197. New York: The Guilford Press

Lue, T. F. (1990). Impotence: a patient's goal-directed approach to treatment. *World Journal of Urology* 8, 67–74.

McCarthy, B. W. (1984). *Male Sexual Awareness*. New York: Carroll & Grag.

McCarthy, B. W. (1992). Treatment of erectile dysfunction of single men. *In Erectile Disorders: Assessment and Treatment*, pp. 313–40, New York: The Guilford Press.

Melman, A. and Tiefer, L. (1992). Surgery for erectile disorders: Operative procedures and psychological issues. In *Erectile Disorders. Assessment and Treatment*, en. R. C. Rosen and S. R.

Leiblum, pp. 255–282. New York: The Guilford Press.

Montague, D. K., Barada, J. H., Belker, A. M., Levine, L. A., Nadig, P. W., Roehrborn, C. G., Sharlip, I. D. and Bennett, A. H. (1996). Clinical guidelines panel on erectile dysfunction: summary report on the treatment of organic erectile dysfunction. *Journal of Urology* 156, 2007–11.

Moos, R. (1977). *Coping with Physical Illness*, New York: Plenum Press.

Morales, A. (1995). Androgen supplementation in practice: the treatment of erectile dysfunction associated with hypotestosteronemia. In *Androgens and the Aging Male*, ed. B. Oddens and A. Vermeulen, pp. 233–46. New York: The Parthenon Publishing Group.

Padma–Nathan, H., Hellstrom, W. G., Kaiser, F. E. et al. (1997). Treatment of men with erectile dysfunction with transurethral alprostadil. *New England Journal of Medicine* 336, 1–7.

Pryor, J. P. (1993). Surgical procedures to correct erectile dysfunction. In *Impotence. An integrated approach to clinical practice*, ed. A. Gregoire and J. P. Pryor, pp. 191–200. Edinburgh: Churchill Livingston.

Reynolds, B. (1991). Psychological treatment of erectile dysfunction of men without partners: outcome results and a new direction. *Journal of Sex and Marital Therapy* 17, 136–46.

Rosen, R. C. (1991). Alcohol and drug effects on sexual response: human experimental and clinical studies. *Annual Review of Sex Research* 2, 119–80.

Rosen, R. C., Leiblum, S. R. and Spector, L. (1994). Psychologically based treatment for male erectile disorder: a cognitive–interpersonal model. *Journal of Sex and Marital Therapy* 20, 67–85.

Rowland, K. F. and Haynes, S. N. (1978). A sexual enhancement program for elderly couples. *Journal of Sex and Marital Therapy* 4, 91–113.

Schiavi, R. C. (1980). Psychological treatment of erectile disorders in diabetic patients. *Annals of Internal Medicine* 92, 337–9.

Schiavi, R. C., White, D., Mandeli, J. and Levine, A. (1997). Effect of testosterone administration on sexual behavior and mood in men with erectile dysfunction. *Archives of Sexual Behavior* 26, 231–41.

Schover, L. R. (1992). Erectile failure and chronic illness. In *Erectile Disorders: Assessment and Treatment*, ed. R. C. Rosen and S. R. Leiblum, pp. 341–67. New York: The Guilford Press.

Schover, L. R. and von Eschenbach, A. C. (1985). Sex therapy and the penile prosthesis: a synthesis. *Journal of Sex and Marital Therapy* 11, 57–66.

Schover, L. R. and Jensen, S. B. (1988). *Sexuality and Chronic Illness: A Comprehensive Approach*. New York: The Guildford Press

Sexton, W. J., Benedict, J. F. and Jarow, J. P. (1998). Comparison of long-term outcomes of penile prostheses and intracavernosal injection therapy. *Journal of Urology* 159, 811–15.

Shabsigh, R. (1998). Penile prosthesis toward the end of the millenium [editorial]. *Journal of Urology* 159, 819.

Soderdahl, D. W., Thrasher, J. B. and Hansberry, K. L. (1997). Intracavernosal drug-induced erection therapy versus external vacuum devices in the treatment of erectile dysfunction. *British Journal of Urology* 79, 952–7.

Tenover, J. L. (1995). Effects of androgen supplementation in the aging male. In *Androgens and the Aging Male*, ed. B. Oddens and A. Vermeulen, pp. 191–204. New York: The Parthenon Publishing Group.

The National Institutes of Health Conference on Impotence (1992). NIH Consensus Statement. December 7–9; **10** (4), 1–31.

Wagner, G., Mayton, M., Smith, M. D. and the multicentre study group. (1998). Analysis of the efficacy of sildenafil (Viagra) in the treatment of male erectile dysfunction in elderly patients. Abstract presented at the 24th Annual Meeting International Academy Sex Research, 3–6 June 1998, Sirmione, Italy, p. 86 (in press).

White, C. B. and Catania, J. A. (1982). Psychoeducational intervention for sexuality with the aged, family members of the aged and people who work with the aged. *International Journal of Aging and Human Development* **15**, 121– 38.

Wiley, D. and Bortz, W. M. II (1996). Sexuality and aging – usual and successful. *Journal of Gerontology* **51A**, M142–M146.

Willke, R. J., Glick, H. A., McCarron, T. J., Erder, M. H., Althof, S. E. and Linet, O. I. (1997). Quality of life effects of Alprostadil therapy for erectile dysfunction. *Journal of Urology* **157**, 2124–8.

Zilbergeld, B. (1992). *The New Male Sexuality*. New York: Bantam.

Aging has emerged as an important area of social concern, first in industrialized countries and now in the less developed regions of the world. Demographic changes caused by increased life expectancy and declines in birth rates have resulted in a dramatic shift, with the proportion of older people increasing rapidly to form a substantial segment of the population. This demographic reality and the growing awareness of the aged as a definable social group have led to gerontology developing as a multidisciplinary endeavor. Initially, much gerontological research was biologically oriented, and only recently has its interaction with psychosocial factors, as they influence health and behavior, become a focus of concentrated attention. While sexological research in the field of aging has made significant advances, moving from the descriptive and epidemiological to the physiological and more recently to the biomedical and clinical, it has yet to fully integrate psychosocial perspectives in its studies. A review of data points to several methodological problems, not all limited to sexological studies, that need to be considered when interpreting the results. Much of the research is cross-sectional in design, confounding the effects of aging with differences in the attitudes, values, and behavior that characterized the different age cohorts as they grew up. Longitudinal studies, on the other hand, are undermined by selective attrition, biasing the results in the direction of the healthier, stable, and cooperative participants. Conclusions are frequently drawn from small, unrepresentative and nonrandom samples of white, middle-class and well-educated volunteers who are probably more liberal in their sexual attitudes than their counterparts who decline to participate in sexological research. Studies of the sexuality of aging males have focused on coital frequencies, neglecting assessment of the motivational, cognitive, and affective dimensions which characterize the sexual experiences of the aged more appropriately.

Behavioral surveys demonstrate that, contrary to popular myths, sexuality remains an important aspect in the lives of a significant segment of the aging population. The frequency of sexual behavior and, to a lesser extent, sexual desire decrease with age and there is an increased prevalence of sexual dysfunctions, primarily erectile problems, as age progresses. Psychophysiological methods provide objective evidence, under controlled conditions, of the effects of aging on male sexual function. The erectile responsiveness to erotic stimuli and nocturnal penile tumescence activity recorded during sleep both significantly decline with age. Frequently ignored, however, is the marked individual heterogeneity in behavioral and physiological measures within age groups, with some men in their 70s and beyond exhibiting levels of sexual function typical of much younger individuals. Contributing to this variability are the persistence of life-long individual differences in sexual behavior, the deleterious effect of medical illness, drugs and psychopathology, and the role of the sexual partner, when available, in the sexual life of aging men. Age-related decreases in male sexual behavior do occur in the absence of pathology, however, and it is important to distinguish the changes intrinsic to aging processes from the consequences of modifiable social, psychological and life-style effects. Neglected in many studies of the sexuality of aging males are noncoital forms of sexual expression and subjective experiences such as sexual enjoyment and satisfaction.

Considerable research has been carried out recently on the hormonal, neural, and vascular processes that mediate the nonpathological effects of aging on male sexuality. Aging is associated with a decrease in total and biologically active circulating testosterone, a gradual decline in testicular function and age-related changes in hypothalamic–pituitary mechanisms controlling gonadal activity. There are wide individual differences in circulating testosterone levels, but hormonal levels, within the normal range, do not account for variations in sexual drive or behavior. There is indirect evidence, however, that the threshold required for the behavioral action of testosterone increases with age, which may result in the hormonal level becoming insufficient to sustain adequate sexual function. Androgens, mainly testosterone, not only play a necessary role in sexual drive, but they may also have effects on general vigor and well-being. Significant anatomical, biochemical and functional CNS changes occur during nonpathological aging, but information about their relationship with changes in male sexuality is limited and indirect. Of particular interest are central monoamines, primarily dopamine, serotonin and noradrenaline, and neuropeptides such as endogenous opioids because of their central role in the regulation of sexual behavior. However, most of the evidence is derived from animal research without a specific focus on the mediation of aging processes. Normal aging may also influence male sexuality by its general effects on sensory systems and, in particular, somatosensory function. Penile sensory vibrotactile sensitivity decreases with age, which may impair sexual behavior by interfering with reflex mechanisms that mediate erections, as well as by modifying the pleasurable quality of the sexual experiences. Of considerable functional significance are age-related vascular changes, including endothelial mechanisms within the corpora cavernosa, that mediate erection. The actions of nitric oxide and other endothelium-derived relaxing factors responsible for vasodilatation decrease with aging, while the activity of endothelin-1, a potent endothelium-generated vasoconstrictor, increases with age. The erectile smooth muscle tone increases with aging, in concert with structural changes within the corpora cavernosa with deposition of subintimal collagen and decreases in vascular elastin, both of which may contribute to decreased penile rigidity in older men.

There are considerable variations in the emotional responses of individuals and couples to age-related decreases in sexual function. Some integrate sexual changes into their overall life without affecting their well-being, some develop coping strategies to adapt to sexual declines and others react with considerable distress, anxiety, loss of self-esteem and relationship difficulties. Sexual attitudes, knowledge, and motivation are important individual dimensions that shape psychological and behavioral reactions to aging. Older men raised in an era of rigid, conservative sexual values and standards have incorporated, to diverse degrees, prejudicial attitudes towards aging sexuality that influence their responses to physiological change. Ignorant that age-related decreases in sexual function normally occur, they may be particularly vulnerable to faulty expectations and performance concerns. The culturally reinforced relationship between sexual ability and feelings of self-worth places aged men at risk of losing self-esteem when faced with decreases in erectile capacity that challenge the denial of aging and the retention of a more youthful self-image. Cognitive appraisal and coping theory provide a useful conceptual framework for understanding personal responses to alterations in sexual functioning. The appraisal of a decrease in penile rigidity as a natural or threatening event is influenced, among other factors, by personal beliefs and expectations, personality disposition and the value of sexual expression within the life history of the individual. Successful coping not only depends on the development of compensatory strategies to maximize adaptation to bodily changes and external circumstances, but also on adjusting personal preferences and expectations to situational constraints. The persistence of well-being and sexual satisfaction despite marked erectile difficulties, noted in several studies, demonstrates the importance of exploring the cognitive and emotional significance of sexuality for the aged, rather than interpreting sexual changes according to performance-oriented agendas.

The second half of the twentieth century has witnessed considerable fluidity in the development and realignment of partnerships encompassing marriage, separation, divorce, extramarital, and same-sex relationships. Most aging men, however, are involved in long-term marriages or remarry soon after divorce. There is a dearth of data on the direct role that relationships play in mediating the effects of aging on male sexuality, despite clinical evidence showing the importance of marital adjustment for sexual satisfaction in late life. Marital relationships are not unchanging, but evolve in keeping with aging and the vicissitudes of life, influencing the well-being of individuals and couples. Marital quality has been reported to decline gradually, to remain unchanged or to improve as couples grow older. Several studies have shown a curvilinear relationship, with good marital satisfaction early on, which then declines because of economic concerns and family pressures, to rise again in late middle age as couples enjoy greater freedom and financial security. Survey data and systematic research have shown an association between marital adjustment and sexual satisfaction regardless of age and duration of marriage. The correlational design of the studies does not permit causality to be identified, although it is likely that both marital and sexual adjustment interact in ways still to be determined to shape the quality of the overall relationship. The congruence of sexual needs and expectations between sexual partners as age progresses appears to be a key ingredient for sexual satisfaction that has not yet been incorporated in aging studies.

The sexuality of older men and couples cannot be distinguished from the social context which, with its implicit values and expectations, conveys individual meaning and significance to life events as people move from one stage of life to the next. 'Male menopause' and 'mid-life crisis' are life-stage-dependent, socially ingrained terms that refer to an elusive constellation of hormonal changes, psychological distress, and sexual difficulties in middle-aged men. The persistence of the notion of a male menopause, despite the lack of validating physiological evidence, may be best explained by cultural forces that promote a sexualized life-style and proficient sexual behavior well into middle-age at a time when sexual capacity begins to decrease. Critical 'turning points' usually occurring at a later stage of life, such as retirement, illness, widowhood and need for institutionalization, can also have profound consequences for sexual identity, gender role, social status, sense of autonomy and control, but the consequences of these events for the sexual life of men and their relationships have yet to be fully explored. Recent social theories, which emphasize active adaptation of the aged when interacting with society and the concept of role change rather than role loss, are clearly relevant to aging and sexuality. There is increasing evidence that old people proactively engage in social interactions that compensate for emotional and physical losses, and optimize the affective and instrumental value of close, intimate relationships. Current social research suggests that older persons are no longer passive recipients of negative sexual biases but that, influenced by their improved knowledge of sexuality, more liberal attitudes and changes in family structure, they are developing intimate relationships more readily, shaping their own sense of sexual worth and identity.

There are distinct socialization differences between the life histories of younger homosexual men influenced by the gay right's movement and the older ones who spent their formative years in a period of social oppression and active discrimination. Older homosexual men are particularly vulnerable to social stigmatization, fear of social disapproval, sexual dysphoria and problems of self-confidence and self-esteem reinforced by the AIDS epidemic. Many of the vicissitudes experienced by aging homosexuals, related to health, retirement, finances and bereavement, are basically the same as those of their heterosexual counterparts, but the consequences for their sexual adjustment can be markedly different. A negative bias towards the sexuality of aging people persists in nursing homes and extended care facilities. The sexuality of the institutionalized aged, both straight and gay, has been ignored or severely restricted, despite evidence that a significant proportion of older residents continue to be interested in sex and would engage in physical expressions of intimacy if the opportunities arose. Health professionals' attitudes to sexual expression and institutional rules have been, in general, repressive. In the USA, new federal regulations concerning older person's rights are now in place and educational programs are being developed to help respond to the sexual expressions of residents in a constructive rather than a punitive manner. However, effective changes responsive to the needs of the institutionalized aged for intimacy are slow to be implemented and much needs to be accomplished in this regard.

Society's increasingly open attitudes to sexual expression and the increasingly sexualized environment reinforced by the Western media in recent years has not been without consequence for the aged. More and more, older men are approaching health-care professionals with sexual concerns, seeking information, reassurance or help. Prevalent concerns reported by older volunteers in our study of healthy aging were unpredictability of erectile function, decreased penile rigidity, loss of sexual attractiveness, fear of sexual rejection, sexual boredom, and distress about their partner's loss of sexual interest. Epidemiological studies such as the Massachusetts Male Aging Study documented, in a random sample of men aged 40–70 years, a 52% prevalence of erectile difficulties, with close to 35% of volunteers rated as moderately or completely impotent. Age emerged as the variable more strongly associated with impotence, but it should be mentioned that 33% of the 70-year-old respondents did not report erectile problems. There were also age-related increases in orgasmic difficulties and coital pain, but the format of their inquiry did not permit a sexual diagnosis to be reached, and we still know little about the prevalence of sexual dysfunctions other than erectile disorders in older men from the general population. The high prevalence of sexual problems in the population at large, and the increasing demand for treatment contributed, during the early 1970s, to the rapid expansion of sex therapy clinics and, more recently, to the establishment of medically based specialized clinics which evaluate and treat erectile problems. Erectile dysfunction – in isolation or, less frequently, in association with hypoactive sexual desire or premature ejaculation – is the most frequent dysfunction with which older men present at sex therapy clinics. Men with loss of sexual desire may not be inclined to seek help unless pressured by their partners, as was the case for most patients with a hypoactive sexual desire disorder evaluated in our clinic. The 'call-for-help' is usually not only motivated by a decline in erectile capacity, but also by the individual's and partner's attitudes and emotional reactions to the sexual change.

Community surveys and the evaluation of patients in medical and sex therapy clinics have disclosed a high prevalence of medical illnesses, postsurgical and drug effects associated with erectile disorders in aging men. The Massachusetts Male Aging Study revealed, for example, that medical conditions and lifestyle factors such as hypertension, heart disease, diabetes, ulcers, arthritis, tobacco and alcohol consumption, medication use, and indices of anger and depression were all related to a higher probability of impotence in the general population, after controlling for age effects. Evaluation of older men with erectile problems in medical clinics confirmed the high prevalence of chronic illness, but diagnoses of 'organogenic impotence' range from 30% to 85%. There is a diverse interpretation of medical findings, depending on whether the specialty or research orientation of the clinic is focused on vascular, hormonal or neurogenic mechanisms. By-and-large, reports from specialized medical centers have minimized the role of psychological factors and, in turn, sex therapy clinics, while acknowledging the role of medical pathology, have given greater emphasis to psychological and relationship determinants. The evaluation of psychological influences in medical clinics is cursory at best and, conversely, medical screening in psychologically based sex programs is limited and equally lacking in sophistication. The high prevalence of chronic disorders associated with erectile dysfunction has led some to the unwarranted statement that impotence has, primarily, an organic basis. Neglected in this conclusion is evidence of a differential referral bias that favors channeling organically disturbed patients to medically based diagnostic centers. The tendency to interpret an association as having causal significance or to view causation as dichotomous (either organic or psychogenic) has lead, frequently, to inaccurate views about the nature of sexual problems in the aged.

Medical disorders may interfere with sexual function through generalized, nonspecific effects and/or by a direct action, mainly on mediating vascular, neural, and endocrine factors. Their sexual effects are frequently multifactorial, involving several physiological mechanisms acting in concert with psychological processes. The effect of chronic illness on individual sexuality may be influenced by stage of life, prior experiences of and attitudes to sex, coping styles, personality characteristics, and the nature of current relationships. Regretfully, there is no empirical information on these aspects, which are critically important for determining the effect of an illness on the sexual satisfaction of older men. Chapter 9 discussed in some detail some of the most prevalent medical disorders that may impair the sexual life of older men. It includes cardiovascular disease, hypertension, diabetes mellitus, Parkinson's disease, endocrine disorders, chronic renal and hepatic failure, chronic obstructive pulmonary disease, arthritis and several postsurgical conditions. The validity of these clinical reports is frequently limited, however, by reliance on retrospective assessment of premorbid sexual function, the reliability of self-reports, lack of consideration of the partner when gathering sexual information, and the absence of age-matched control groups.

The role of psychopathology in changes in the sexual behavior of aging men has received attention infrequently. Despite the high prevalence of dementia among the aged and the concerns expressed by spouses and care-givers, there are limited data on the impact of cognitive disorders on sexual function and marital life. Among the reported problems in ongoing relationships are inadequate sexual advances, disrupted sex play, increased sexual demands or difficulties because of loss of sexual desire by the demented patient or the care-giving partner. Sexual acting out, such as masturbation in public or inappropriate sexual talk, is occasionally reported, but there is no evidence that sexually disinhibited or aggressive behaviors are common manifestations of dementia. Depression, as a nosological entity or as a psychological symptom, is common among older patients and is frequently noted in ambulatory medical settings associated with a wide range of medical problems. Results from the Massachusetts Male Aging Study showed that depression strongly predicts sexual difficulties and low sexual satisfaction, correlating with a higher probability of erectile dysfunction in aging men. Clinical studies, mostly uncontrolled and retrospective, report that depression has a negative effect on male sexuality, but the results are frequently confounded by the deleterious effect of antidepressants on sexual function. Prospective research on unmedicated depressed patients has shown a decrease in sexual satisfaction, which improves after behavioral treatment of the mood disorder, but no reduction in sexual drive or behavior. These findings challenge the notion that the frequency of sexual behavior is necessarily impaired in depression and emphasizes the importance of the patient's cognitive appraisal of their own sexuality. Although older patients have been included in several studies, lack of stratification of results by age prevents conclusions specific to the aged to be drawn.

Prescription drugs should be considered, along with medical and psychiatric illness, as a significant risk factor for sexual dysfunction in the aged. A disproportionately large amount of prescription and nonprescription drugs are consumed by older populations. Multiple pathology, higher medication dosage, long duration of treatment, polypharmacy, and drug interactions all contribute to the increased prevalence of noxious drug effects in the elderly population. Numerous publications, mainly case reports or uncontrolled clinical series, implicate a wide range of pharmacological agents as having adverse effects on male sexual function. Most frequently reported in aging populations are antihypertensive medications, mainly thiazide diuretics, sympatholytic agents and beta-adrenergic blockers, other cardiovascular drugs such as digoxin and antiarrhythmic agents, psychotropic medications, cancer chemotherapy agents, histamine-2 antagonists, carbonic anhydrase inhibitors and drugs with hormonal action such as antiandrogens for the treatment of benign prostatic hypertrophy or prostatic cancer. Not to be overlooked are alcohol and nicotine, two drugs of abuse with significant sexual effects, that continue to be prevalent among the aged. However, information on rates of sexual side-effects of specific medications within drug classes varies widely. Reports of adverse reactions have frequently failed to adequately characterize the components of the sexual response impaired by the drug and have ignored interactive influences such as the effects of aging itself, underlying medical conditions, psychological status and relationship factors. Drug intake may also influence sexuality through generalized adverse actions on well-being, energy level and mood, and be an important, and frequently ignored, factor in medication noncompliance.

The determinants of help-seeking behavior for sexual problems in aged men have received little research attention. Clinical experience shows that, in addition to a decline in sexual capacity, psychological and relationship factors frequently trigger the decision to contact health-care professionals about sexual complaints. Marital difficulties, emotional depression and life events that compromise a sense of autonomy or self-esteem commonly contribute to destabilize sexual adjustment and satisfaction. The evaluation of a sexual problem, primarily of erectile capacity, is frequently flawed by the tendency to reach categorical (either psychogenic or organic) and mechanistic (single cause–single effect) diagnostic conclusions. Modern views about causation have resulted in a paradigm shift, where traditional boundaries between disciplines are being bridged and new interdisciplinary fields, such as behavioral medicine, are emerging. This multidimensional, interactive approach to problems of health and illness have yet to be fully adopted by sexual medicine. Ideally, a comprehensive evaluation of a sexual disorder is best implemented in multidisciplinary clinics where integrated access to medical, urological and psychological expertise is available. In practice, patients with sexual disorders, mainly erectile dysfunction, are frequently referred to specialized centers which, depending on their orientation, may follow markedly divergent evaluation pathways.

The primary care practitioner is well placed to address the sexual concerns of older men, identify the existence of sexual dysfunctions and eventually provide limited sexual counseling. A problem-oriented sexual, medical and psychosocial history, involving the partner where appropriate, a physical examination and routine laboratory tests most often suffice to identify clinically significant psychological determinants, relevant medical conditions, risk factors and drug effects. Depending on the nature of the problem, and the patient's/couple's expectations and motivation, appropriate referrals for further evaluation and diagnostic testing may be made. Patients with evidence of psychological determination, mood disorders or relationship difficulties may be offered additional psychological assessment and therapy. Clinical evidence of hypogonadism and loss of sexual drive requires endocrine screening which includes total and bioavailable testosterone and, possibly, measurement of prolactin and luteinizing hormone. Nocturnal penile tumescence (NPT) and rigidity monitoring, best carried out in a sleep laboratory, and audiovisual sexual stimulation methods have value in objectively assessing erectile capacity. When interpreting abnormal NPT findings, we must consider age-related normative information, the individual's affective state, such as depression or excessive anxiety, and abnormalities in sleep architecture. When the clinical pattern of the dysfunction suggests organic involvement, particularly in patients with a history of cardiovascular difficulties, intracavernosal testing of vascular function is indicated. The development of adequate erections following intracavernosal injection of vasoactive agents, although not ruling out arteriogenic factors, indicates normal veno-occlusive function and suggests the option of penile injection therapy. An inadequate erectile response, however, has no diagnostic significance since it may be because of psychological inhibition. Specialized vascular assessments, such as color Duplex ultrasonography and pulsed Doppler analysis, cavernosometry, cavernosography and angiography, are tests usually carried out on younger patients before vascular surgery. Their clinical value necessitates further validity studies, age-related normative information and uniform diagnostic criteria across laboratories. Neurological testing, with the exception of penile biothesiometry, has limited value for dysfunctional men without clinical neurological evidence, because of their lack of specificity concerning the autonomic control of genital vasocongestion.

The comprehensive treatment of sexual problems of aging men, most frequently erectile difficulties, should aim at improving sexual satisfaction for the patient, alone or with his partner, and not be limited to the restoration of erectile capacity. The therapeutic strategy requires an integrated approach with balanced attention given to medical and psychological issues. Medically, it includes managing underlying chronic disorders and addressing reversible conditions such as hypogonadism, drug effects, alcohol abuse and cigarette smoking. Psychologically, it involves addressing unrealistic expectations about sexual performance, motivation for treatment and the pathogenic role of emotional and interpersonal problems. Older men have been socialized to avoid open discussion of emotional or relationship aspects, particularly of a sexual nature. They approach the family doctor with the belief that their erectile difficulties have a medical cause and the expectation that a medical intervention, hopefully 'a pill', will solve the problem. They are reluctant to implement a psychological referral, preferring a medically oriented specialist who, if not sensitive to emotional issues, frequently carries out a cursory psychological evaluation and suggests medical or invasive interventions. It is critically important for the diagnostician to provide an unbiased view of the nature of the sexual difficulty, and to discuss the advantages and limitations of relevant therapeutic options so that the patient can reach a fully informed decision.

Sexual counseling, behavioral or marital therapy should be offered first to patients and couples with significant psychological involvement in the pathogenesis of the sexual dysfunction. Educational, cognitive, behavioral and interpersonal therapeutic components may be combined based on the patient's/couple's characteristics and needs, therapist's theoretical orientation and treatment setting. Medical intervention includes a wide array of approaches such as hormonal treatment, oral agents, intracavernosal pharmacotherapy, external vacuum devices, penile prosthetic implants, and vascular reconstructive surgery. The patients' pre ferred medical treatment is usually oral medication but, until recently, the effectiveness of agents such as yohimbine or trazodone for the treatment of erectile disorders has been disappointing. This situation is rapidly changing with the recent availability of drugs such as sildenafil, a peripherally acting type-5 phosphodiesterase inhibitor that appears to facilitate erections in response to erotic stimulation in patients with erectile difficulties. More information is required about the clinical indications and long-term efficacy and safety of this and similar agents still in the process of development. Intracavernosal pharmacotherapy or vacuum devices may be recommended, alone or in association with sexual counseling, to patients with significant organic pathogenesis or those who are unmotivated to engage in psychological treatment. Penile prostheses should be reserved for selected patients after careful screening and counseling. Vascular surgery remains an exceptional procedure for sexually dysfunctional older men. There is a need for outcome studies on the long-term treatment efficacy of psychological and medical interventions on the sexual function and satisfaction of aging men with sexual difficulties.

Over the last 25 years we have witnessed two convergent developments: the heightened awareness by professionals and the general public of the prevalence of erectile problems among the aged, and the availability of an ever-expanding panoply of therapeutic approaches to correct erectile failure. Knowledge that a large number of medical illnesses and drugs contribute to sexual difficulties, the development of sophisticated diagnostic methods and a more realistic view about the effectiveness of sex therapy all contributed to the increased interest in medico-surgical treatments for male sexual dysfunction. These methods, valuable as they are, have shifted attention to the penis, neglecting the significance of the individual and the context of his life. Aging men and their partners, depending on their expectations and motivation, may benefit from these therapeutic gains, but if not adequately evaluated and informed may be misled by interpreting a natural or psychologically induced, age-related decrease in erectile firmness as a medical issue. The emergence of sexually active oral medications for erectile dysfunction has blurred the distinction between specific therapeutic needs and unrealistic social expectations and demands for enhanced sexual performance. New pharmacological approaches represent potential advances in the overall treatment of sexually dysfunctional older men. However, their value needs to be considered judiciously, together with other psychosexual and medical interventions, within an integrated view that takes into account psychological and relationship aspects which are important to sexuality and contentment as we grow old.

Index